THE GOLD'S GYM™ TRAINING ENCYCLOPEDIA

Other Gold's Gym books published by Contemporary:

Gold's Gym Book of Bodybuilding
Gold's Gym Nutrition Bible
Solid Gold: Training the Gold's Gym Way

THE GOLD'S GYM™ TRAINING ENCYCLOPEDIA

Peter Grymkowski, Edward Connors, Tim Kimber and Bill Reynolds

CB
CONTEMPORARY BOOKS

Library of Congress Cataloging-in-Publication Data

The Gold's gym training encyclopedia.

    Includes index.
     1. Bodybuilding.   2. Exercise.   I. Grymkowski, Peter.
   GV546.5.G65   1984   646.7′5
   ISBN 0-8092-5446-8   84-09611

All exercises were photographed by John Balik at Gold's Gym, Venice, California.

Cover photos and miscellaneous illustrations courtesy of Joe Weider, Publisher, *Muscle & Fitness* magazine.

Selected Nautilus exercises were photographed at the Brentwood Fitness Center, Brentwood, California.

Exercise models: Lee Haney, Inger Zetterqvist, Tom Platz, Sue Ann McKean, Charles Glass, Cindy Lee, Lesley Koslow, Andreas Cahling, Maria Gonzalez, Matt Mendenhall, Chris Glass, Dale Ruplinger, Boyer Coe, Vickie Schiff, Tim Belknap, Julie Stangl, Ann Slater, Cheryl Platz, Joe Bucci, Janaire O'Hara, Rachel McLish, Bob Jodkiewicz, Tina Plakinger, Mike Christian, Janice Regan, Rick Valente, Dawn Marie Gnaegi, and Bronston Austin, Jr.

All suggestions and recommendations in this book are made without warranty or guarantee, express or implied, and the author and publisher disclaim all liability in connection with the use of this information. The material presented herein is not a substitute for the advice of a physician before taking or administering any drug, including steroids, or undertaking any exercise program.

Published by Contemporary Books
A division of The McGraw-Hill Companies
4255 West Touhy Avenue, Lincolnwood (Chicago), Illinois 60712-1975 U.S.A.
Copyright © 1984 by Bill Reynolds and Gold's Gym Enterprises, Inc.
Printed in the United States of America
International Standard Book Number: 0-8092-5446-8
01 02 03 04 05 06 ML 47 46 45 44 43 42 41 40 39 38 37 36 35 34 33 32 31

CONTENTS

THE GOLD'S GYM™
TRAINING ENCYCLOPEDIA

Other Gold's Gym books published by Contemporary:

Gold's Gym Book of Bodybuilding
Gold's Gym Nutrition Bible
Solid Gold: Training the Gold's Gym Way

1

BASIC INFORMATION

Many of you reading this book can skip over the information in this chapter. You are either a seasoned bodybuilder who has long since mastered the basics of the activity, or you have already read and assimilated the vast store of information found in *The Gold's Gym Book of Bodybuilding* (Contemporary, 1983). But for many readers new to bodybuilding, the information presented in this chapter is an essential requisite to safe and productive weight workouts.

The following topics are discussed in this chapter: basic bodybuilding terminology; how resistance training works; resistance progression; proper exercise form; when and where to work out; what to wear when you train; breathing patterns during weight-training exercise; safety procedures; training frequency; rep ranges; rest intervals between sets; break in to heavy exercise and how to cope with muscle soreness; the use of a training diary; and how to warm up correctly prior to a heavy weight workout. And we also present three progressively more intense training programs for those of you who are new to bodybuilding.

We will also briefly discuss a variety of advanced-level training principles and methods in Chapter 10. These principles will help you to make good gains from your bodybuilding workouts, but they should not be misconstrued as a replacement for reading *The Gold's Gym Book of Bodybuilding*.

Basic Terms

Over the years, a small dictionary of unique and specialized bodybuilding terms has evolved. If you aren't familiar with at least the most fundamental bodybuilding terms, you will grow confused when you read any of the proliferation of bodybuilding books and magazines on the market. There are eleven fundamental terms defined in this section, and once mastered they will allow you to talk bodybuilding on an equal footing with the biggest champions training at Gold's Gym.

An *exercise* is each individual movement (e.g., a Bench Press or Squat) that you do when you train. Indeed, an exercise is often referred to as a *movement*. Literally hundreds of bodybuilding exercises are described in great detail and clearly illustrated in chapters 2–9 of this book, as well as in all three previous Gold's Gym books.

A *repetition* (which is often called a *rep*) is

1

every individual, distinct, and full cycle of an exercise. For example, in a Bench Press movement, you would start your repetition with your arms straight, bend your arms and lower the barbell to lightly touch your chest, then complete the rep by again bringing your arms to a fully straightened position.

Groupings of reps (usually in the range of 8–15) are called *sets*. The word "set" is a mathematical term referring to a grouping of any entity. Each set is followed by a brief *rest interval* of about 60 seconds. This rest interval allows you to catch your breath and partially recuperate before beginning a new set. In normal bodybuilding training, you will do multiple sets (usually between 3–5) of each exercise.

The full list of exercises, sets, and reps that you perform in one training session is called a *workout, routine, program,* or *training schedule.* Sometimes the term "workout" refers to the training session itself. When you actually perform your routine, you are *working out* or *training.* A workout is also sometimes referred to as a *training session.*

How Bodybuilding Training Works

Bodybuilding is a strict stimulus–response activity. When you subject a muscle to a load that it is not used to handling, it is forced to increase in mass and strength in order easily to handle that weight the next time you lift it. This increase in muscle mass and strength is referred to as *muscle hypertrophy.*

The object in bodybuilding training is to put a greater load on the muscles by gradually increasing the weight you use or the number of reps that you perform with a particular weight. Normally, you will increase the number of reps you perform with a weight over a set range (e.g., between 6–10 reps) until you can do the higher number of reps. Then you drop back to the lower number of reps with a slightly heavier weight and begin to work your way back up in reps.

If you look at the exercise routines listed for various bodybuilders in one of the workout chapters, you will see a range of reps listed for most exercises. These are called *guide numbers,* the smaller figure being the *lower guide number*

and the larger figure the *upper guide number.* Assuming that you do one set of 6–10 reps in the Bench Press, you will find a sample of how you would progress in resistance in Figure 1-1 below. You should note that "60 × 6" is a form of bodybuilding shorthand meaning "six reps with 60 pounds."

	Mon	Wed	Fri
Week 1	60 × 6	60 × 7	60 × 8
Week 2	60 × 9	60 × 10	65 × 6
Week 3	65 × 7	65 × 8	65 × 9
Week 4	65 × 10	70 × 6	70 × 7
Week 5	70 × 8	70 × 0	70 × 10
Week 6	75 × 6	75 × 7	75 × 8

Figure 1-1: Example of Simple Resistance Progression.

The amount of weight you add to the bar once you have reached the upper guide number for reps depends on your sex, your relative strength level, and the body part you are working. On leg and back exercises, men can add 20–30 pounds and women can add 10–15 pounds to each movement when they've reached the upper guide number. On exercises for other muscle groups, men can add 5–10 pounds and women can add 2½–5 pounds to each movement when they are ready to move up the resistance in an exercise.

The first example of resistance progression was for a bodybuilder doing only one set of a movement. However, you will usually do multiple sets (3–5) of each exercise. In that case, you should reach the upper guide number for reps on each set before increasing the weight and dropping back to the lower guide number. There is an example of this more complex form of progression in Figure 1-2 on page 3 (assuming three sets of 8–12 reps in the Seated Pulley Row movement).

You can't expect to add new reps to a movement every workout because your body is subject to natural up-and-down energy cycles and on a "down" day you will feel weaker-than-normal. However, when you are on an "up"

	Mon	Wed	Fri
Week 1	70 × 8	70 × 10	70 × 10
	70 × 8	70 × 9	70 × 10
	70 × 8	70 × 8	70 × 9
Week 2	70 × 11	70 × 12	70 × 12
	70 × 10	70 × 11	70 × 12
	70 × 10	70 × 10	70 × 10
Week 3	70 × 12	80 × 9	80 × 11
	70 × 12	80 × 9	80 × 10
	70 × 12	80 × 8	80 × 8
Week 4	80 × 11	80 × 12	80 × 12
	80 × 10	80 × 10	80 × 11
	80 × 9	80 × 10	80 × 10
Week 5	80 × 12	80 × 12	90 × 9
	80 × 12	80 × 12	90 × 8
	80 × 10	80 × 12	90 × 8
Week 6	90 × 10	90 × 11	90 × 12
	90 × 9	90 × 10	90 × 11
	90 × 8	90 × 9	90 × 10

Figure 1-2: Example of Complex Resistance Progression.

cycle, you will be able to make up lost ground by adding more reps than you normally can.

Correct Exercise Form

There are two primary reasons why you should always use scrupulously strict exercise form—to avoid injury, and to place the greatest possible stress on your working muscles. Injuries are usually caused when you either attempt to lift a very heavy weight with poor form, or you go too heavy before you are fully warmed up. So, taking time for a proper warm-up and maintaining strict form in all your exercises will drastically decrease the incidence of progress-halting injuries, giving you better long-term gains from your training.

Most novice bodybuilders use poor form (which is called "cheating") in order to avoid working truly hard at an exercise. By bending your back or jerking your legs at an opportune time, you can make an exercise much easier to perform. However, this is unfortunately not the object of bodybuilding training. Your goal every workout should be to stress each muscle group with maximum intensity, the only way of ensuring optimum muscle hypertrophy.

What is proper exercise form? Good biomechanics (form) first involves maintaining the body position recommended for each exercise and moving only the specified joints and parts of your body. It also involves using a full range of motion in each exercise, extending the working muscles completely, contracting them to the limit, then again extending them on each repetition. And strict form involves moving the weight slowly enough during each repetition to keep bar momentum from robbing your muscles of a bit of the stress they should receive from an exercise.

When and Where to Work Out

It makes little difference what time of the day you train, as long as you set a regular time to work out and don't miss any training sessions. The peak use hours at Gold's Gym/Venice are in the mid-morning, late-afternoon, and early evening hours. However, you will find champion bodybuilders working out at all hours of the day and night. At the time he reached his zenith as a bodybuilder, Pete Grymkowski (Mr. World and an original Gold's Gym owner) trained in the middle of the night after a 15-hour business day.

Where you train is governed by the options you have available. It would be nice if every bodybuilder could train in one of the more than 100 Gold's Gym facilities worldwide, but everyone does not have access to such a well-equipped gym. You may have no other alternative but to work out at home in your garage or basement with only an adjustable barbell and dumbbell set and a couple of benches.

In choosing where to work out when you have viable alternatives, you should always seek to train at the facility that is best equipped. In the early days of your bodybuilding involvement, you can get along well with a minimum of equipment; but when you are an advanced bodybuilder, you will need the widest possible variety of equipment in order to develop a massive, highly detailed physique. Matters of expense should always be secondary to the functional qualities of a gym.

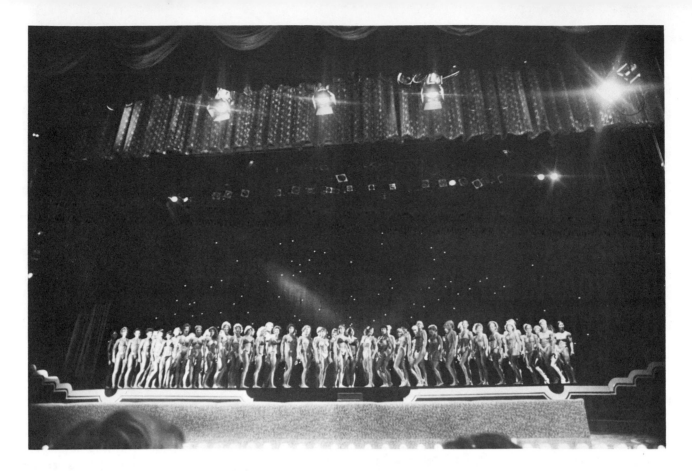

The end result of proper training and gut-hard work could put you on stage. For women, above is the overall lineup for the 1981 America and below are the finalists for the 1983 Pro World Championship.

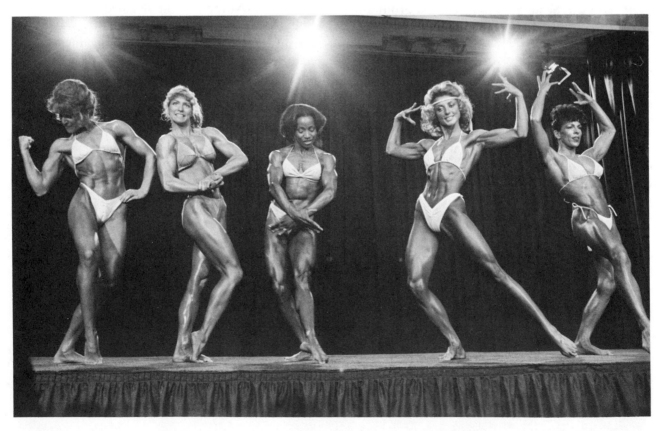

Candy Csencsits   Sherry Atton   Carla Dunlap   Kike Elomaa   Julie Baumgartner

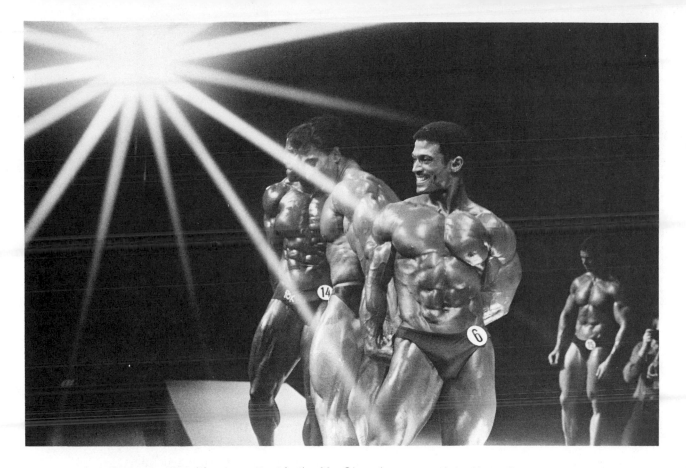

For men, the ultimate contest is the Mr. Olympia competition. Above is a dramatic shot of Mohamed Makkawy (front), Samir Bannout (middle), and Bertil Fox during comparison rounds.

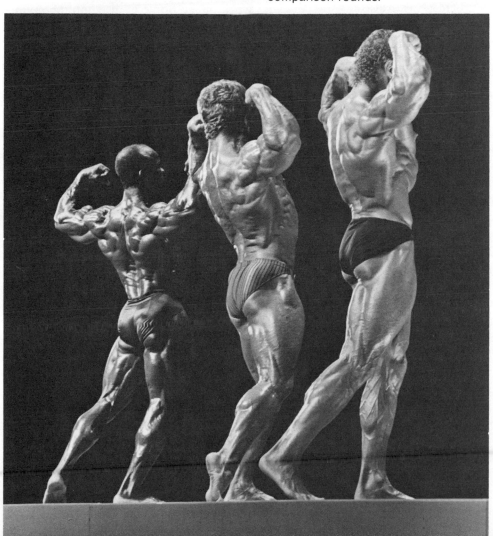

What to Wear

You should dress according to climate. If it is warm in the gym, you can probably get along fine wearing only shorts and a t-shirt or tank top (men, of course, can train just in shorts if they like). But when the weather is cool, you should wear a warm-up suit, or perhaps even more clothing. Remember that two or three light layers of clothing will keep you warmer than one thick layer.

While you will see many bodybuilders training with bare feet, it's a better practice to wear running shoes during a workout. These shoes have a built-in arch support that will protect your feet from injury. And the sole on running shoes will assure you of a nonslip foot placement when you do your calf work.

Whether or not you wear socks, or an athletic supporter or bra are matters of personal preference.

Breathing Patterns

There are three schools of thought regarding how to breathe as you perform an exercise:

- You should inhale during the exertion phase of each repetition and exhale during the recovery cycle.
- You should exhale during the exertion phase of each repetition and inhale during the recovery cycle.
- You need not concern yourself about when to inhale and exhale because you will naturally breathe correctly as you do an exercise.

One thing is clear about breathing during bodybuilding training: *You must never hold your breath as you exert.* Doing so cuts off the flow of blood to and from your brain, and can cause you to black out. Physiologists call this reaction the *Valsalva maneuver* and if it occurs in the middle of a set you could be seriously injured.

While you will eventually breathe correctly (unconsciously) during a set, you should initially adhere to a breathing rule: Exhale during the exertion phase of each repetition and inhale during the recovery cycle. This rule will prevent you from incurring the Valsalva maneuver, and

it will permit you to use maximum weights in every exercise with total safety.

Safety Procedures

We don't wish you to conclude that bodybuilding training is not a safe activity because there are far fewer serious injuries in our sport than in most others. However, this safety record is largely due to bodybuilders knowing, understanding, and applying commonly accepted weight-training safety rules. The best list of safety rules that we have seen was provided to us by Lou Ferrigno (Mr. America, Mr. International, Mr. Universe, and a successful film actor). Here are Louie's 12 safety rules and brief discussions of each rule:

1. *Always use spotters.* One or two safety spotters should be standing by to prevent a heavy barbell from falling on you whenever you perform limit or near-limit lifts, especially in the Bench Press and Squat exercises. Needless to say, these spotters must be alert.

2. *Never train alone.* If you train alone, you won't have a spotter available. Those bodybuilders who work out in home gyms should convince a family member to sit in on their workouts whenever heavy training is planned.

3. *Use catch racks.* Many bench-pressing benches and squat racks have safety-catch racks attached, and they should always be used to protect you from injury. If your bench or rack doesn't have built-in catch racks, you can improvise them by strategically positioning sturdy boxes or thick blocks of wood where the barbell plates can descend onto them and rest in a safe position should you fail to complete a repetition with a heavy poundage.

4. *Use collars on your barbell.* One common cause of injury is having the plates slide off one end of a barbell bar during a heavy set. When this happens, the temporarily heavier end will whip violently downward, potentially wrenching your lower back, knee, shoulder, or other joints. It will sometimes seem inconvenient to secure collars on the end of the bar each time you change weights, but fastening those collars securely in place will prevent injuries.

5. *Never hold your breath during an exercise.* (The reasoning behind this rule was explained in

the previous section of this chapter.)

6. *Maintain good gym housekeeping.* Even if you are simply walking from one end of a gym to the other, you can trip over barbells, dumbbells, or loose plates lying on the gym floor. Therefore, it's a good practice always to place loose equipment in proper storage areas or racks as soon as you finish using them. And when barbells and dumbbells are returned to the correct racks, you won't need to search all over the gym for the mate to a 25-pound dumbbell that you wish to use in your next exercise.

7. *Train under competent supervision.* Many injuries occur when a bodybuilder uses poor exercise form, something that can't happen when you work out in a large, public gym with alert instructors who immediately correct poor biomechanics in an exercise.

8. *Don't train in an overcrowded gym.* If you are forced to wait more than a couple of minutes between sets to use a certain piece of equipment, your body can cool off enough to cause an injury. In overcrowded gyms this can happen relatively easily. It's better to change your workout hours to a time when the gym is less crowded.

9. *Always warm up thoroughly.* Just as a cooled off body can be injured, it's possible to suffer an injury when you fail to warm up properly prior to a heavy training session. (One good way to warm up thoroughly before a workout is presented at the end of this chapter.)

10. *Use proper form in all exercises.* This rule was suggested in #7 above. Correct biomechanics are stressed in each exercise description in this book, and it's important for you to take these suggestions seriously.

11. *Use a weightlifting belt.* When you do heavy Squats, back work, and overhead lifts, you can protect your lower back and abdomen from injury by wearing a weightlifting belt tightly cinched around your waist. And if you need to protect an old joint injury, you should use elastic gauze bandages wrapped tightly around the joint.

12. *Acquire as much knowledge as possible about weight training and bodybuilding.* The more you know about your sport, the more intelligently you can avoid injuries. You should read every possible book and magazine related to the sport in an effort to improve and update your knowledge of bodybuilding training.

How to Learn an Exercise

If you are a novice to bodybuilding training, you must be careful that you learn to correctly perform each exercise from the first day you step into a gym. The longer you train with poor biomechanics, the harder it will be to change these poor habits.

The best way to master each exercise begins with a careful comparison of the written description of the movement with the exercise photos provided for it. This should give you a good image of how the movement is performed. You can next do the exercise with a broomstick or an unloaded barbell to begin building up a knowledge of the correct path of each movement. And finally, you can gradually use heavier weights in each movement.

After a few weeks of practice, each exercise will become automatic. But before that, you can improve your exercise performance by thinking through the complete movement and mentally rehearsing it before you attack the actual weight.

Although we firmly believe that you can master each exercise just by using the descriptions and illustrations in this book, it is a good practice to have an experienced bodybuilder or gym instructor review your form in each movement. With such critical feedback, it is impossible to learn incorrect biomechanics in each movement.

Workout Frequency

When you complete a heavy training session, your muscles require at least 48 hours of rest before they can be stressed again. This rest period allows your body time to completely recuperate—remove fatigue toxins from the muscles and restore supplies of oxygen and muscle glycogen—and increase their hypertrophy

In the first weeks of your bodybuilding training, you should work out three nonconsecutive days per week. Normally, you will train on Mondays, Wednesdays, and Fridays, but any other combination of three nonconsecutive days each week will be acceptable. This scheme gives you 48 hours of rest to allow for complete physical recuperation and muscle growth to occur.

One early method of increasing workout intensity is to gradually increase the total number of sets that you do for each muscle group. After three or four months, however, you will be doing so many sets for each body part that you may not have sufficient energy available to train your full body with maximum poundages in a single training session. At that point, you will begin to divide your body program into two equal parts and train each part on a different day.

In the most basic type of *split routine,* you will work half of your body on Mondays and Thursdays, the other half on Tuesdays and Fridays. Two examples of four-day split routines are presented in Figure 1-3 below.

	M	T	W	T	F
Week 1	1	2	1	2	1
Week 2	2	1	2	1	2
Week 3	1	2	1	2	1
Week 4	2	1	2	1	2
Week 5	1	2	1	2	1

Figure 1-4: Five-Day Split Routine.

"1" on Figure 1-4) of your program on Monday, Wednesday, and Friday, the second half (indicated by "2" on Figure 1-4) on Tuesday and Thursday. And the second week you will do the second half on Monday, Wednesday, and Friday, the first half on Tuesday and Thursday. Week Three repeats Week One, Week Four repeats Week Two, and so on.

Moving up again in intensity, we come to the six-day split routine. There are two types of six-day splits, and the least intense form of six-day split is one in which you train each major muscle group twice per week. The more intense form of six-day split includes three weekly workouts for each major muscle group. Examples of both types of six-day split routine are presented in Figure 1-5 below.

Alternative A

Mon-Thur	Tues-Fri
Abdominals	Abdominals
Chest	Thighs
Back	Upper Arms
Shoulders	Forearms
Calves	Calves

Alternative B

Mon-Thur	Tues-Fri
Abdominals	Abdominals
Chest	Thighs
Shoulders	Back
Upper Arms	Forearms
Calves	Calves

Note: Both calves and abdominals can be worked more than three days per week without overtraining either muscle group.

Figure 1-3: Examples of Four-Day Split Routines.

One step up the intensity ladder from four-day split routines is the five-day split routine. With this routine, you will again split your body program into halves, but this time you work the halves on alternate days. The first week you work out, you will do the first half (indicated by

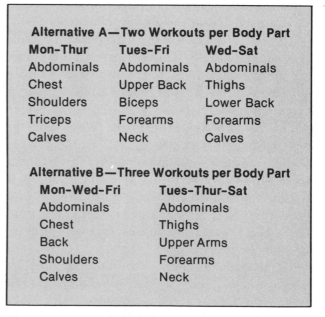

Alternative A—Two Workouts per Body Part

Mon-Thur	Tues-Fri	Wed-Sat
Abdominals	Abdominals	Abdominals
Chest	Upper Back	Thighs
Shoulders	Biceps	Lower Back
Triceps	Forearms	Forearms
Calves	Neck	Calves

Alternative B—Three Workouts per Body Part

Mon-Wed-Fri	Tues-Thur-Sat
Abdominals	Abdominals
Chest	Thighs
Back	Upper Arms
Shoulders	Forearms
Calves	Neck

Figure 1-5: Examples of Six-Day Split Routines.

Halfway between a five-day and six-day split routine in intensity is the popular four-day training cycle in which you split your body into three parts, then train each one on consecutive days, resting the fourth day and beginning the cycle anew on the fifth day. For example, you can do your chest and back the first day, work legs the second day, hit shoulders and arms the third day, and take the fourth day to rest.

Rep Ranges

Considerable scientific research has been conducted to determine what rep ranges are best for developing power, building muscle mass, and improving local muscular endurance. Very low reps (with poundages that only allow 1–3 reps) are best for developing raw power, moderately low reps (4–6) are best for building great muscle mass, medium reps (8–12) will give you a good combination of mass and muscularity, and high reps (over 15) are good for building muscle endurance.

One chief advantage of weight training is that you can selectively stress individual muscles—and even just a part of a muscle—in relative isolation from the rest of the body. But you can also stress each individual muscle with a specific number of reps to develop whatever physical quality you wish. Combined, these two factors make bodybuilding training one of the best ways to develop physical fitness as you improve your physique.

Rest Intervals

In normal training, you should rest approximately 60 seconds between sets to allow your body to partially recover from the exertion of the previous set before starting another. However, this length of rest interval should be considered an "average" one because you can take shorter rest intervals when working small muscle groups like the biceps and triceps. Conversely, you will need to rest more between sets for large body parts like thighs and back in order to catch your breath sufficiently to do justice to the next set.

Prior to a competition, you will use a tech-nique called *quality training* in which you intentionally reduce the rest intervals down to an average of about 30 seconds between sets. When your energy reserves have been depleted by a strict precontest diet and you complicate matters by quality training, you will inevitably discover that you can't handle your usual heavy training poundages. But as long as you push very quickly and deliberately through your workout, you can maintain good muscle mass and rip your physique to shreds while handling lighter weights.

Break-In and Muscle Soreness

If you aren't used to the heavy exercise of bodybuilding training, you will end up with incredibly sore muscles should you attempt to jump right into a full-scale workout schedule without a gradual break-in to heavy resistance training. Therefore, you should initially do only one set of each recommended movement in the beginning-level training program listed at the end of this chapter. After three workouts at this intensity level, you can comfortably move up to performing two sets of each exercise. And after three more workouts, you can perform the entire program.

Each time you switch to a new training program—which should be each 4–6 weeks—you will also experience a mild degree of muscle soreness if you fail to take it a little easy for the first one or two workouts. This is because your muscles will be stressed from new angles and require a workout or two to become used to the different exercises that you are using.

Even if you adhere strictly to the recommended break-in procedure, you might experience a mild degree of muscle soreness. If you feel any discomfort, you can alleviate the pain by soaking for 15–20 minutes in a hot bath once or twice a day for a day or two.

Training Diaries

Most of the best bodybuilders keep detailed training diaries in which they record their workouts and sometimes their diet, mental attitude, quality and amount of sleep, energy levels, things that account for a particular mental state or energy level, and any other factor that can have an effect on their bodybuilding progress. The more detailed your records, the better you will be able to use them to determine which exercises, routines, training techniques, nutritional practices, and so forth, have the most beneficial influence on your bodybuilding results.

At best, bodybuilding is a hit-and-miss proposition. We can give you general rules about how your body *should* react to various stimuli, but every body is so uniquely structured that it will react differently than every other body. As a result, your first few months and years of bodybuilding training should be treated as one grand experiment in which you try out every exercise, training program, workout technique, and diet in an effort to develop an optimum training philosophy for your own body.

Since bodybuilding results cannot be seen over a short term measured in days, your experiments should each last for 4–6 weeks. And over this longer term, you can most easily determine your progress by reviewing your training log. Where did you experience a muscle growth spurt? When did your strength levels improve most rapidly? What caused your body fat percentage to diminish? Answer these and a variety of similar questions, correlate this evaluation with your records of what you have been doing in each workout, and you will come closer to an answer to which training program and techniques work best for you.

You can use one of several commercially produced training diaries, the best of which is the *Muscle & Fitness Training Diary* (Contemporary, 1982). Or, you can use any bound ledger or record book that you find in an office supply or stationery store. Some bodybuilders even jazz up their diaries by using hand-tooled leather covers for the book, but any permanently bound book with blank pages will serve excellently as a workout log.

At a minimum, you should record the date of each workout and the exact exercises, weights, sets, and reps performed in that training session. Using the form of bodybuilding shorthand presented earlier in this chapter, in the next column is a sample of such a diary entry.

10-22-84

1. Hanging Leg Raises: 0 × 15 × 15 × 12
2. Roman Chair Sit-Ups: 0 × 30 × 30 × 30
3. Hyperextensions: 0 × 15; 10 × 12; 20 × 10
4. Seated Pulley Rows: 160 × 12; 170 × 10; 190 × 8; 210 × 6
5. Front Lat Pulldowns: 120 × 12; 140 × 10; 150 × 8; 160 × 6
6. One-Arm Dumbbell Bent Rows: 60 × 12; 70 × 10; 80 × 8; 85 × 6
7. Barbell Shrugs: 205 × 15; 225 × 12; 245 × 10; 255 × 8
8. Incline Barbell Press: 135 × 12; 165 × 10; 185 × 8; 205 × 6
9. Parallel Bar Dips: 0 × 15; 25 × 10; 45 × 8; 55 × 6
10. Flat-Bench Flyes: 45 × 10; 50 × 8; 55 × 6
11. Cross-Bench Pullovers: 50 × 15; 60 × 12; 70 × 10
12. Dumbbell Wrist Curls: 40 × 15; 50 × 12; 60 × 10
13. Barbell Reverse Wrist Curls: 55 × 15; 65 × 12; 70 × 10
14. Seated Calf Raises: 100 × 12; 120 × 10; 130 × 9
15. Donkey Calf Raises: 225 × 20 × 18 × 14

For a more complete diary, you should add in your meals, supplements, the times of day at which you work out and eat, energy levels, and so forth. And if you are on an anabolic drug therapy program, you should enter your dosages in your diary as well.

Monthly physical progress records can also be helpful. A daily record of your body weight at the time you work out can give you graphic information about how quickly you are gaining muscle mass or losing body fat stores. At the beginning level of bodybuilding, you can also take various anthropometric measurements (upper arm girth, chest girth, thigh girth, etc.), but after about six months of training the quality of your muscle mass becomes much more important than the girth of a particular limb or part of your torso. Then, it's best to have photos taken of your physique in standard poses each month and affix the photos to the pages of your diary with glue or tape.

Samir Bannout (1983 Mr. Olympia) sums up the value of a training diary: "I am able to chart my progress over a six-month or one-year period of time using my training diaries. And whenever I am feeling less than enthusiastic about an impending workout, I can gain considerable inspiration from reviewing my older diaries. It's difficult to see progress over the short term, but when I look at my training poundages a year ago, I can see marked improvements. The heavier I go in my workouts, the larger my muscles, so this graphic indication of my rate of progress can really fire me up for a workout!"

Warming Up

A proper 10–15 minute warm-up prior to a heavy session with the weights is essential as a means of preventing injuries. Exercise physiologists have determined that a proper warm-up will increase your pulse rate, augment blood circulation, refine motor coordination, make the muscles and connective tissues more supple and resistant to injury, and actually help to generate more forceful muscle contractions.

Your initial warm-up should include aerobic exercise, calisthenics, and stretching, but the stretching exercises should be of low intensity until you are completely warm. Your warm-up should conclude with a series of two or three light, high-rep (15–20 repetitions) sets of a basic exercise for the area that you will train first. So if you are doing a chest and shoulder workout, you can finish up your warm-up with two or three light, but progressively heavier, sets of Bench Presses. Following is a suggested warm-up program that you can use prior to a heavy weight workout:

Jogging in Place or *Skipping Rope:* You can do either of these forms of aerobic exercise for 3–5 minutes, starting with a slow cadence and

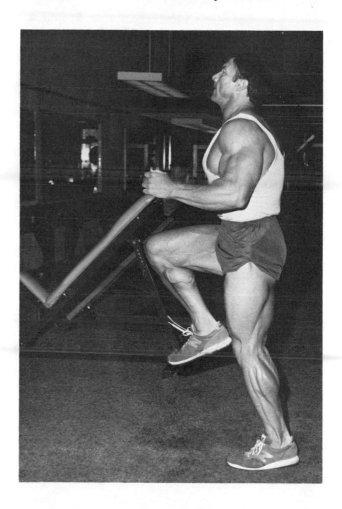

Jogging in Place, above; Skipping Rope, below.

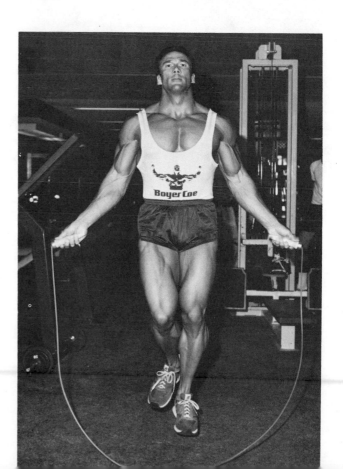

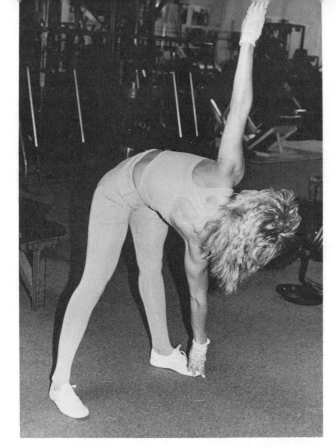
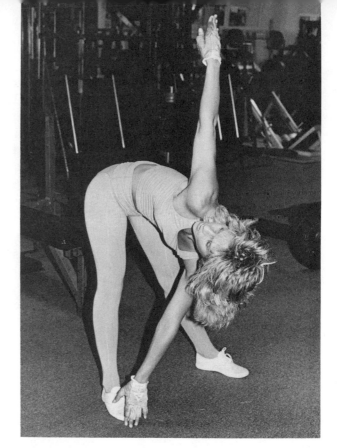

Alternate Toe Touch to left and right.

Push-Up—start/finish, left; midpoint, right.

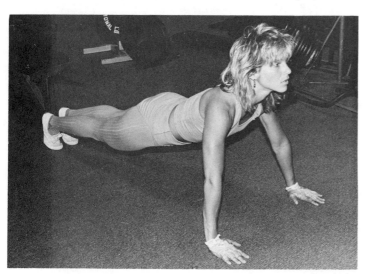
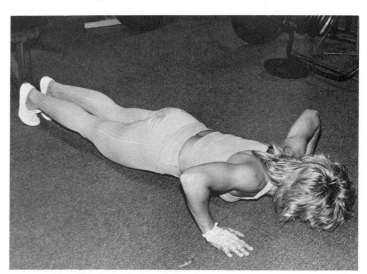

working up to a relatively quick pace for the last minute or so.

Alternate Toe Touches: Place your feet a bit wider than shoulder width and extend your arms straight out to the sides and parallel to the floor. Bend forward and twist to your left so you can touch your left foot with your right hand. Return to the starting position and repeat the movement to the other side. Alternate sides until you have done 12–15 reps to each side.

Push-Ups: Support your weight on straight arms with your body straight as illustrated. Lower your body down until your chest touches the floor by bending your arms. Push yourself back to straight arms' length. Repeat the movement until you have either done as many as you can or you have done 25 repetitions.

Jumping Jacks: Stand erect with your feet

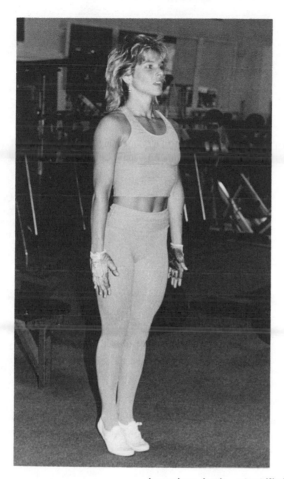
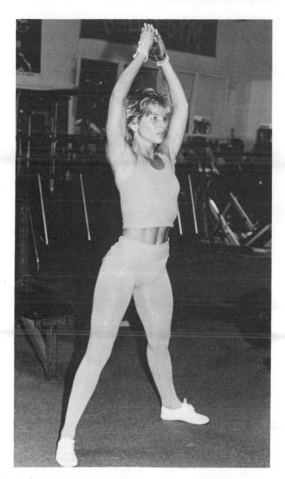

Jumping Jack—start/finish, left; midpoint, right.

Hamstring Stretch.

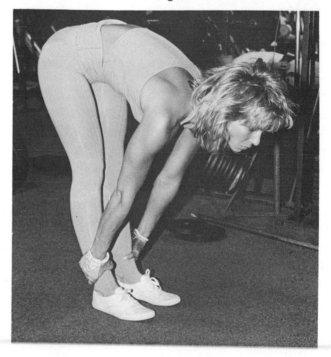

together and your arms straight down at your sides. Bend your legs slightly and jump into the air, simultaneously moving your arms directly out to the sides and upward until your hands touch each other above your head just as your feet contact the floor. As you move your arms upward, you must spread your legs apart so when you touch the floor again with your feet they are a little wider than shoulder-width on each side. Immediately jump back in the air again and return to the starting point. Repeat this movement 25–30 times.

Hamstrings Stretch: Stand erect with your arms down at your sides and your feet about six inches apart. Bend forward at the waist, reaching downward to grasp your ankles with your hands. Pull your torso toward your legs until you feel a painful sensation in your hamstrings. Back off an inch on the stretch and hold this fully stretched position for 30–60 seconds.

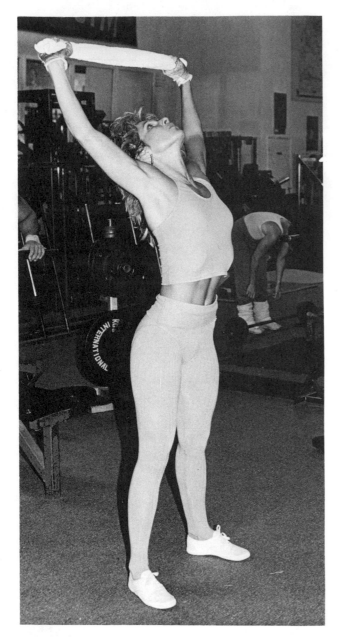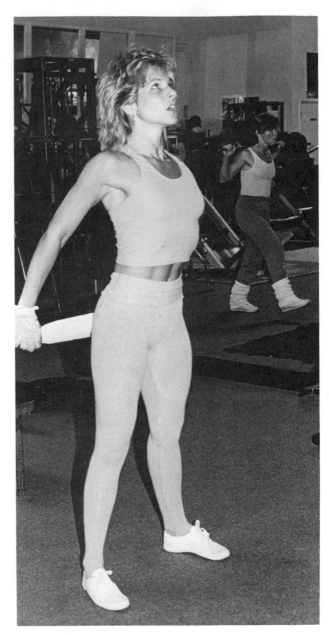

Shoulder Stretch—start, left; finish, right.

Shoulder Stretch: Grasp the ends of a towel and stand erect with your arms straight and the towel resting across your upper thighs. Slowly move your hands upward and to the rear, "dislocating" your shoulders and allowing the towel to come to rest across the backs of your thighs. Return to the starting point and repeat the movement 5–8 times.

Torso Circles: Stand erect with your feet set about shoulder-width apart and place your hands on your hips. Keeping your legs straight throughout the movement, bend forward at the waist until your torso is parallel to the floor. Rotate your torso to the right side, around to the rear, to the left side, and then back forward, attempting to keep your torso parallel to the floor throughout the movement. Do 3–5 repetitions in this direction, then repeat the movement 3–5 times in the opposite direction.

Head Circles: Stand erect with your feet set

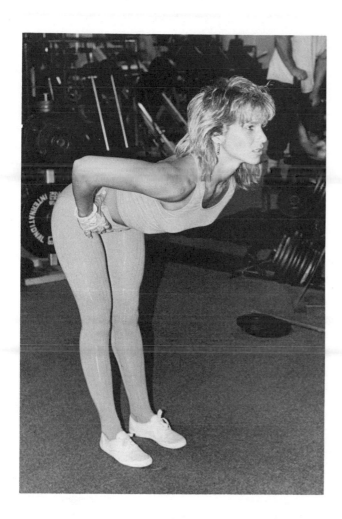
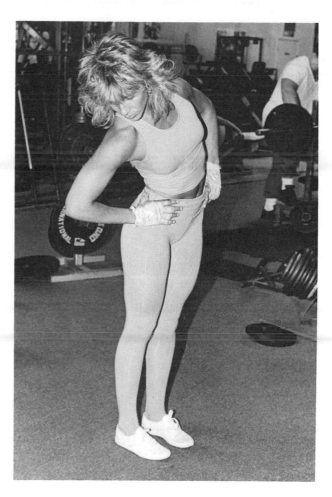

Torso Circle—forward, above left; right side, above right; back, below left; left side, below right.

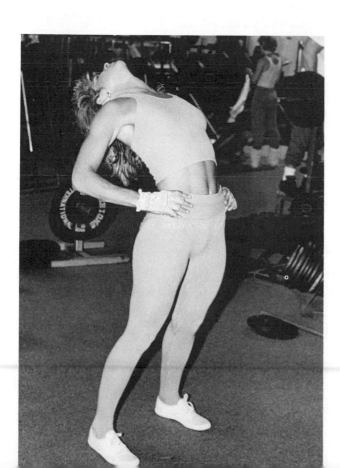
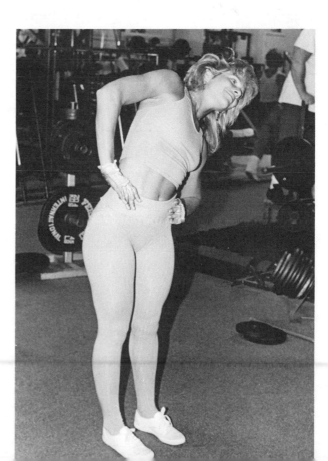

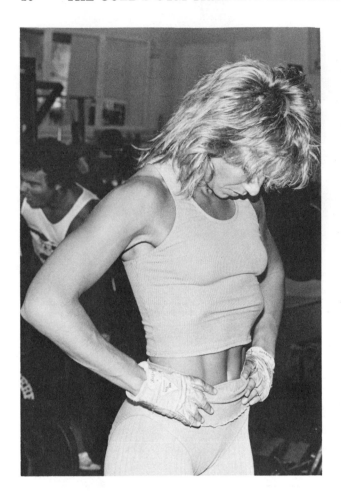

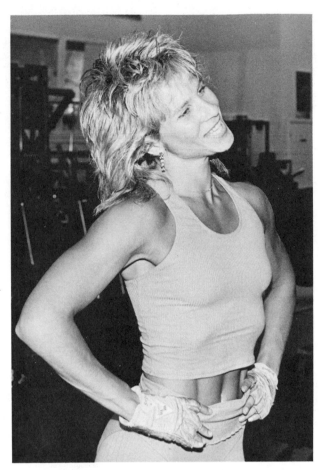

Head Circle—forward, above left; right side, above right; back, below left; left side, below right.

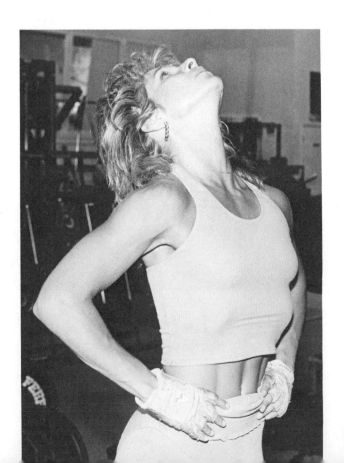

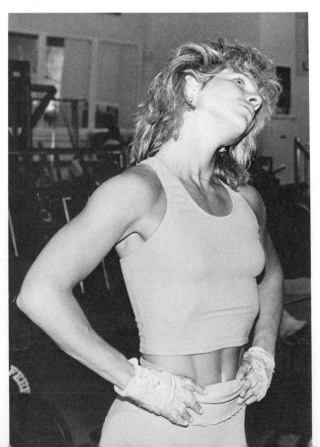

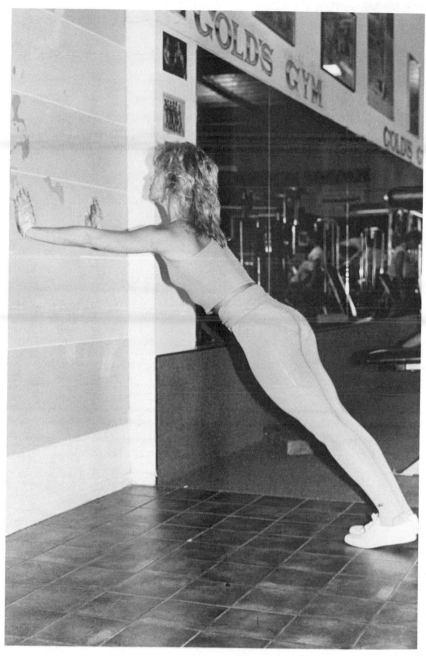

Calf Stretch.

shoulder-width apart and your hands on your hips. Relax your neck and drop your head forward to your chest. Move your head to the right in a circle to the side, back, left side, and again to the front. Continue this circular movement for 3–5 repetitions. Reverse and do the same number of repetitions in the opposite direction.

Calf Stretches: Stand about two feet away from a wall facing toward the wall. Place your feet about shoulder-width apart, keep your torso and legs in one straight line, and reach forward to place your hands on the wall at shoulder height and shoulder-width apart. Try to move your heels toward the floor to stretch your calves. If you can comfortably place your heels on the floor in this position, you should move your feet about 6–8 inches more away from the wall. Hold this stretched position for 30–60 seconds.

Full-Body Workouts

Many readers will be highly experienced body-builders who follow high-intensity workouts. However, others will be novices to the activity. They should follow the series of progressively more intense workouts that follows.

LEVEL ONE
(first six weeks of training)

Exercise	Sets	Reps
Sit-Ups	2–3	20–30
Leg Presses	3	10–15
Leg Curls	2	10–15
Seated Pulley Rows	3	8–12
Upright Rows	2	8–12
Bench Presses	3	8–12
Military Presses	2	8–12
Standing Barbell Curls	2	8–12
Lying Triceps Extensions	2	8–12
Barbell Wrist Curls	2	10–15
Standing Calf Raises	3	15–20

LEVEL TWO
(second six weeks of training)

Exercise	Sets	Reps
Bench Leg Raises	3	20–30
Roman Chair Sit-Ups	2	20–30
Hyperextensions	2	10–15
Squats	3	10–15
Leg Extensions	2	10–15
Leg Curls	3	10–15
One-Arm Dumbbell Bent Rows	3	8–12
Front Lat Pulldowns	2	8–12
Barbell Shrugs	2	10–15
Incline Dumbbell Press	3	8–12
Bench Presses	2	8–12
Press behind the Neck	2	8–12
Side Laterals	2	8–12
Standing Dumbbell Curls	3	8–12
Incline Triceps Extensions	3	8–12
Dumbbell Wrist Curls	2	10–15
Barbell Reverse Wrist Curls	2	10–15
Seated Toe Raises	3–4	10–15

LEVEL THREE
(third six weeks of training)

Monday–Thursday

Exercise	Sets	Reps
Hanging Leg Raises	2–3	10–15
Incline Sit-Ups	2–3	15–20
Seated Twisting	2–3	50
Incline Barbell Press	4	6–10
Flat-Bench Flyes	3	8–12
Dumbbell Presses	3	8–12
Side Laterals	2	8–12
Bent Laterals	2	8–12
Upright Rows	3	8–12
Seated Pulley Rows	4	8–12
Pulldowns behind the Neck	3	8–12
Cross-Bench Pullovers	2	10–15
Seated Calf Raises	3	8–12
Calf Presses	2	15–20

Tuesday–Friday

Exercise	Sets	Reps
Roman Chair Sit-Ups	2–3	20–30
Bench Leg Raises	2–3	20–30
Squats	4	10–15
Leg Extensions	3	10–15
Leg Curls	3–4	10–15
Stiff-Leg Deadlifts	2–3	10–15
Barbell Curls	3	8–12
Barbell Preacher Curls	2	8–12
Pulley Pushdowns	3	8–12
Standing Dumbbell Extensions	2	8–12
Barbell Wrist Curls	3	10–15
Barbell Reverse Wrist Curls	3	10–15
Standing Calf Raises	3	10–15
Donkey Calf Raises	2	15–20

Looking Ahead

In Chapter 2, we will discuss one of the favorite topics of virtually all bodybuilders—biceps training. Our discussion will include descriptions and illustrations of more than 25 commonly used biceps movements and a listing of the favorite biceps training programs of a wide variety of champion male and female bodybuilders from Gold's Gym.

2 BICEPS TRAINING

In 1842 the great American poet, Henry Wadsworth Longfellow, penned these immortal lines in his classic work, *The Village Blacksmith:*

> Under the spreading chestnut tree
> The village smithy stands;
> The smith a mighty man is he
> With large and sinewy hands.
> And the muscles of his brawny arms
> Are strong as iron bands.

There has been a timeless fascination with huge, muscular, powerful upper-arm development. Indeed, among men, large and powerful arms have been a symbol of masculine strength and physical prowess for centuries. And with the recent emergence of women's bodybuilding has come a very healthy interest in awesome female arm development as well.

Although the triceps muscles make up far more than half of the upper-arm muscle mass, the biceps receive the bulk of attention among champion bodybuilders. Everyone marvels at the biceps development of a Lou Ferrigno, Boyer Coe, Sergio Oliva, Arnold Schwarzenegger, Mike Christian, Casey Viator, or Mike Mentzer. And even though women's bodybuilding is a very new sport, the biceps development

of Laura Combes, Lesley Koslow, Mary Roberts, Carla Dunlap, and Rachel McLish are also talked about with reverence.

Anatomy and Kinesiology

There are two muscle groups on the front of the upper-arm—the *biceps* and *brachialis.* The brachialis lies beneath the biceps and is most easily seen in a highly muscular bodybuilder as a band of muscle lying between the biceps and triceps in a back arm pose. The brachialis helps to bend the upper arm, particularly when the hand is in a pronated position (i.e., when the palm is down). The brachialis is directly stressed in the Reverse Curl movement and indirectly stressed in many back exercises, such as Chins, Lat Pulldowns, Barbell Rows, and Seated Pulley Rows.

The biceps are a two-headed muscle that serve two functions—to bend the arm from a straight position, and to supinate the hand. All bodybuilders understand that bending the arm under stress, as in a Barbell Curl, directly affects the biceps muscles, but very few bodybuilders fully understand the supination function of the biceps muscles.

You can visually confirm the effect of supinating your hand by observing a couple of arm poses in the mirror. First, do a biceps shot with your wrist rotated so your palm is away from your body. You will see that your biceps muscles appear long and flat. But if you rotate your wrist so your palm is toward your body, your biceps will peak upward, indicating that more biceps muscle fibers are under tension.

Since your hands are locked into position when you do Curls with a barbell or EZ-Curl bar—as well as with all exercise machines—you can't supinate your hands in any long-bar or machine movements. You can best supinate your hand while curling a dumbbell upward. As you curl a dumbbell upward from the side of your leg, your palm is initially facing toward your leg, but it is rotated upward (or supinated) as you curl the dumbbell to your shoulders. Therefore, you should never neglect dumbbell movements in your biceps programs.

Biceps Exercises

In this section you will find nearly 30 major biceps movements, each fully described and illustrated. Add in the numerous variations of each basic exercise, and you will have more than 50 biceps exercises in your basic pool of bodybuilding movements.

If you are relatively unfamiliar with bodybuilding exercises, you should carefully review both the written description and exercise photos of each movement before first trying it, and then, with a very light weight. Only when you are confident that you are correctly performing the exercise, should you use a weight that taxes the muscles you are trying to work. And any time you aren't fully confident that you are correctly performing an exercise, you should ask an experienced bodybuilder or gym instructor to check out your exercise form.

Standing Barbell Curls

Emphasis: This is the most basic of all biceps movements. Not only does it strongly stress the biceps muscles, but also places significant stress on the powerful *flexor muscles* on the inner sides of the forearms.

Starting Position: Take a shoulder-width un-

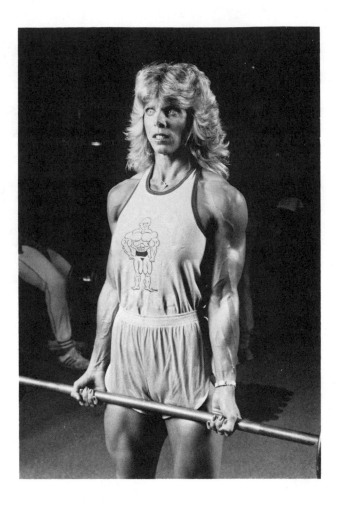

der-grip on a moderately weighted barbell (with this grip, your palms will be facing away from your body in the correct starting position of the movement). With your feet set about shoulder-width apart, stand erect with your arms hanging straight down at your sides and the barbell resting across your upper thighs. Press your upper arms against the sides of your torso and hold them in this position throughout the movement. (If you have well-developed lats, it will be extremely difficult to press your upper arms against the sides of your torso as you do Barbell Curls; in such a case, you should merely attempt to hold your upper arms motionless as you perform the exercise.)

Movement Performance: Moving only your forearms, use biceps strength to move the barbell from the starting position across your upper thighs in a semicircular arc to a point just beneath your chin. For the first half of the

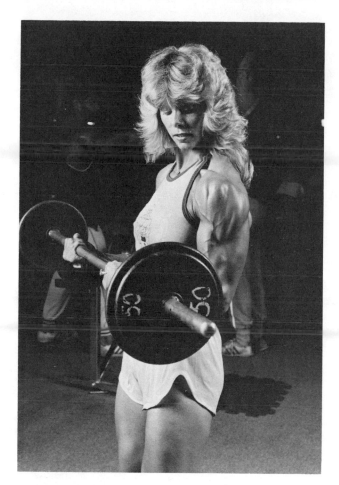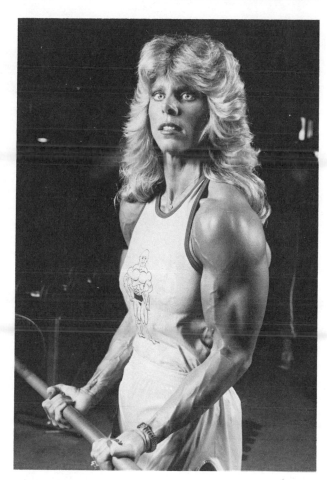

Standing Barbell Curl—start, opposite page; near finish, above left. Standing Barbell Curl with narrow grip, above right.

movement, you should keep your wrists straight; and at the finish of the movement, you can flex your wrists. Lower the weight slowly back to the starting point and repeat the movement.

Training Tip: If you have too much trouble keeping your torso from moving back and forth as you do Standing Barbell Curls, you should perform the movement with your back resting against a wall or upright post in the gym. With your back restrained in this manner, it's impossible to cheat when you do Barbell Curls.

Exercise Variations: You can vary your grip over quite a wide range when doing Standing Barbell Curls. You can use any width of grip from a very narrow one with your hands touching in the middle of the bar to one as wide as the length of the bar will permit. Wide-Grip Barbell Curls were a favorite of the man with the Mount Everest biceps, Arnold Schwarzenegger (seven times Mr. Olympia). You can also use an EZ-

Curl bar in this movement. This "wiggly bar" puts your wrists in a position of great comfort, but it actually moves your biceps *away* from a supinated position. As a result, many top bodybuilders avoid using an EZ-Curl bar in their biceps programs.

Cheating Barbell Curls

Comment: This is one of the first movements in which you can effectively use the cheating principle of training. By continuing a set of Barbell Curls to the point where you can no longer complete a full rep (this is called *training to failure*), you can effectively use Cheating Barbell Curls to force your biceps to continue working past the point of normal failure. And, this is a great way to push them to even faster-than-normal growth. Once you have failed a rep, use just enough torso swing to boost the bar past

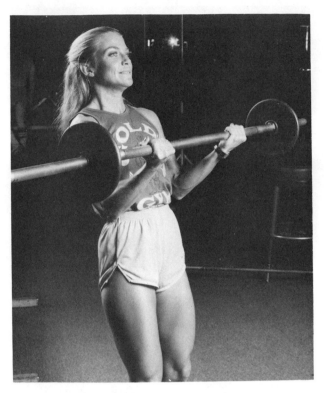

Cheating Barbell Curl at midpoint.

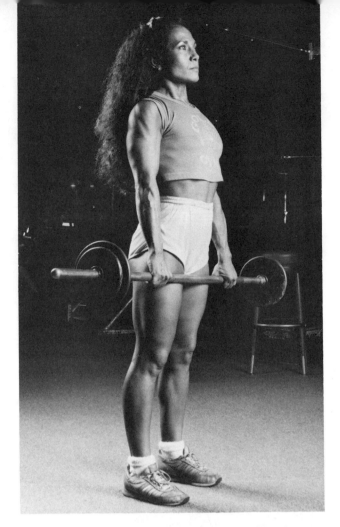

Barbell Reverse Curl—start, above; finish, below.

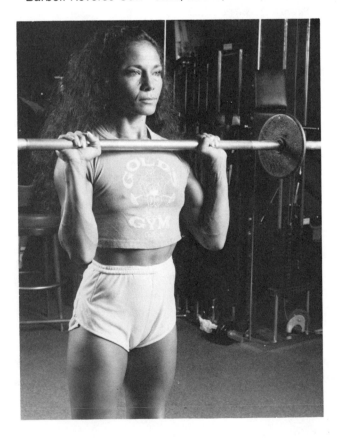

the point at which it would normally fail to continue up to the finishing point. From there, you should use the biceps strength you have left to finish the curl, then resist the downward momentum of the bar as powerfully as possible as you lower the bar. In general, you will never need to do more than two or three cheating reps in any movement.

Barbell Reverse Curls

Emphasis: Reverse Curls place primary emphasis on the brachialis muscles and the powerful *supinator muscles* on the upper and outer parts of the forearms. Secondary stress is placed on the biceps.

Starting Position: Take a shoulder-width over-grip (your hands will be facing in the opposite direction as for Standing Barbell Curls) on a barbell. Place your feet a comfortable distance apart and stand erect with your arms hanging straight down at your sides and the barbell resting across your upper thighs. Press your upper arms against the sides of your torso and hold them in this position throughout the movement. You should also keep your wrists

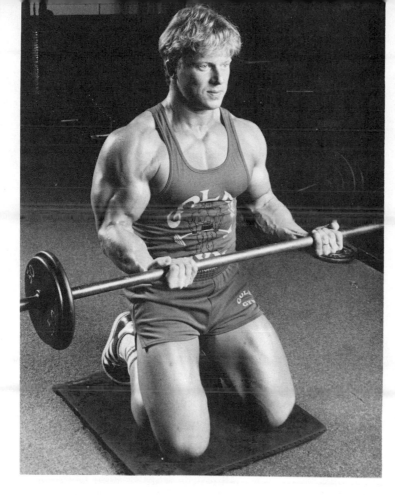

Kneeling Barbell
Curl at midpoint.

held straight throughout the exercise.

Movement Performance: Moving only your forearms, slowly curl the barbell in a semicircular arc from the starting position across your upper thighs to a position just beneath your chin. Slowly lower the barbell back along the same arc to the starting point and repeat the movement for the suggested number of repetitions.

Training Tip: As with Barbell Curls, you can perform Reverse Curls with your back resting against a wall or upright post to prevent cheating.

Exercise Variations: The same grip variations used for Barbell Curls also apply to Reverse Curls, although it is anatomically difficult to use a grip much wider than shoulder-width in this movement. Very few bodybuilders use a cheating movement when they perform Barbell Reverse Curls.

Kneeling Barbell Curls

Emphasis: As with Standing Barbell Curls, this movement places very strong stress on the biceps and forearm flexor muscles and secondary stress on the brachialis muscle group.

Starting Position: Kneel on a pad placed on the floor of the gym to protect your knees during the movement. Take a shoulder-width undergrip on a moderately weighted barbell and assume an erect body position on your knees, your arms running down the sides of your torso and the bar resting across your upper thighs. Press your upper arms against the sides of your torso throughout the movement.

Movement Performance: Moving only your forearms, use biceps strength to curl the barbell in a semicircular arc from the starting point to a position directly beneath your chin. Lower the weight slowly back to the starting point and repeat the exercise.

Comment: It is exceedingly difficult to cheat when you do Barbell Curls in a kneeling position, so this exercise is gaining popularity among "heavily armed" bodybuilders.

Exercise Variations: You can use the wide variety of grips suggested for Standing Barbell Curls in this kneeling variation of the exercise. And you can use a reversed grip in the exercise if you wish to place greater stress on your brachialis and forearm muscles.

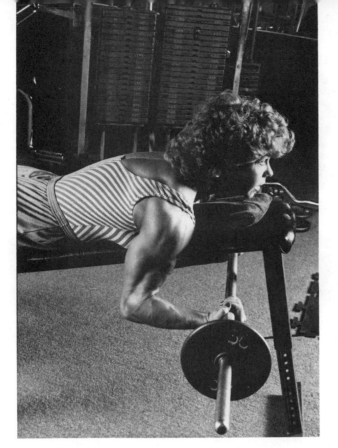

Prone Incline Barbell Curl at midpoint.

Spider Bench Barbell Curls

Comment: This exercise is the same movement as Prone Incline Barbell Curls, except that it is performed lying facedown on a high, flat exercise bench. Spider Bench Barbell Curls are another great biceps-peaking movement.

Barbell Slide Curls

Emphasis: This unique variation of Standing Barbell Curls stresses the biceps from a new angle. It places less stress on the brachialis and forearm flexors than the normal version of Standing Barbell Curls.

Starting Position: Take a shoulder-width under-grip on a moderately weighted barbell. Place your feet about shoulder-width apart and stand erect with your arms hanging straight down your sides and the bar resting across your upper thighs. Incline your torso slightly backward at the waist.

Movement Performance: Slowly curl the barbell up the front of your torso, actually sliding it up your waist and chest and allowing your elbows to travel to the rear. You probably won't be able to get the bar much higher than the lower edge of your pectorals, but this will be a sufficient range of motion for your biceps to benefit greatly from the movement. Return the bar to the starting point and repeat the movement.

Comment: This is a favorite biceps movement of Mohamed Makkawy, winner of numerous professional bodybuilding titles.

Barbell Concentration Curls

Emphasis: Performed with a barbell, Concentration Curls strongly stress the biceps in relative isolation from the rest of the body. Barbell Concentration Curls are an excellent exercise for enhancing the natural peak of your biceps.

Starting Position: Take a narrow under-grip in the middle of a barbell handle (there should be about 4–6 inches of space between your little fingers when you have the correct grip width). Set your feet about shoulder-width apart and bend your torso forward until it is held parallel to the floor throughout the movement. Hang your arms directly downward from your shoulders, and try to keep your upper arms motionless throughout the movement.

Prone Incline Barbell Curls

Emphasis: This unique movement very strongly stresses the biceps muscles, particularly in the peak-contracted position. Prone Incline Barbell Curls are not performed that frequently by bodybuilders, but this is nonetheless one of the best exercises for building an Everest peak on your biceps.

Starting Position: Take a shoulder-width under-grip on a light barbell and lie facedown on a 30–45-degree incline bench. Your arms should be straight and hanging directly down from your shoulders. It is essential that you keep your upper arms motionless throughout this movement.

Movement Performance: Slowly bend your arms to curl the weight in a semicircular arc from the starting point to as high a position as possible (preferably up to touch the underside of the bench just beneath your face). Lower the weight slowly back to the starting point and repeat the movement.

Exercise Variations: You can change your grip width on this movement, but you'll probably discover that you get the best quality of contraction in your biceps if you use a medium-to-relatively narrow grip on the bar.

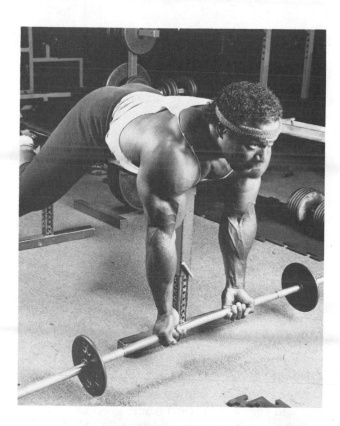
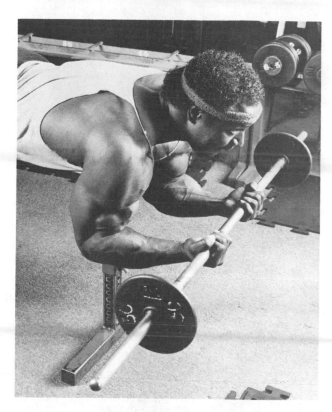

Spider Bench Barbell Curl—start, left; finish, right.

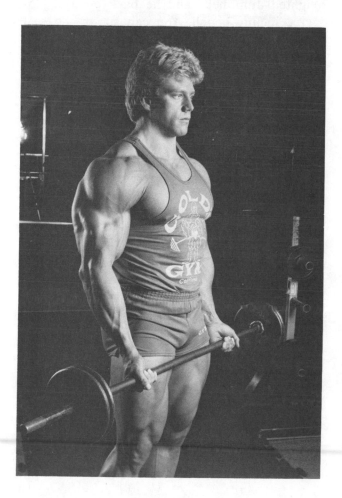
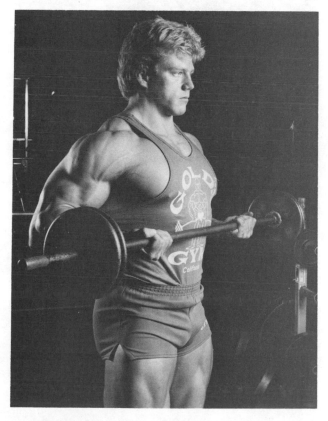

Barbell Slide Curl—start, left; finish, right.

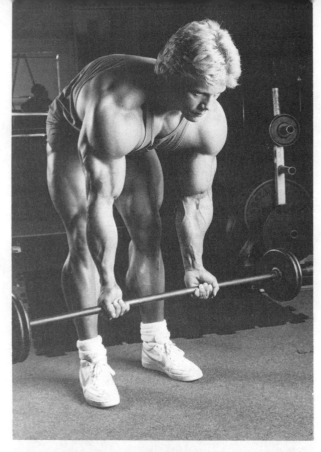

Movement Performance: Without moving anything but your forearms, slowly curl the bar upward from the starting point in a semicircular arc to the base of your neck. Hold this peak-contracted position for a moment, lower the barbell back to the starting point, and repeat the movement for the desired number of repetitions.

Comment: This is a favorite biceps-shaping movement of Robby Robinson, winner of virtually every bodybuilding title but Mr. Olympia.

Exercise Variations: You can use different grip widths, and even an over-grip, on this movement. You can also perform it in relative comfort by resting your elbows on your knees as you curl the bar upward.

Incline Dumbbell Curls

Emphasis: This is a good, general biceps movement which particularly hits the full belly of the muscle group. Secondary stress is on the brachialis and forearm flexor muscle groups.

Starting Position: Grasp two moderately weighted dumbbells and lie back on a 30–45-degree incline bench. You can sit on the seat bench if one is provided; otherwise, you should simply stand on the foot platforms provided with the bench. Hang your arms directly downward from your shoulders and rotate your wrists so your palms are facing each other. Try to keep your upper arms motionless throughout the movement.

Movement Performance: Slowly curl the dumbbells forward and up to your shoulders, simultaneously rotating your wrists so your palms are upward at least during the last half of the movement. Reverse the procedure to return the dumbbells to the starting point. Repeat the movement.

Exercise Variations: Normally, you will curl the dumbbells directly forward, but they can be curled somewhat out to the sides, or even directly out to the sides. Each new angle at which you curl the dumbbells produces a unique new stress on your biceps. For full development, you should try every variation possible.

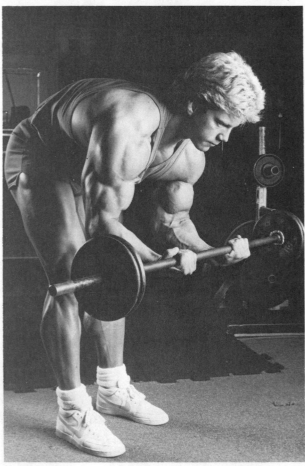

Barbell Concentration Curl—start, top; finish, bottom.

Prone Incline Dumbbell Curls

Emphasis: This version of Incline Curls places a strong peak contraction effect on your biceps.

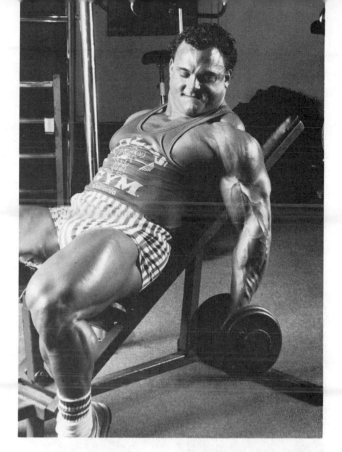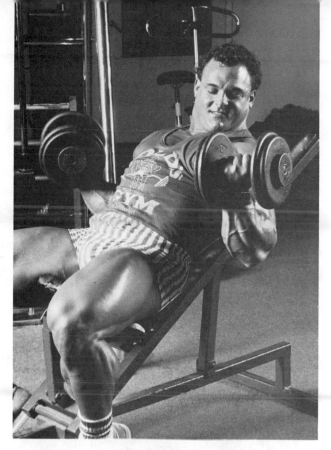

Incline Dumbbell Curl—start, left; near finish, right.

Prone Incline Dumbbell Curl—start, left; finish, right.

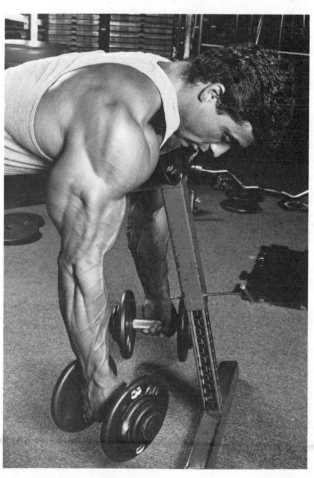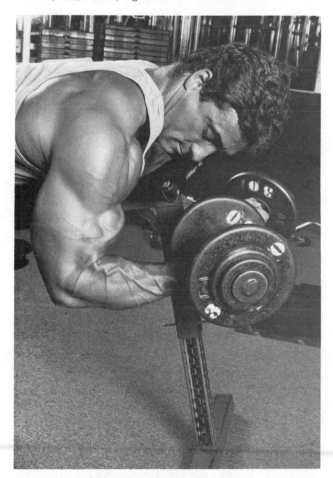

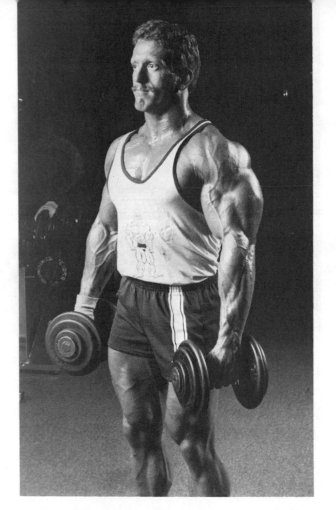
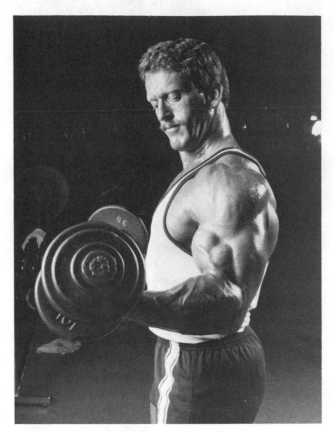

Standing Dumbbell Curl—start, left; midpoint, right.

Secondary stress is placed on the brachialis and forearm flexor muscles.

Starting Position: Grasp two light dumbbells and lie face-down on a 30–45-degree incline bench. Hang your arms straight down from your shoulders and rotate your wrists so your palms face each other. Keep your upper arms motionless throughout the movement.

Movement Performance: Slowly curl the dumbbells up to your shoulders, simultaneously rotating your wrists so your palms are facing upward during at least the last half of the movement. Reverse the procedure to lower the weights back to the starting point. Repeat the movement.

Comment: This was a favorite biceps peaking movement of the great Boyer Coe, winner of numerous IFBB pro titles over the years.

Standing Dumbbell Curls

Emphasis: Dumbbell Curls very effectively place major stress on the biceps muscles and secondary emphasis on the brachialis and forearm

flexor muscles.

Starting Position: Grasp two moderately weighted dumbbells, place your feet a comfortable distance apart, and stand erect with your arms straight down at your sides and your wrists rotated so your palms are facing the sides of your legs. Keep your upper arms motionless during the exercise.

Movement Performance: Slowly curl the dumbbells forward and up to your shoulders, simultaneously supinating your wrists so your palms are facing upward during at least the last half of the movement. Reverse the procedure to lower the dumbbells back to the starting point, and repeat the movement.

Exercise Variations: You can curl the dumbbells alternately, one being curled upward as the other is lowered. This is a good method of preventing torso swing from helping you to complete each rep. And rather than always curling the weights directly forward, you can curl them outward at various angles to stimulate your biceps somewhat differently with each new angle.

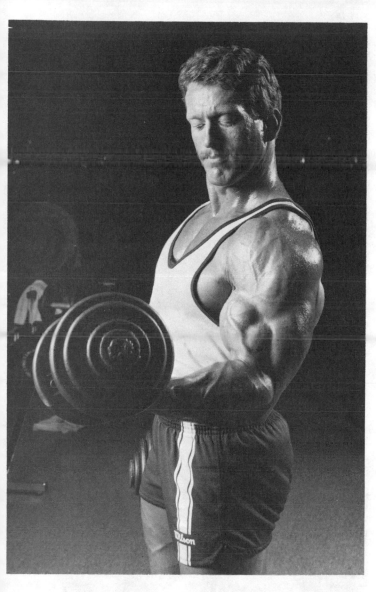

Standing Dumbbell Curl
—alternating arms.

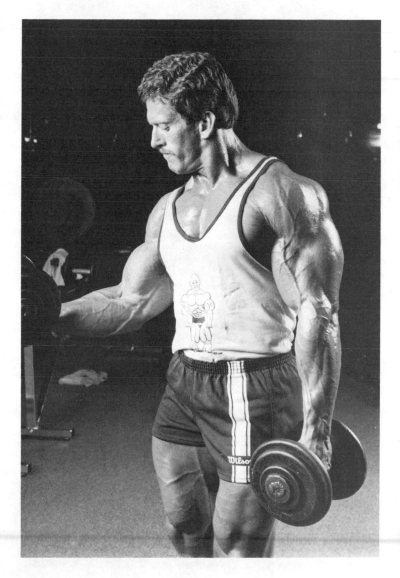

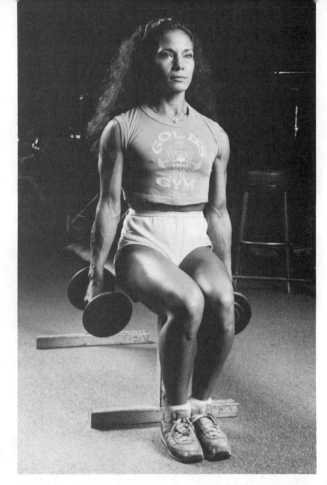
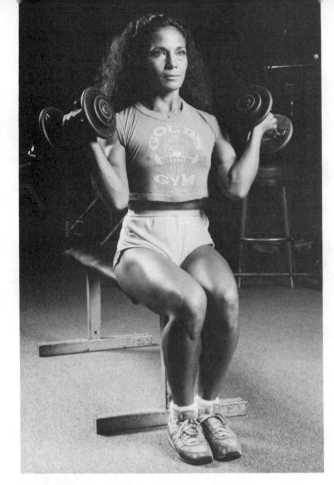

Seated Dumbbell Curl—start, left; finish, right.

Kneeling Dumbbell Curl—start, left; finish, right.

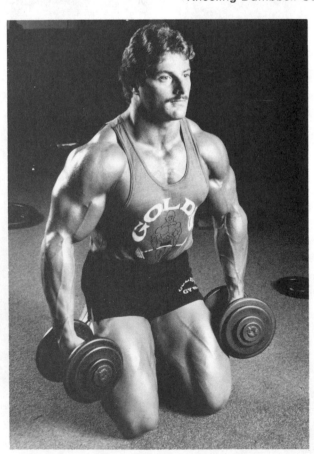
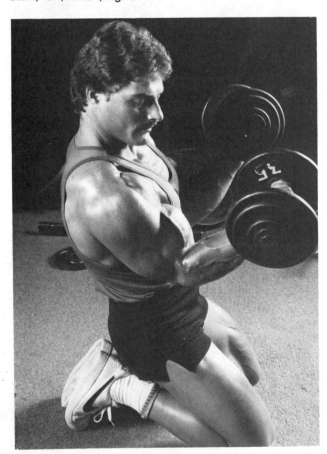

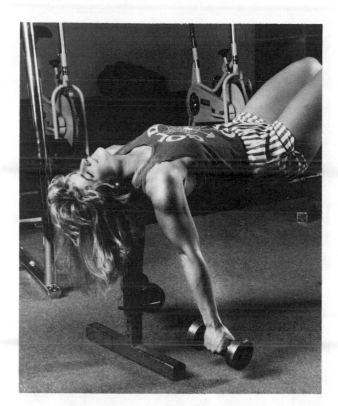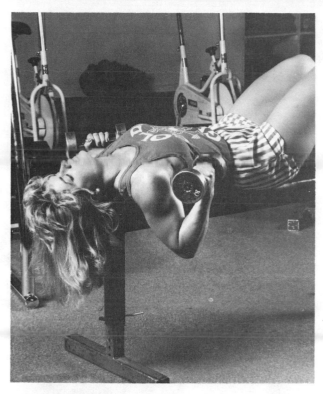

Lying Dumbbell Curl—start, left; finish, right.

Seated Dumbbell Curls

Comment: This is the same movement as Standing Dumbbell Curls, except that it is performed seated at the end of a flat exercise bench, which isolates your legs from the movement and makes it somewhat more strict than the standing version. While seated, you can curl the dumbbells either simultaneously or alternately.

Kneeling Dumbbell Curls

Comment: Again, this is a very similar movement to Standing Dumbbell Curls, except that it is performed while kneeling on a pad placed on the gym floor. Kneeling very effectively isolates your legs from the movement, making this version of Dumbbell Curls significantly more strict than Standing Dumbbell Curls. In a kneeling position, you can curl the dumbbells either simultaneously or alternately.

Lying Dumbbell Curls

Emphasis: Dumbbell Curls performed lying on your back on a high, flat exercise bench very directly stress the biceps muscles, particularly the lower biceps. Secondary emphasis is on the brachialis and forearm flexor groups.

Starting Position: Grasp two moderately weighted dumbbells and lie back on a flat exercise bench that is high enough off the floor for the weights to clear the floor when you have your arms extended directly downward from your shoulders. You can either place your feet flat on the floor on either side of the bench to balance your body in position, or you can curl your legs up over your torso to isolate them from the movement. Keep your upper arms motionless throughout the exercise.

Movement Performance: Moving only your forearms, slowly curl the dumbbells directly forward and upward to your shoulders. Your palms should be facing each other at the starting point of the movement, and you should supinate your hands during the curl so your palms are facing upward during at least the last half of the movement. Reverse the procedure and lower the weights back to the starting point. Repeat the movement.

Exercise Variations: Rather than always curling the dumbbells directly forward, you can curl them outward away from the bench at varying angles.

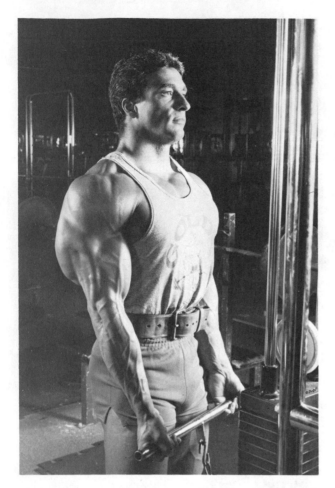
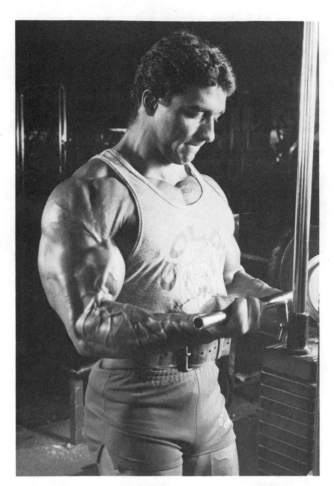

Standing Cable Curl—start, left; midpoint, right.

Standing Cable Curls

Emphasis: The several variations of this movement all stress the biceps quite strongly and place secondary stress on the brachialis and forearm flexor muscle groups.

Starting Position: Attach a short bar handle to the cable running through a floor pulley and grasp the handle with a relatively narrow undergrip. Place your feet about shoulder-width apart one or two feet back from the floor pulley and stand erect with your arms straight and your upper arms pinned against the sides of your torso.

Movement Performance: Moving only your forearms, slowly curl the handle from the starting point to a position just beneath your chin. Return your hands to the starting point and repeat the movement for an appropriate number of counts.

Exercise Variations: You can perform a very effective variation of this movement by simply lying on your back with your feet toward the floor pulley and doing your curls in this position. Since the floor restrains your upper arms from moving in a way that would help you cheat up your reps, this movement is a very direct way to stress your biceps. Both the standing and lying variations of this Cable Curl movement can be performed with a reversed grip to place a greater degree of stress on your brachialis and forearm muscles.

Loop-Handle Cable Curls

Emphasis: This is an excellent biceps-shaping exercise that a lot of champs prefer to include in their routines just prior to a competition.

Starting Position: Attach a loop handle to the

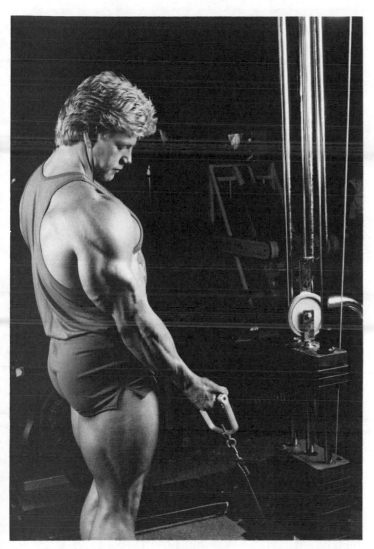
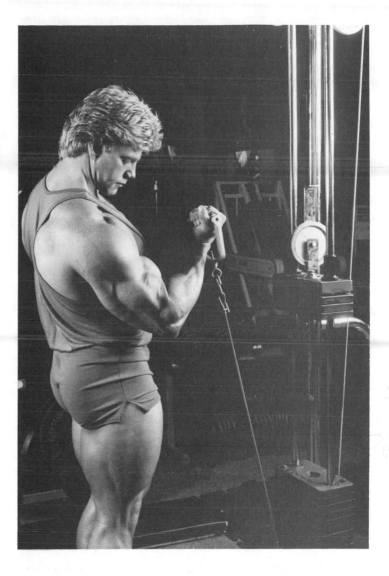

Loop-Handle Cable Curl—start, above; finish, right.

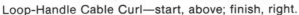

end of a cable running through a floor pulley and grasp the handle in your left hand. Stand about two feet back from the pulley with your right side turned slightly away from the pulley. Anchor your left elbow against your side and fully straighten your arm.

Movement Performance: Moving nothing but your forearm, slowly curl the loop handle up to your shoulder. Hold this peak-contracted, top position for a moment, lower back to the starting point, and repeat the movement. Be sure to perform the same number of sets and repetitions with each arm.

Comment: This is a favorite exercise of Rachel Mclish, whose well-shaped biceps have won her two IFBB Miss Olympia titles.

Exercise Variations: With two adjacent floor pulleys, you can do this movement with both arms at a time, either curling both hands up simultaneously or alternately.

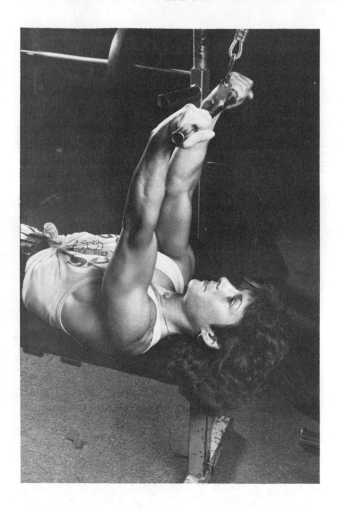

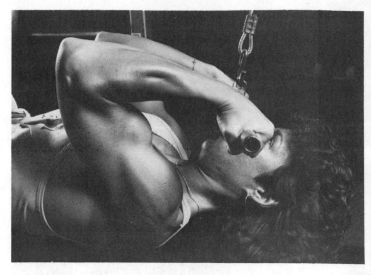

Lat Machine Curl—start, left; finish, above.

Exercise Variations: You can also do this exercise one arm at a time with a loop handle attached to the overhead pulley. And with the straight-bar handle, you can use an over-grip to place greater stress on your brachialis and forearm muscles.

Barbell Preacher Curls

Emphasis: Barbell Preacher Curls build a long, full biceps. All variations of Preacher Curls are excellent for filling in the lower biceps. Secondary stress is on the brachialis and forearm flexor muscle groups.

Starting Position: Take an under-grip on a barbell with your hands set slightly wider on each side than the width of your shoulders. Bend your arms fully, then lean over the top of a preacher bench, wedging your armpits over the top edge of the bench and running your upper arms directly down the angled surface of the bench. Your forearms should be placed on the bench a little narrower than the width or your grip on the bar. Fully straighten your arms.

Movement Performance: Use your biceps strength to slowly curl the barbell from the starting point to a position just at the base of your throat. Lower the weight deliberately back to the starting point and repeat the movement for the suggested number of repetitions.

Lat Machine Curls

Emphasis: This is a good biceps-peaking exercise that places fairly strong, secondary stress on the brachialis and forearm flexor muscles.

Starting Position: Attach a straight-bar handle to an overhead lat machine and move a flat exercise bench in position beneath the pulley so you can lie on your back on the bench with your shoulders directly beneath the pulley. Take a narrow under-grip on the pulley bar and lie on your back on the bench, extending your arms directly upward toward the pulley. It's essential that you keep your upper arms motionless during the movement.

Movement Performance: Moving only your forearms, slowly curl the lat machine handle down to touch the base of your neck. Hold this peak-contracted position for a moment, allow the bar handle to return to the starting point, and repeat the movement.

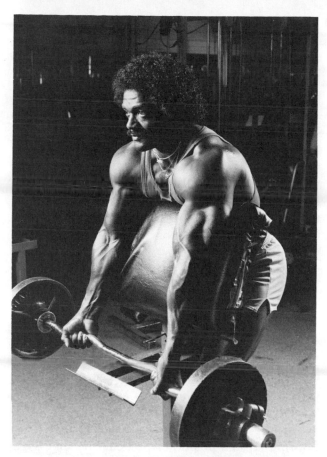
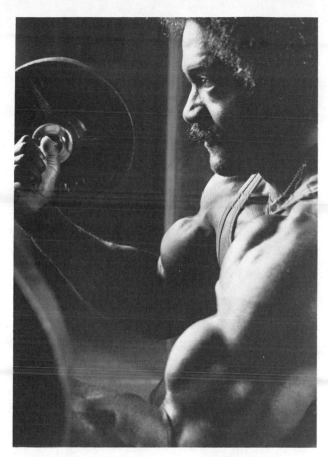

Barbell Preacher Curl—start, left; finish, right.

Reverse-Grip Barbell Preacher Curl—start, right; finish, left. Note narrow grip and use of EZ-Curl bar.

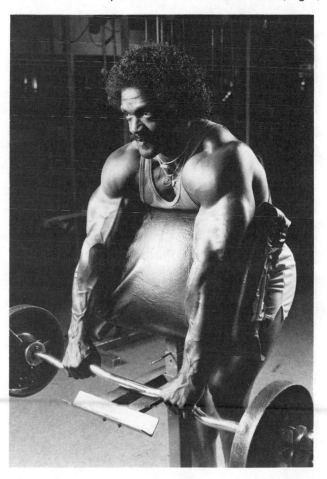
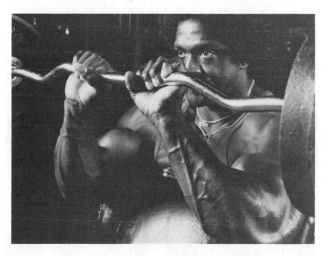

Training Tip: It's essential that you lower the barbell slowly back to the starting point with your arms straight. If you forcefully dropped the weight, attempting to get a rebound at the bottom of the movement, you could conceivably rupture either the biceps muscle itself or a biceps tendon.

Exercise Variations: Many bodybuilders like

to use an EZ-Curl bar (particularly with a narrow grip) on this movement. Regardless of the type of bar used, you can vary the width of your grip from very narrow to as wide as the length of the bar will permit. You can also do this exercise with a reversed grip to strongly stimulate your brachialis and forearm muscles.

Dumbbell Preacher Curls

Emphasis: As with Barbell Preacher Curls, Dumbbell Preacher Curls develop a long, full biceps, with a particularly full, lower-biceps development.

Starting Position: Grasp two moderately weighted dumbbells and position yourself over the preacher bench as you did for the barbell version of this movement. Your upper arms should run parallel to each other down the angled surface of the bench. Fully straighten your arms.

Movement Performance: Slowly curl the dumbbells up to your shoulders, being sure to curl them along an arc slightly outside the line of

your upper arms on the padded surface of the bench. Slowly straighten your arms to return to the starting point of the exercise and repeat it for an appropriate number of repetitions.

Training Tip: Again, never bounce the dumbbells at the bottom of the movement.

Exercise Variations: Most commonly, you can vary this movement by performing it with one arm at a time. This can be done by running your upper arm down the angled pad of the bench. Or if you don't have a preacher bench in your gym, you can run your upper arm down the angled surface at the top of an incline bench.

Cable Preacher Curls

Emphasis: As with Barbell and Dumbbell Preacher Curls, this exercise builds a long, full biceps. And when you do Preacher Curls with cables, you can keep a more continuous form of tension on your working biceps muscles.

Starting Position: Attach a bar handle to a floor pulley and position a preacher bench about two feet back from the pulley. Take a narrow

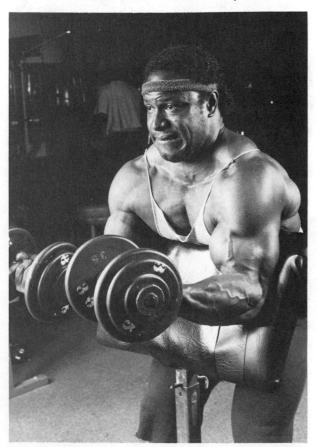

Dumbbell Preacher Curl at midpoint.

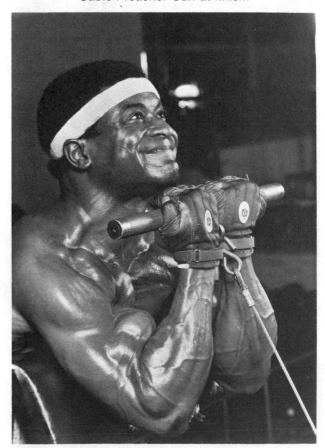

Cable Preacher Curl at finish.

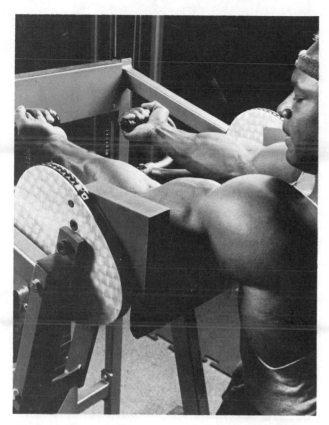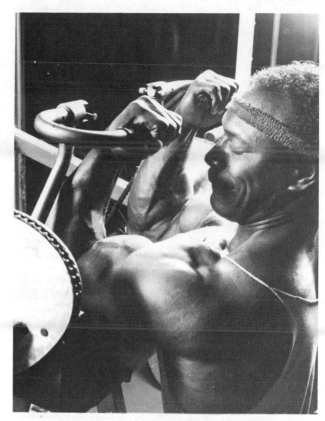

Nautilus Curl—start, left; finish, right.

under-grip on the bar handle and position yourself over the preacher bench so the top of it is wedged beneath your armpits and your upper arms run down the angled surface of the bench more or less parallel to each other. Fully straighten your arms.

Movement Performance: Slowly curl the handle upward in a semicircular arc until it touches your neck. Return slowly and deliberately to the starting point and repeat the movement.

Exercise Variations: By attaching a loop handle to the floor pulley cable, you can do this movement with one arm at a time. And with the bar handle, you can use an over-grip to place greater stress on your brachialis and forearm flexors.

Nautilus Curls

Emphasis: This is a very direct and balanced, stress-producing machine that builds high-quality biceps muscle tissue. Minimal secondary stress is placed on the brachialis and forearm flexor muscle groups.

Starting Position: The height of the machine's seat must be adjusted so your upper arms can be extended upward from your shoulders at precisely the angle of the arm-support pad once you are seated in the machine. There are two types of weight-transfer arrangements on the various Nautilus biceps machines. In the first type, you merely grasp two handles in your hands. In the second, you rest your wrists against two pads. In either case, your palms must be facing upward during the movement. Straighten your arms fully.

Movement Performance: Slowly bend both arms as completely as possible, pause for a moment in this peak-contracted position, return to the starting point, and repeat the movement.

Exercise Variations: You can do this exercise with one arm at a time, Casey Viator's favorite variation. Casey was the youngest man to ever win the Mr. America title (he was 19.) Or, you can do it in alternate-arms fashion by first curling both arms completely, then lowering and recurling each one alternately until you have fully fatigued your biceps.

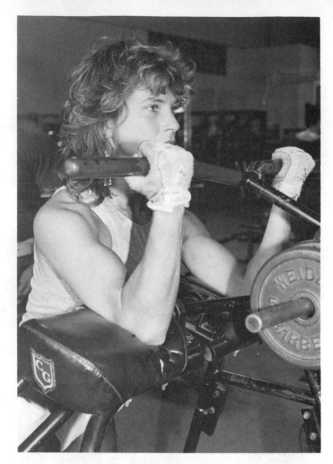

Corbin-Pacific Curl at finish.

Machine Curls

Emphasis: There are several other biceps-curling machines in common usage, and they all operate on the same principles to stongly stress the biceps muscles over a full range of motion.

Starting Position: These machines generally have a preacher-bench-like padded surface over which you lean and run your upper arms down the angled pad of the machine. With your palms up, grasp the handle of the machine and fully straighten your arms.

Movement Performance: Slowly curl the handle up to your neck, pause for a second in the peak-contracted position, return to the starting point, and repeat the movement.

Comment: The main reason why Machine Curls are superior to other types of free-weight curls is that they offer continuous tension throughout the full range of motion. In Barbell Curls, you only feel strong resistance during the middle third of the movement's range of motion, in contrast to feeling strong stress over the full range of motion in Machine Curls.

Seated Dumbbell Concentration Curls

Emphasis: Seated Dumbbell Concentration Curls emphasize the peak on your biceps. The movement is relatively worthless for building biceps mass, however.

Starting Position: Sit at the end of a flat exercise bench and position your feet slightly wider than shoulder-width apart. Grasp a relatively light dumbbell in your left hand and rest the back of your left arm against the inside of your left thigh. With your palm fully supinated, straighten your arm. You can either place your right arm behind your left arm to brace it in position, or you can rest your right hand on your right knee during the exercise.

Movement Performance: Slowly curl the weight up to your shoulder, pausing for a moment at the top of the movement. Lower the dumbbell back to the starting point and repeat the movement. Do an equal amount of work with your right arm.

Standing Dumbbell Concentration Curls

Emphasis: Standing Dumbbell Concentration Curls also emphasize the peak on your biceps.

Starting Position: Grasp a relatively light weight in your left hand. Stand near a high, flat exercise bench or a dumbbell rack and place your right hand on the bench or rack to brace your torso at about a 45-degree angle in relation to the floor. Hang your left arm directly down from your shoulder and straighten it completely. Be sure to keep your left upper arm motionless throughout the movement.

Movement Performance: Being sure to fully supinate your hand, curl the dumbbell slowly up to your shoulder. Pause for a moment in the peak-contracted position, lower the weight slowly back to the starting point, and repeat the movement. Do an equal amount of work for both arms.

Hammer Curls

Emphasis: This is a Dumbbell Curl that more strongly stresses the brachialis and forearm muscles than the biceps.

Starting Position: Grasp two moderately weighted dumbbells, place your feet about

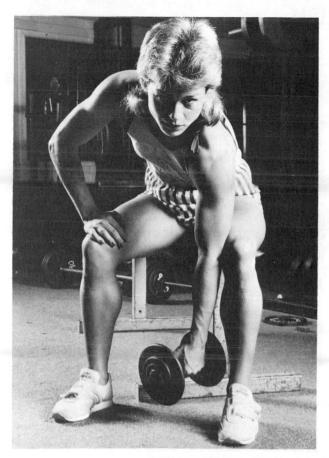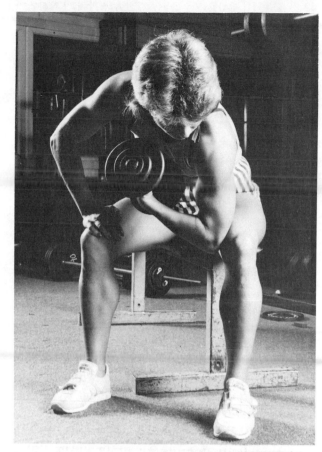

Seated Dumbbell Concentration Curl—start, left; finish, right.

Standing Dumbbell Concentration Curl at midpoint.   Hammer Curl at midpoint.

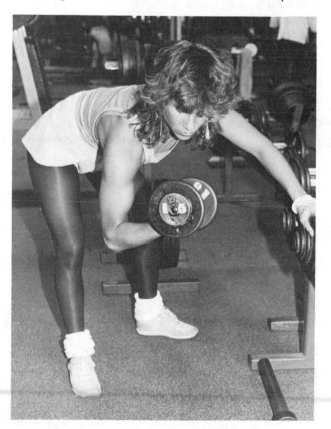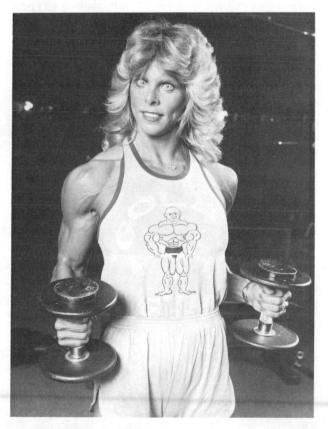

shoulder-width apart, and stand erect with your arms running straight down at your sides. You should rotate your hands so your palms are facing inward toward each other throughout the movement.

Movement Performance: Slowly curl the weights up to your shoulders, lower them back to the starting point, and repeat the movement.

Exercise Variations: As long as you don't supinate your hands during the movement, you can do Hammer Curls in alternate fashion if you prefer. They can also be performed seated.

Zottman Curls

Emphasis: This excellent movement places equal stress on the biceps, brachialis, and forearm muscle groups.

Starting Position: Grasp two moderately weighted dumbbells, place your feet about shoulder-width apart, and stand erect with your arms running straight down at your sides. Turn your wrists so your palms are facing inward toward each other at the beginning of the movement.

Movement Performance: Begin curling the dumbbell in your left hand upward, supinating your hand as you complete the movement. Then

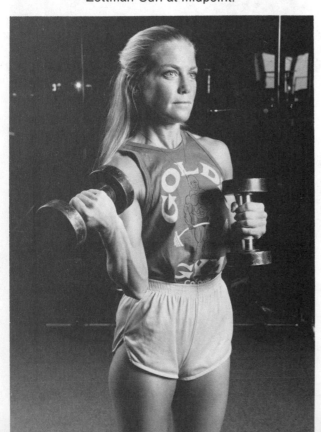

Zottman Curl at midpoint.

at the top of the movement, rotate your left hand so your palm is down as you lower the dumbbell. As soon as you begin lowering the dumbbell in your left hand, start to curl up the dumbbell in your right hand, supinating it as you finish the curl, then turning your palm down as you lower the weight. Continue curling alternately in this fashion until you have performed the required number of repetitions with each arm.

Suggested Biceps Routines

If you have less than a few weeks of training behind you, the following biceps routine can profitably be performed three nonconsecutive days per week:

Exercise	Sets	Reps
Standing Barbell Curls	3	6–10
Seated Dumbbell Curls	2	6–10

After 4–6 weeks of steady training on the forgoing program, you can use this biceps routine three days per week:

Exercise	Sets	Reps
Standing Barbell Curls	3	10–6*
Barbell Preacher Curls	2	6–8
Seated Dumbbell Concentration Curls	1–2	8–12

* All exercises marked with an asterisk should have the weights and reps pyramidded. With each succeeding set, the weight on the bar should be increased and the number of reps performed decreased.

After about three months of steady training, you should switch to a four-day split routine in which you train each major muscle group (including the shoulders) twice per week. This is typically how a lower-level competitive bodybuilder will work out in the off-season. Following is a sample biceps training program for off-season competition training:

Exercise	Sets	Reps
Barbell Preacher Curls	4	12–6*
Alternate Dumbbell Curls	3	6–10
Wide-Grip Barbell Curls	3	6–10
Barbell Concentration Curls	2	8–12

Every advanced bodybuilder trains differently from all others prior to a competition, as you will see in the following section listing the biceps routines of a wide variety of men and women who either train or have trained at Gold's Gym.

Biceps Routines of the Gold's Champs

In this section, you will find a variety of biceps training programs used by many of the Gold's Gym superstars who have won the sport's highest titles. Keep in mind as you examine these training programs that these men and women have been training for many years and have developed enormous recuperative abilities. It is unlikely that you can make good gains using their full routines. Instead, you should use these training programs as examples of how to work your own biceps. In all likelihood, you can do the same exercises as your favorite champion, but scale down the number of sets that he or she does of each movement to meet your own abilities.

Exercise model and American Championship runner-up, Lesley Koslow.

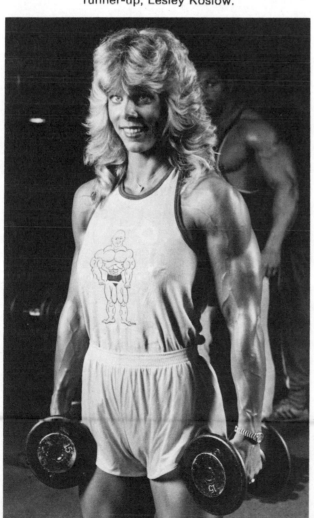

LOU FERRIGNO (MR. UNIVERSE)

Exercise	Sets	Reps
Barbell Preacher Curls	4	8–10
Incline Dumbbell Curls	4	8–10
Seated Dumbbell Curls	4	8–10
Dumbbell Concentration Curls	4	8–10

LAURA COMBES (MS. AMERICA)

Exercise	Sets	Reps
EZ-Curl Bar Curls	3	8–10
Alternate Dumbbell Curls	3	8–10
Cable Preacher Curls	3	8–10
Machine Curls	3	8–10
Seated Dumbbell Concentration Curls	3	8–10

KAY BAXTER (GOLD'S CLASSIC CHAMPION)

Exercise	Sets	Reps
Cable Preacher Curls	4	12–15
Standing Barbell Curls	4	10–12
Incline Dumbbell Curls	4	10–12
Dumbbell Concentration Curls	4	15–20

ED CORNEY (MR. UNIVERSE)

Exercise	Sets	Reps
Standing Barbell Curls	3–4	8–10
Barbell Preacher Curls	3–4	8–10
Wide-Grip Machine Curls	3–4	8–10
Dumbbell Concentration Curls	3–4	8–10
Barbell Reverse Curls	3–4	8–10

LANCE DREHER (MR. UNIVERSE)

Exercise	Sets	Reps
Incline Dumbbell Curls	5	6–10
Dumbbell Concentration Curls	5	6–10
Nautilus Curls	5	6–10

GEORGIA MILLER FUDGE (PRO WOMEN'S CHAMP)

Exercise	Sets	Reps
Incline Dumbbell Curls	4	6–7
High-Pulley Preacher Curls	4	6–7
Low-Pulley Preacher Curls	4	6–7

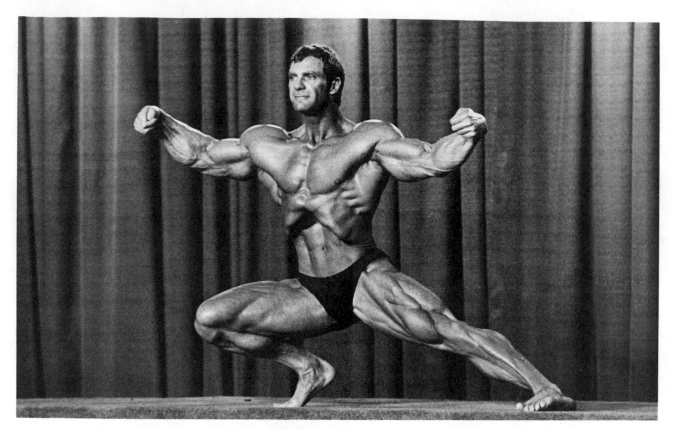

Scott Wilson.

CHARLES GLASS
(MR. UNIVERSE)

Exercise	Sets	Reps
Standing Barbell Curls	4	8–10
Nautilus Curls	4	8–10
Seated Dumbbell Curls	4	8–10
Barbell Concentration Curls	4	10–12

SCOTT WILSON
(PRO MR. AMERICA)

Exercise	Sets	Reps
Standing Barbell Curls	4–5	8–10
Alternate Dumbbell Curls	4–5	8–10
Cable Preacher Curls	4–5	8–10

BERTIL FOX
(MR. UNIVERSE)

Exercise	Sets	Reps
Cheating Curls (EZ-Curl bar)	6	6–8
Incline Dumbbell Curls	6	6–8
Dumbbell Concentration Curls	6	6–8
Barbell Preacher Curls	6	6–8
One-Arm Cable Curls	6	6–8

TOM PLATZ
(MR. UNIVERSE)

Exercise	Sets	Reps
Alternate Dumbbell Curls	4–5	8–10
Standing Barbell Curls	5–6	8–10

DANNY PADILLA
(MR. UNIVERSE)

Exercise	Sets	Reps
Dumbbell Curls	5	6–8
Dumbbell Concentration Curls	4	10
Incline Dumbbell Curls	4	8–10
Standing Barbell Curls	4	8–10

DENNIS TINERINO
(MR. UNIVERSE)

Exercise	Sets	Reps
Alternate Dumbbell Curls	4	5–6
Barbell Preacher Curls	4	5–6
Standing Barbell Curls	4	5–6

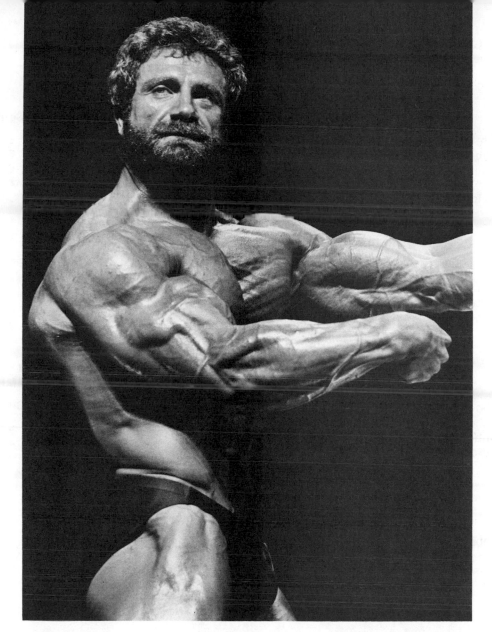

Jusup Wilkosz.

CASEY VIATOR
(MR. AMERICA)

Exercise	Sets	Reps
Dumbbell Concentration Curls	4-5	10-12
One-Arm Standing Cable Curls	4	10-12
Standing Barbell Curls	4	10-12
Alternate Dumbbell Curls	4	10-12

TIM BELKNAP
(MR. AMERICA)

Exercise	Sets	Reps
Standing Barbell Curls	3	10
Seated Dumbbell Curls	3	10
One-Arm Cable Curls	3	10

JUSUP WILKOSZ
(MR. UNIVERSE)

Exercise	Sets	Reps
Incline Dumbbell Curls	5	10-12
Barbell Preacher Curls	5	10 12
Dumbbell Concentration Curls	5	10-12

RICK WAYNE
(MR. WORLD)

Exercise	Sets	Reps
Barbell Cheat Curls	3-4	8-10
Seated Dumbbell Curls	3-4	8-10
Close-Grip Barbell Curls	3	8-10
Incline Dumbbell Curls	3	8-10

MIKE CHRISTIAN
(MR. CALIFORNIA)

Exercise	Sets	Reps
Alternate Dumbbell Curls	3–4	8–12
Incline Dumbbell Curls	3–4	8–10
Barbell Curls	3–4	8–10
Seated Dumbbell Concentration Curls	3–4	10–12

BILL GRANT
(MR. WORLD)

Exercise	Sets	Reps
Nautilus Curls	3	8–10
Incline Dumbbell Curls	3	8–10
Barbell Preacher Curls	3	8–10

GARY LEONARD
(MR. AMERICA)

Exercise	Sets	Reps
Incline Dumbbell Curls	5	6–8
Barbell Preacher Curls	5	6–8
Seated Dumbbell Concentration Curls	5	6–8

PAT NEVE
(MR. USA)

Exercise	Sets	Reps
Incline Dumbbell Curls	4	8–12
Standing Barbell Curls	4	8–12
Barbell Preacher Curls	4	8–12

JOE NISTA
(PAST-40 MR. UNIVERSE)

Exercise	Sets	Reps
Incline Dumbbell Curls	4	6–8
Barbell Preacher Curls	4	8
Dumbbell Concentration Curls	3	10–12

DALE RUPLINGER
(MR. UNIVERSE)

Exercise	Sets	Reps
Standing Barbell Curls	3–4	6–10
Incline Dumbbell Curls	3–4	6–10

SERGIO OLIVA
(MR. OLYMPIA)

Exercise	Sets	Reps
Barbell Curls	6	8
EZ-Curl Bar Preacher Curls	6	8
Dumbbell Preacher Curls	6	8
Dumbbell Concentration Curls	4	8

MANUEL PERRY
(MR. USA)

Exercise	Sets	Reps
Barbell Curls	5	12–15
Standing Dumbbell Curls	5	12–15
Dumbbell Concentration Curls	5	12–15
Cable Concentration Curls	5	12–15

ROBBY ROBINSON
(PRO GRAND PRIX CHAMP)

Exercise	Sets	Reps
Standing Barbell Curls	4	10–12
Barbell Concentration Curls	4	10–12
One-Arm Cable Curls	4	10–12

KAL SZKALAK
(MR. UNIVERSE)

Exercise	Sets	Reps
Incline Dumbbell Curls	5	8–9
Barbell Preacher Curls	5	8
Nautilus Curls	5	12
Cable Concentration Curls	5	12
Barbell Reverse Curls	5	12

Looking Ahead

In Chapter 3, we'll discuss how to train your chest, including descriptions and photographs of nearly 30 exercises, plus more routines of the top men and women who train at The Hall of Champions, Gold's Gym!

3 CHEST TRAINING

Next to the biceps, which were discussed in the preceeding chapter, the pectoral muscles of the chest are the showiest body part. And a deep, full-appearing chest is one indication of buoyantly excellent health. So, it is little wonder that so many male and female bodybuilders are preoccupied with developing a deep, thickly muscled chest.

Most champion male bodybuilders have deep ribcages and thick, striated pectorals. Some bodybuilders with particularly awesome chest development are Lou Ferrigno, Charles Glass, Bertil Fox, Samir Bannout, Tom Platz, Robby Robinson, Dr. Franco Columbu, Arnold Schwarzenegger, Roy Callender, Chris Dickerson, Casey Viator, Scott Wilson, Andreas Cahling, and Tim Belknap.

Many female bodybuilders also have superior pectoral development, although only the upper and inner pecs are visible when a woman poses at a major competition. Some of the best female chest developments belong to Rachel McLish, Carla Dunlap, Laura Combes, Claudia Wilborn, Kay Baxter, Carolyn Cheshire, Lynn Conkwright, and Lisa Elliott-Kolakowski.

Anatomy and Kinesiology

The large, fan-shaped *pectoralis* muscle group lies over the upper rib cage. Originating from attachments on the rib cage, it attaches via a large tendon to the *humerus,* or upper-arm bone. The pectoral muscles contract to pull the humerus from a position with the elbow well behind the body to one in which the elbow is forward and well across the midline of the body. By pulling the humerus across the body at various angles, you can selectively stress different parts of your pectoral muscles. For example, pulling your arm across your torso below shoulder level stresses the lower pectorals, while pulling it across your torso above shoulder level places greater stress on your upper pecs.

Ribcage Expansion

One school of bodybuilding experts insists that it is possible to enlarge the volume of your ribcage by stretching and lengthening the cartilages that attach your ribs to your *sternum* (breast bone). While there is no conclusive proof

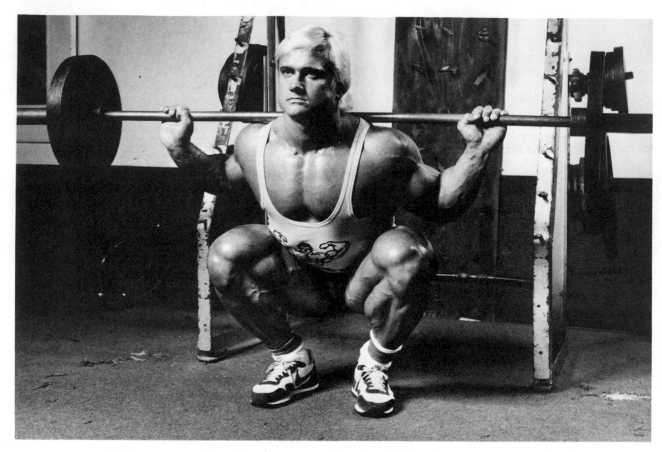

Tom Platz demonstrates breathing squats.

that this can be accomplished, it is worth a try at doing the exercises suggested in this section.

Theoretically, it is easiest to stretch the cartilages of your ribcage if you are still in your teens. During your growth years, these cartilages are soft and pliable; later in life when you have stopped growing in height, they are harder and less easily stretched to a new length.

Ribcage expansion is accomplished by supersetting a deep breathing exercise with one that stretches the ribcage. The first movement is called Breathing Squats. It is a normal Squat, but with a pattern of deep breaths between each repetition. And it is done with no more than your body weight on the bar, since you should be concentrating on your breathing patterns rather than on developing more thigh muscle mass.

Load up the bar, take it off the rack, and prepare yourself to squat. Before each of the first 10 reps in your set, you should take three very deep breaths, squeezing out all possible air as you exhale and then pulling in as much air as

possible when you inhale. For the next 10 reps of your set, you should take four deep breaths between each count. And for the final five repetitions of your 25-rep set, you should take five breaths before each squatting motion.

Without resting, you should proceed immediately to doing light Cross-Bench Pullovers with a dumbbell weighing about half as much as the one you use for pectoral development. This exercise is described in detail later in this chapter, but when you use it for ribcage expansion, you should do the movement with relatively straight arms. And, you must take a deep breath during each repetition, starting to inhale as you begin to drop the weight from straight arms' length in a semicircular arc down behind your head.

Beginning-level bodybuilders can do one or two of these supersets of Breathing Squats and Breathing Cross-Bench Pullovers. Intermediate-level bodybuilders can do three supersets, and advanced-level athletes can do four or five su-

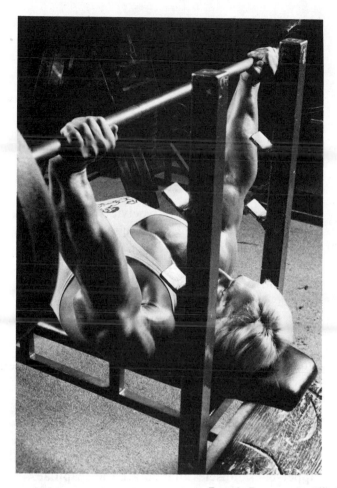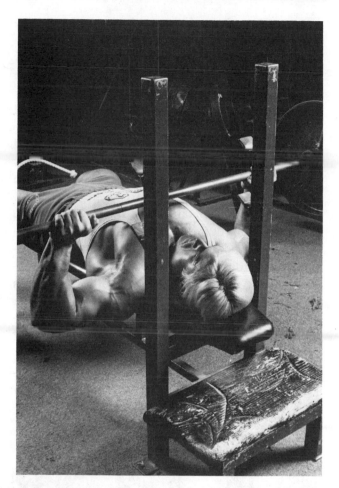

Bench Press—start/finish, left; midpoint, right.

persets in an effort to further expand their ribcages.

Chest Exercises

You will find approximately 30 major chest movements in this section, each of which is fully described and depicted. Add in the numerous variations of each basic movement, and you will have more than 60 chest exercises in your basic pool of bodybuilding exercises. That should be a sufficient variety of chest exercises to satisfy any bodybuilder.

Bench Presses

Emphasis: Bench Presses are considered to be one of the best basic exercises for the upper body. Benches strongly stress the pectorals (particularly the lower and outer sections of the

muscle group), anterior deltoids, and triceps. Secondary emphasis is on the medial heads of the deltoids, the latissimus dorsi, and other upper-back muscles that impart rotational force on the *scapulae*.

Starting Position: Place a barbell on the rack of a pressing bench and adjust the weight on the bar to an appropriate poundage. Lie back on the bench with your shoulder joints 3–4 inches toward the foot end of the bench from the rack supports. Place your feet flat on the floor to balance your body on the bench as you do the movement. Take an over-grip on the bar with your hands set 3–5 inches wider on each side than shoulder width. Straighten your arms to remove the barbell from the rack and move it to a supported position directly above your shoulder joints.

Movement Performance: Making sure that your elbows travel directly out to the sides, bend your arms and slowly lower the barbell from the supported position downward to lightly touch your chest two or three inches above the lower edge of your pectorals. Without bouncing the weight, slowly push it back to straight arms' length. Repeat the movement for the suggested number of repetitions.

Training Tips: You'll see some badly informed bodybuilders who place a rubber pad on their chests and bounce the bar off the pad to gain momentum at the bottom part of the movement. This is not only unsafe, but unwise because the object of bodybuilding is to place maximum resistance on the working muscles, not to use ego-boosting poundages. Another cheating technique used by bodybuilders is to allow their hips to come off the bench so the body is in a bridge position. This little cheat shifts stress to the more powerful lower pectoral muscles, which can lead to a bad balance in your chest musculature.

Exercise Variations: The most common variation in this movement is moving the grip either

inward or outward. When you use a grip of less than shoulder-width, you shift stress more to the inner pectorals and triceps. A very wide grip places more stress on the outer pectorals and anterior deltoids. One of the best ways to involve the pecs with optimum intensity is to lower the weight to the base of your neck rather than to your chest, a motion that allows a longer range of movement. On most exercises done lying on your back, you can isolate your legs from the movement by lifting them off the floor and curling them up over your pelvic structure.

Comment: This is one exercise in which it is extremely dangerous to handle near-limit weights without a safety spotter standing at the head end of the bench. And when you have a spotter standing in this position, he or she can give you forced reps easily and conveniently.

Incline Presses

Emphasis: Incline Presses performed with either a barbell, two dumbbells, or on a machine strongly stress the upper pectorals, anterior deltoids, and triceps. Significant secondary stress is on the lower pecs, medial deltoids, and the upper-back muscles that rotate the scapulae.

Starting Position: Place a barbell on the support rack at the head end of an incline bench and adjust the weight on the bar to an appropriate poundage. Lie back on the bench and sit on the seat provided. Some incline benches don't have a seat, in which case you should keep your feet on the platforms provided for them and fully straighten your body as you lie back on the bench. Take an over-grip on the bar with your hands set 3–5 inches wider on each side than the width of your shoulders. Straighten your arms to remove the barbell from the rack and bring it to a supported position directly above your shoulder joints.

Movement Performance: Being sure to keep your elbows back as you do the exercise, slowly bend your arms and lower the barbell down to lightly touch your upper chest at the base of your neck. Without bouncing the bar off your chest or arching your back, steadily push the barbell back to the starting point. Repeat the exercise for the required number of repetitions.

Exercise Variations: As with Bench Presses, you should vary the width of your grip when you

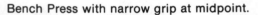

Bench Press with narrow grip at midpoint.

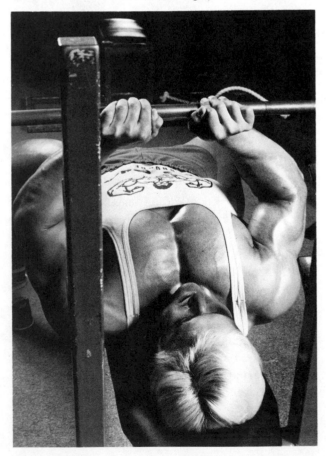

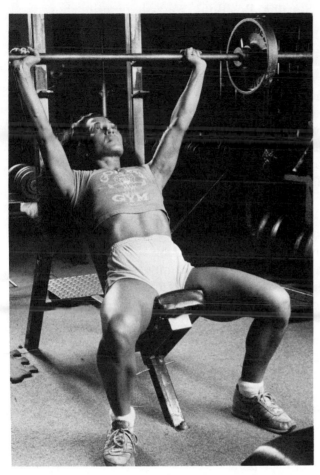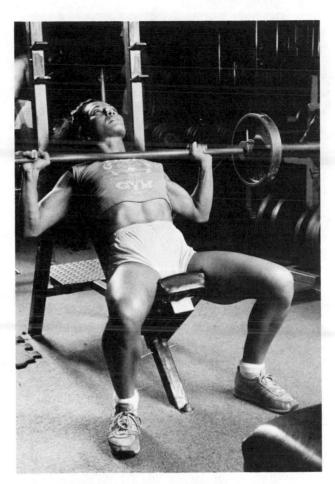

Barbell Incline Press—start/finish, left; midpoint, right.

do Incline Presses with a barbell. Most body-builders do Inclines on a 45-degree angled bench, but you can and should vary the angle of the bench down to as low as about 30 degrees. Each new bench angle stresses the pecs somewhat differently.

Decline Presses

Emphasis: Decline Presses performed with either a barbell, two dumbbells, or on a machine strongly stress the lower and outer pectorals, anterior deltoids, lats, and triceps. Secondary stress is on the upper pecs, medial deltoids, and the upper-back muscles that rotate the scapulae.

Starting Position: Place a decline bench with the head end between two support racks. Rest a barbell on the rack and adjust its weight to an appropriate level. Hook your toes under the restraint bar of the bench and recline on it with your head at the lower end. Take an over-grip on the bar with your hands set 3–5 inches wider than your shoulders on each side. Straighten your arms to lift the weight from the rack to a supported position at straight arms directly above your shoulder joints.

Movement Performance: Keeping your elbows back, slowly bend your arms and lower the barbell down to touch the lower part of your chest at your pec line. Without bouncing the weight, slowly push it back to straight arms' length. Repeat the movement for an appropriate number of repetitions.

Training Tip: Be sure to have a spotter standing at the head end of the bench to protect your face and neck from injury if you lose control of the weight.

Exercise Variations: To increase the range of motion on this exercise, you can lower the barbell to the base of your neck. On all varia-

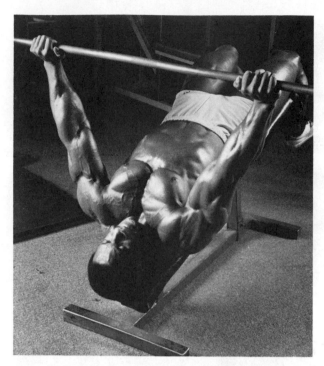

Barbell Decline Press—start/finish, above;
midpoint, below.

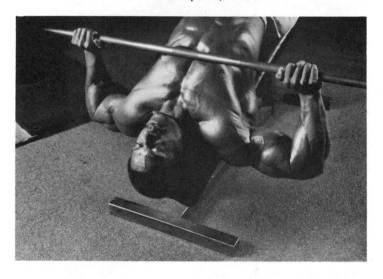

Starting Position: We will describe how to perform this exercise on a flat bench and then give you highlights of the incline and decline variations. Place a flat bench so the head end of it is perpendicular to the pressing handles of the machine. Lie back on the bench and position your body so your shoulder joints are directly below the pressing handles. Take an over-grip in the middle of the pressing handles, which will force you to fully bend your arms. Rotate your elbows downward until they are directly beneath the handles.

Movement Performance: Slowly straighten your arms and push the handles upward until your arms are straight. Lower back to the starting point and repeat the movement. On this and the incline/decline variations of the movement, you can adjust the width of your grip.

Exercise Variations: At Gold's/Venice we developed an incline bench that places your butt almost on the floor. You can place this sort of short incline bench beneath the pressing handles of a Universal Gym machine and do Universal Incline Presses. Similarly, you can position a decline bench between the handles and do Decline Presses.

Smith Machine Flat/Incline/Decline Bench Presses

Emphasis: As with a Universal Gym machine, you can do Benches, Inclines, and Declines on a Smith machine to stress the appropriate areas of your pectorals, deltoids, and triceps.

Starting Position: Place a flat, incline, or decline bench in the Smith machine and adjust the height of the weight to a position so it is just short of where you would hold it at straight arms' length when lying on the bench. Lie back on the bench and take an over-grip on the bar with your hands set 3–5 inches wider on each side than the width of your shoulders. Straighten your arms and rotate the stop hooks attached to the bar to release them.

Movement Performance: Keeping your elbows back, slowly bend your arms and lower the barbell down to lightly touch your chest. Without bouncing the bar off your chest, slowly push it back to straight arms' length. Repeat the exercise for the recommended number of repetitions.

tions of Decline Presses with a barbell, you can vary the width of your grip and use different angles of bench declines.

Universal Flat/Incline/Decline Bench Presses

Emphasis: You can do Benches, Inclines, and Declines at the Bench Press station of a Universal Gym machine to stress appropriate areas of your pectorals, deltoids, and triceps.

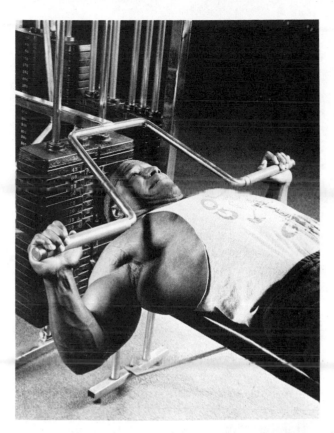
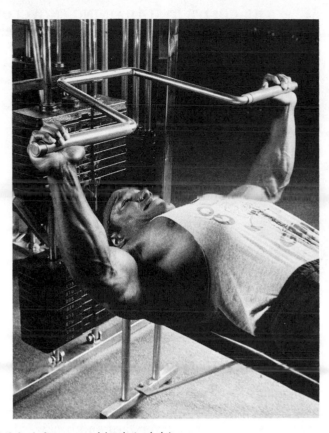

Universal Bench Press—start/finish, left; near midpoint, right.

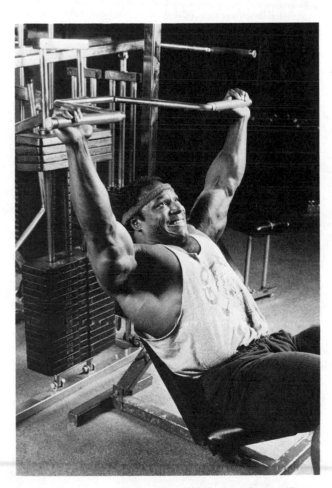
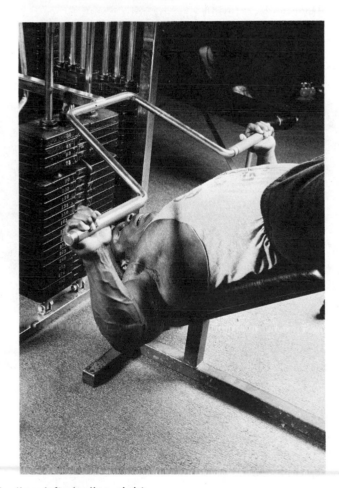

Universal Bench Press—incline, left; decline, right.

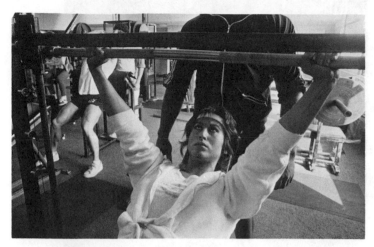

Smith Machine Press performed by Rachel McLish on an incline bench.

Exercise Variations: Of course, you can vary the width of your grip in this exercise, regardless of the angle of bench that you use. You can also place uniquely different stresses on your pectorals by moving the bench forward and backward 2–3 inches so you are forced to lower the bar down to a different part of your chest. Since the weight is on a sliding track, there is no danger of losing your balance when you do this exercise.

Nautilus Bench Presses

Emphasis: The effect of this movement is similar to that of a Decline Press. It strongly stresses the lower and outer pectorals, anterior deltoids, and triceps. Secondary stress is on the upper pectorals, medial deltoids, lats, and the upper back muscles that rotate your scapulae.

Starting Position: Sit in the machine and recline back against the angled bench. Place your feet on the foot peddle and push against it to bring the pressing handles into a position where you can conveniently grasp them. Grasp the handles with your palms facing each other, release pressure on the foot pedal, and allow the weight of the machine to push your hands as far past the front of your torso as is comfortably possible.

Movement Performance: Push forward on the handles until your arms are straight. Slowly return to the starting point and repeat the movement.

Training Tips: You can use a technique called *negative emphasis* on the movement. With negative emphasis, you will push the weight out to straight arms' length with both arms, remove your right hand from the lever arm, and slowly

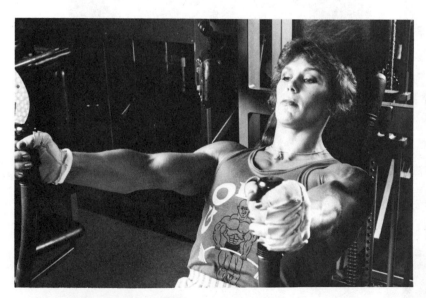

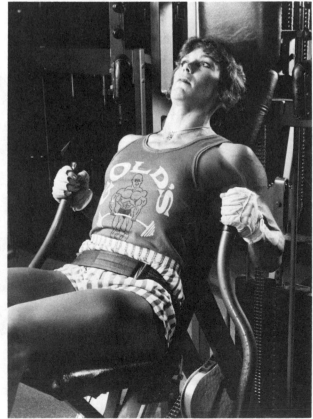

Nautilus Bench Press—start/finish, above; midpoint, right.

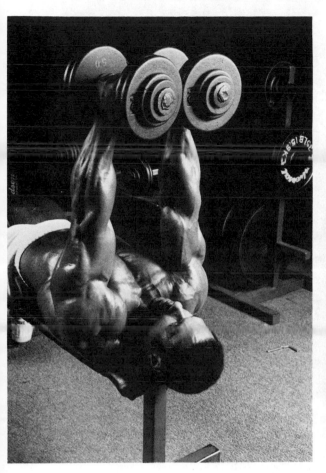

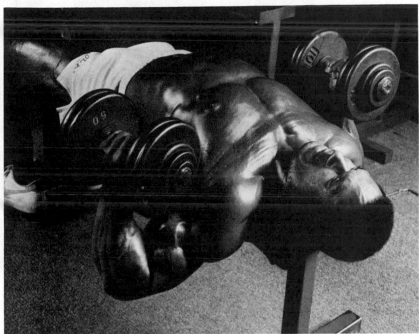

Dumbbell Press (flat bench)—start/finish, left; midpoint, below.

lower the weight while resisting it with the muscles on the left side of your body. Replace your right hand, push the weight back out with both hands, and this time lower it with only your right hand. Alternate hands until you have fully fatigued your chest, shoulder, and arm muscles.

Exercise Variation: By raising and lowering the seat on which you sit, you can place differing stresses on your pecs, delts, and triceps.

Dumbbell Flat/Incline/Decline Presses

Emphasis: As with a barbell or any of several types of exercise machines, you can do Flat, Incline, and Decline Bench Presses while holding two heavy dumbbells in your hands. And you can select the angle of bench that stresses the area of your pectorals that you wish to hit. You also stress your anterior delts and triceps when doing all forms of Dumbbell Bench Presses, plus place secondary stress on your medial deltoids, lats, and the muscles of your upper back that rotate your scapulae.

Starting Position: The hard part about doing this exercise is getting the dumbbells into position at straight arms' length above your shoulder joints. One common way of doing this is to have training partners hand you the weights, although this can be a very clumsy process if they fail to release their grips on the weights at the same instant. On a flat bench, you should start out sitting at the end of the bench with the dumbbells resting on end against your thighs. Keeping your legs flexed toward your torso, roll backward onto the bench with your arms straight. This will bring the dumbbells easily to straight arms' length. To return to the starting point, you simply curl up your legs, place your knees against the ends of the weights, and roll back to a sitting position.

On a decline bench, you can grasp the weights lying on the floor behind your head. Then, keeping your arms straight, you can have a training partner deadlift the dumbbells in a semicircular arc up to straight arms' length for you.

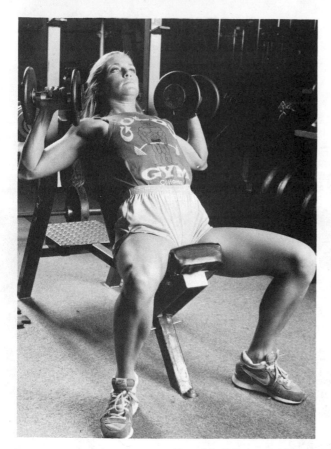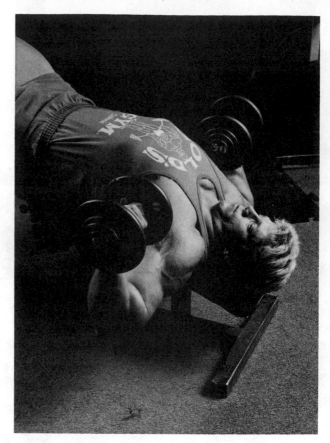

Dumbbell Press (midpoint)—incline, left; decline, right.

It's a little more difficult to get the weights to the starting point on an incline bench. The best technique that we've seen was used by Ken Waller. Ken started with the dumbbells resting on his knees, then lifted one knee at a time up to shoulder height to bring the weights to his shoulders. Then at the end of a set, he would lower them one at a time by reversing the process.

Movement Performance: Keeping your elbows back and your palms facing forward, slowly lower the dumbbells down to at least shoulder level. And if you can lower them to a point below shoulder level, it's much better to do so. Push the weights back up to straight arms' length, bringing them together directly over your chest until they touch each other. Repeat the movement for the desired number of reps.

Exercise Variations: You can also do this movement with your palms facing inward, toward each other. And keep in mind the wide variety of bench angles that you can use when performing Incline and Decline Dumbbell Presses. Sometimes you can improvise a low incline or decline bench simply by placing a 4″ × 4″ block of wood under the head or foot end of a flat bench.

Flat/Incline/Decline Dumbbell Flyes

Emphasis: When you do Flyes, you can isolate your triceps from the movement and place very direct stress on your pecs and anterior delts. Minor secondary stress is on your medial deltoids and triceps. You can select the area of your pectorals that you wish to stress by the angle of bench that you use for this movement.

Starting Position: Grasp two light dumbbells and lie on your back on your choice of exercise bench. Bring the weights to straight arms' length directly above your shoulder joints and rotate your wrists so your palms are facing each other. Bend your arms about 10 degrees and maintain this rounded-arm position throughout the movement.

Movement Performance: Being sure that your upper arms travel directly out to the sides, slowly lower the dumbbells in semicircular arcs to as low a position as is comfortably possible. At the bottom part of the movement, your elbows should be below the level of your torso. Using pectoral strength, slowly return the weights back along the same arcs to the starting point. Repeat the movement for the suggested number of repetitions.

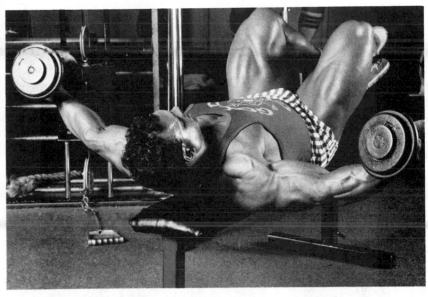

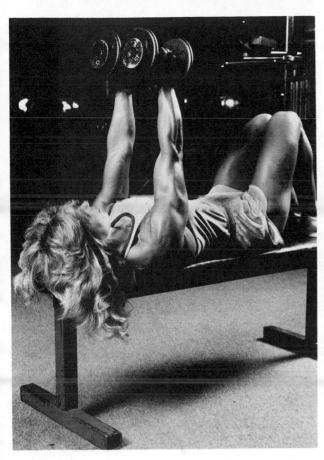

Dumbbell Flyes—start, left; finish, right.

Dumbbell Flyes—stiff-arm (midpoint), left; decline (start), right.

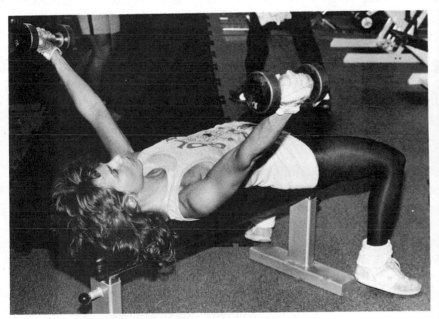

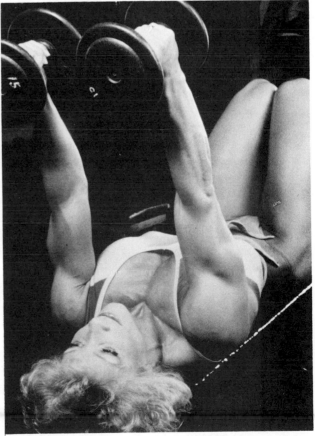

Exercise Variations: You can also do Stiff-Arm Flyes on a flat, incline, or decline bench. You shouldn't use weights quite as heavy as when you keep your arms slightly bent, because Stiff-Arm Flyes can place harmful stress on your elbows if you use maximum poundages.

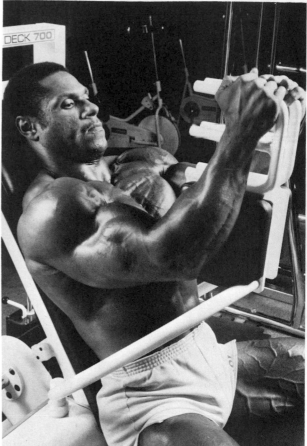

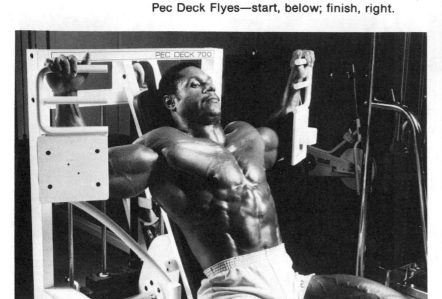

Pec Deck Flyes—start, below; finish, right.

Pec Deck Flyes

Emphasis: This movement has evolved only in the past 10 years. Pec Deck Flyes allow you to isolate stress on your pectorals with only minimal involvement of your anterior deltoid muscles. You'll particularly find this movement good for adding mass to the inner edges of the pectorals where they originate from the *sternum* (breast bone). And because Pec Deck Flyes place direct stress on the pecs even in the fully contracted position of the movement, this is an excellent exercise for using peak-contraction reps for your chest.

Starting Position: Adjust the seat to a height that puts your upper arms parallel to the floor when you are sitting in the seat and have your fingers resting over the top edge of the movement pads attached to the machine. Sit on the seat facing away from the weight stack and place your elbows against the padded surfaces, your forearms running straight up the pads and your fingers curled over the top edges of the pads. Allow the weight to pull your elbows as far as comfortably possible to the rear, stretching your pectorals prior to initiating each repetition.

Movement Performance: Use pectoral strength to push with your elbows against the pads, moving the pads forward until they touch each other directly in front of your chest. Hold this contracted position for a moment, return to the starting point, and repeat the movement for the suggested number of repetitions.

Training Tip: For a more intense stress on your pectorals, you can do this exercise with one arm at a time. Whenever you do movements with one arm or leg rather than with two limbs, you can place greater mental concentration on the working muscles. This is due to the fact that you needn't split your focus between two working limbs.

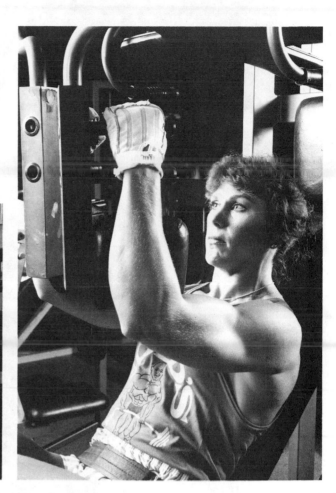

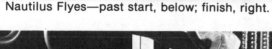
Nautilus Flyes—past start, below; finish, right.

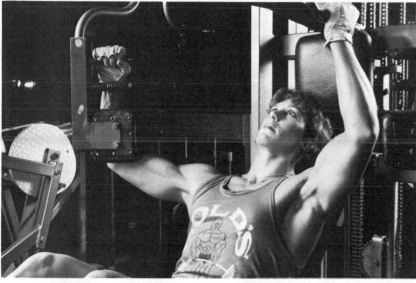

Exercise Variations: You can adjust the height of the seat both upward and downward 3–5 inches to place different angles of stress on your working pectorals. And Charles Glass (Mr. Universe) does a Pec Crunch movement on the pec deck with his elbows held high on the pads, doing short movements mainly in the peak-contracted position of the exercise.

Nautilus Flyes

Emphasis: This movement is similar in effect to Pec Deck Flyes, except that there is more stress placed on the lower and outer pectorals.

Starting Position: Adjust the height of the machine's seat so your upper arms are parallel to the floor when you are in the starting position of the movement. Place your elbows against the pads attached to the movement arms of the machine, resting your fingers lightly over either

the upper or lower handles attached to the movement arm. Allow the weight of the machine to push your elbows back to a position with your pectorals fully stretched.

Movement Performance: Use pectoral strength to push the pads forward until they touch each other directly in front of your chest. Hold this fully contracted position for a moment, return to the starting point, and repeat the exercise for the required number of reps.

Training Tip: You can easily do this movement with one arm at a time while holding on to the handle above your chest with your free hand.

Exercise Variation: The Brother Company also markets a chest machine that gives you a movement very similar to Nautilus Flyes.

Pulley Flyes

Emphasis: Depending on the angle of the

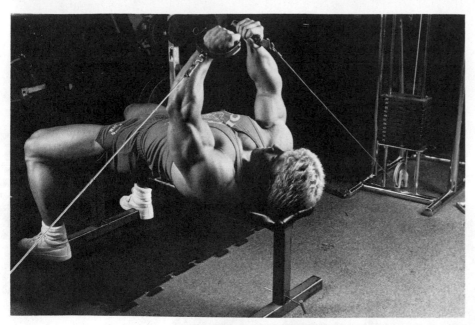

Pulley Flyes—start, above; finish, right.

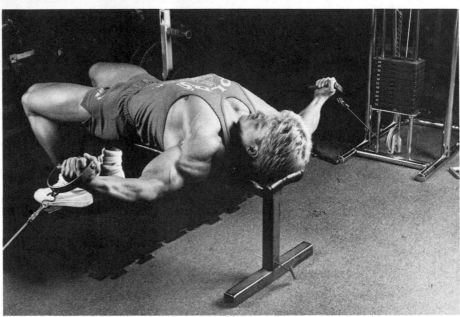

bench on which you perform Pulley Flyes, you can stress any section of your pectorals. Incline Pulley Flyes place maximum stress on your upper and inner pectorals; Decline Pulley Flyes stress the lower and outer pecs; and Flat-Bench Pulley Flyes put emphasis on the remainder of the pectoral muscle mass.

Starting Position: We will describe Incline Pulley Flyes, and you can easily learn how to do the movement on a flat or decline bench from carefully reviewing this exercise description. Place an incline bench between two floor pulleys in such a position that, in the low point of the movement, your arms are at a 90-degree angle with your torso and your hands point directly at the pulleys. Attach loop handles to the cables, grasp the handles, and lie back on the bench. With your palms toward each other and your arms slightly bent, bring your hands together directly above the middle of your chest.

Movement Performance: Keeping your arms slightly bent throughout the movement, slowly lower your hands in semicircular arcs directly out to the sides and downward to as low a position as comfortably possible. Use pectoral strength to return your hands back along the same arcs to the starting position and repeat the movement for the suggested number of repetitions.

Exercise Variations: To stress your pecs from

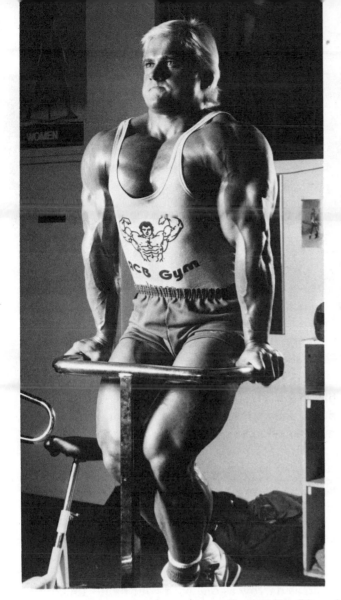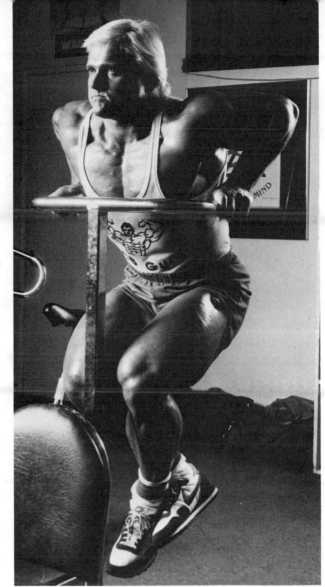

Parallel Bar Dip—start, left; finish, right.

new angles, you can adjust the bench forward or backward from the recommended position. And you can use a wide variety of incline and decline bench angles.

Parallel Bar Dips

Emphasis: This is an excellent upper body movement that stresses the pectorals, anterior deltoids, and triceps with great intensity. The pectoral emphasis is primarily on the lower and outer sections of the pecs. Secondary emphasis is on the medial deltoids and the upper back muscles that rotate the scapulae.

Starting Position: There are two types of parallel bars, one in which the bars are actually parallel and another in which the bars are wider apart on one end than at the other end. Regardless of the bars used, take a grip that will have your palms facing toward each other and jump up to support your body at straight arms' length above the bars. Bend your legs for body stability, place your chin on your chest, and incline your torso forward. (There is also a type of dip used primarily for triceps development in which you hold your torso upright during the movement, but when training to stress your pecs you must incline your torso forward into the movement.)

Movement Performance: Allowing your elbows to travel a bit out to the sides, bend your arms and lower your body down as far below the bars as possible. Slowly push back up to the starting point and repeat the movement.

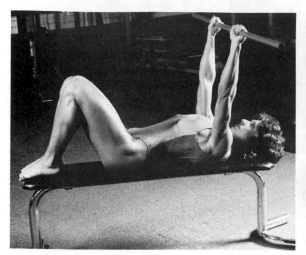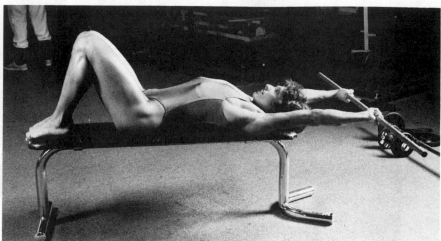

Stiff-Arm Barbell Pullover—start, left; finish, right.

Training Tips: Some dipping bars have a weight stack attached to one end of a cable and a hip belt attached to the other end that allows you to add resistance to the movement. Otherwise, you can attach a dumbbell to your waist with a loop of rope or nylon webbing, or with a special weight-supporting belt.

Exercise Variations: The angled set of parallel bars allow you to take a variety of grip widths on the bars when you do Parallel Bar Dips. With a wider grip, you can reverse your grip to place a more intense form of stress on your pectorals. You can also do Parallel Bar Dips on the Nautilus multi unit.

Stiff-Arm Barbell Pullovers

Emphasis: This exercise intensely stresses the pecs, lats, and serratus muscles. The movement is often used to stretch the ribcage when attempting to expand the volume of the chest.

Starting Position: Take a shoulder-width over-grip on a light barbell. Lie back on a flat exercise bench with your feet flat on the floor on either side of the bench to balance your body during the movement. Extend your arms directly upward from your shoulders, as at the start of a Bench Press movement, and keep your arms held straight throughout the movement.

Movement Performance: Allow the weight to travel in a semicircular arc down and back behind your head to as low a position as possi-

ble. Slowly return the weight to the starting point and repeat the movement for the desired number of repetitions.

Training Tips: When you do this exercise for ribcage expansion, you should begin taking in as deep as possible a breath as the bar descends. Exhale as you return to the starting point.

Exercise Variations: Some bodybuilders tell us that they get a better feel in the movement if they lie on the bench with their heads off the end. You can also vary the width of your grip from as narrow as one with your hands touching each other in the middle of the bar to as wide as the length of the bar will permit. And you can even do the exercise lying across a flat bench with only your torso in contact with the bench.

Stiff-Arm Dumbbell Pullovers

Emphasis: This movement has exactly the same effect on your body as Stiff-Arm Barbell Pullovers.

Starting Position: Grasp two light dumbbells and lie back on a flat bench with your feet flat on the floor to balance your body on the bench. Extend your arms directly upward from your shoulders with your palms toward your feet as if for the start of a Dumbbell Bench Press. Keep your arms straight throughout the movement.

Movement Performance: Lower the dumbbells down to the rear in a semicircular arc to as low a position as is comfortably possible. Return

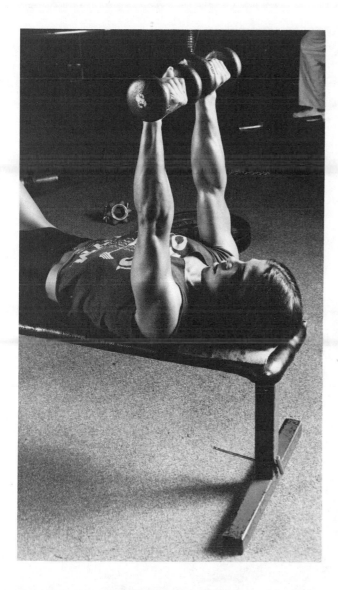

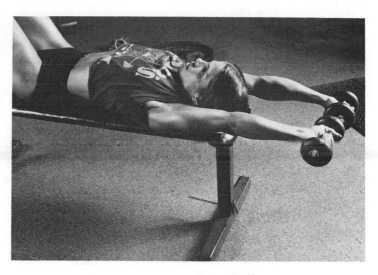

Stiff-Arm Dumbbell Pullover—start, left;
finish, above.

the weights slowly to the starting point and repeat the exercise.

Exercise Variations: You can also do this movement with a single dumbbell held in both hands, your palms flat against the upper plates and your thumbs encircling the handle of the dumbbell. And to particularly stress your serratus muscles, you can do the barbell version of this movement while lying back on an incline bench.

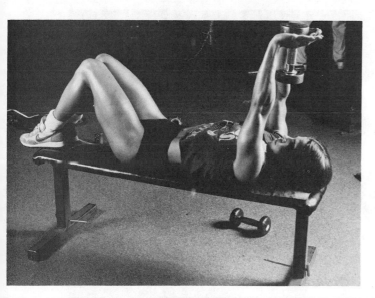

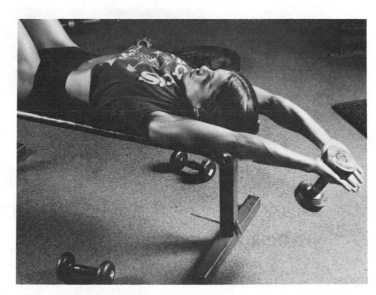

Stiff-Arm Dumbbell Pullover (using one dumbbell)—start, left; finish, right.

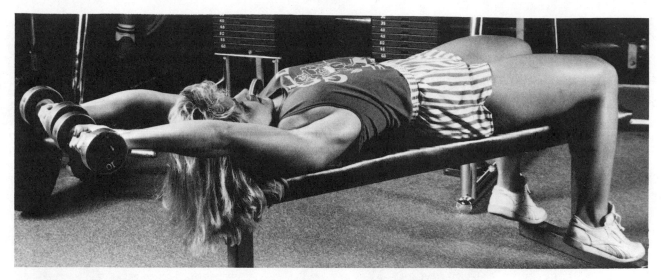

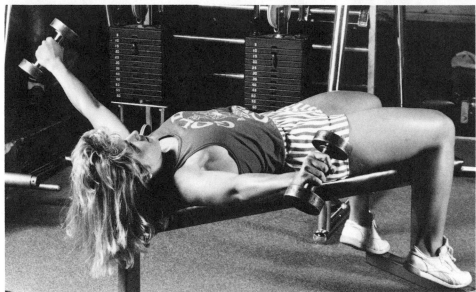

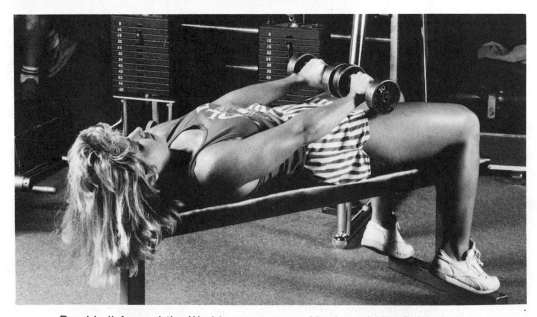

Dumbbell Around-the-Worlds—start, top; midpoint, middle; finish, bottom.

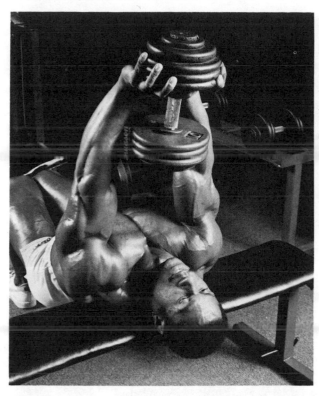 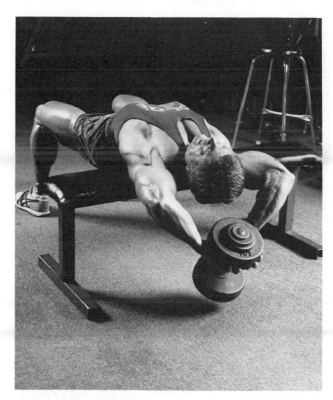

Cross-Bench Dumbbell Pullover—start, left; finish, right.

Dumbbell Around-the-Worlds

Emphasis: This light, dumbbell exercise can be performed on flat, incline, and decline benches to stress every section of your pectorals from unique angles.

Starting Position: Assume the same starting position as for Dumbbell Flyes on your choice of bench, but use dumbbells that weigh approximately 25% less than the weight you use for Flyes.

Movement Performance: Lower the dumbbells down in semicircular arcs to the rear, as if you were doing the first part of a Pullover movement. Then when the dumbbells contact an imaginary line drawn through the length of the middle of your body, start moving the weights in a wide arc on each side along this through-body plane until the dumbbells are at your thighs. Finally, do a Front Lateral Raise movement upward from your thighs, and continue the motion back to the starting point.

Exercise Variations: You can also do this exercise in the opposite direction, lowering it in a forward direction rather than to the rear. You can also do only half of the movement, lowering

the weights to the rear, moving them toward your feet only until your arms are at 90-degree angles with your torso, then doing the finish of a Dumbbell Flye movement to return the dumbbells to the starting point.

Cross-Bench Dumbbell Pullovers

Emphasis: This movement strongly stresses the pectorals, lats, and serratus muscles.

Starting Position: Lay a moderately heavy dumbbell on its end about two feet from the center of a flat exercise bench. Lie crosswise on the bench with just your upper torso in contact with the bench. Your feet should be about shoulder-width apart and placed flat on the floor to steady your body in position during the exercise. Reach over and place your palms flat against the inner sides of the top sets of plates, your thumbs around the dumbbell bar to keep the weight from slipping out of your hands. Pull the dumbbell up off the bench and bring it to a position supported at straight arms' length directly above your chest.

Movement Performance: Simultaneously lower the dumbbell in a semicircular arc downward

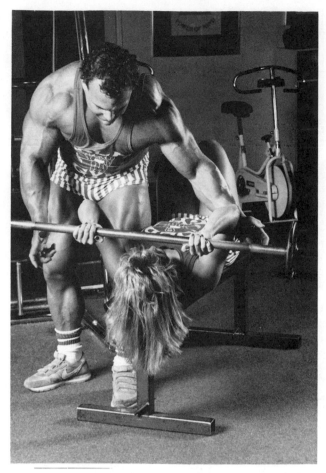
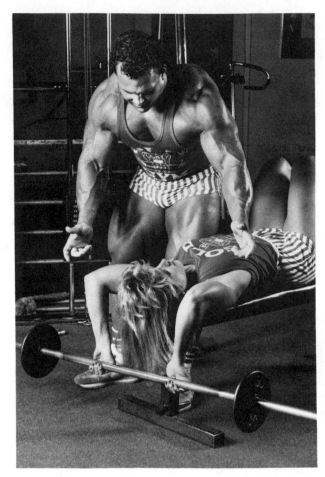

Bent-Arm Barbell Pullovers—start, left; finish, right.

behind your head and bend your arms about 15 degrees. As soon as you have lowered the weight to as comfortably low a position as possible, return it back along the same arc to the starting point while straightening your arms. Repeat the exercise for an appropriate number of reps.

Training Tip: You can get a better stretch in the bottom position of the movement by lowering your hips about six inches as the dumbbell nears the low point of the exercise.

Exercise Variation: This movement can also be performed while lying lengthwise along the bench and with your head off the end of the bench.

Bent-Arm Barbell Pullovers

Emphasis: With Bent-Arm Pullovers, you can place very intense stress on your pectorals, latissimus dorsi, and serratus muscles.

Starting Position: Take a narrow over-grip (about six inches between your index fingers) in the middle of a barbell bar and lie back on a flat exercise bench with your feet placed flat on the floor to balance your body on the bench as you do the movement. Your arms should be fully bent and the weight should be resting on your chest.

Movement Performance: Slowly move the barbell in a semicircular arc past your face and down to as low a position behind your head as is comfortably possible. Pull the bar back along the same arc to the starting point and repeat the movement for the desired number of repetitions.

Training Tip: It's essential that you keep your elbows as close together as possible as you lower and raise the barbell in this movement. Allowing them to travel out to the sides puts your shoulders in an unfavorable mechanical position.

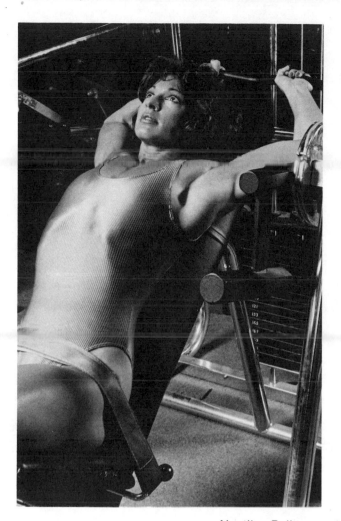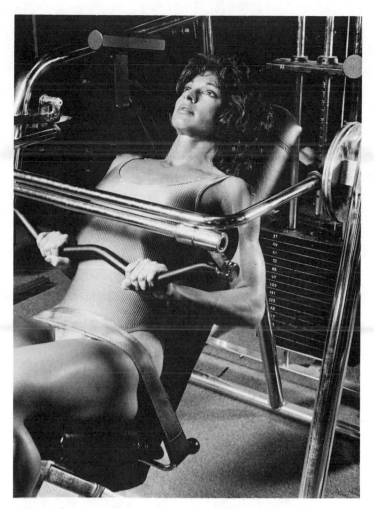

Nautilus Pullover—start, left; finish, right.

Exercise Variation: You can do Bent-Arm Pullovers either with your head resting on the bench or with it hanging off the end of the bench.

Nautilus Pullovers

Emphasis: As with Bent-Arm Pullovers, Nautilus Pullovers strongly stress the pectorals, lats, and serratus muscles. This particular movement also places significant stress on the upper-abdominal muscles.

Starting Position: Adjust the seat height so your shoulder joints are even with the pulley pivot point when you sit in the seat. Sit down and fasten the seat belt over your lap. Push down with your feet on the pedal in front of you to bring the lever arm down to a position where you can place your elbows against the pads.

Grasp the handles attached to the lever arms with a light grip. Take your feet off the pedal and allow the weight on the machine to pull your elbows upward and backward as far as is comfortably possible.

Movement Performance: Use chest and back strength to push with your elbows against the pads. This will move the pads in a semicircular arc downward until the cross bar on the arm touches your abdomen. You should lean slightly into the movement in this position and hold the fully contracted position for a moment before returning to the starting point. Repeat the movement for the required number of repetitions.

Training Tip: To fully stress your chest and back muscles, you can do partial reps at the finish position of the movement, allowing your elbows to travel only 3–5 inches.

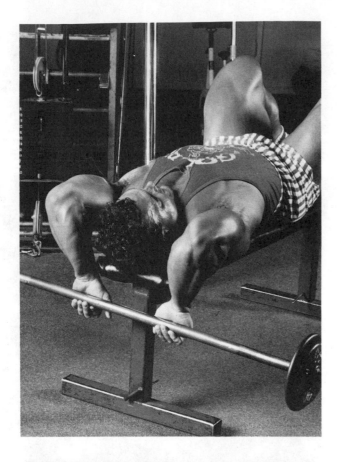

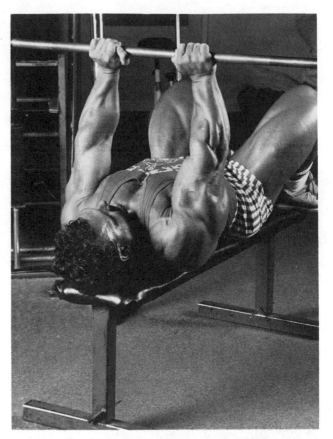

Pullover and Press—start, above left; midpoint, below left; finish, above right.

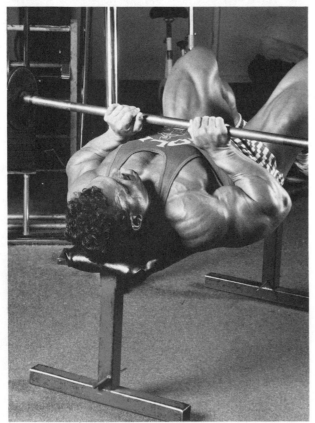

Pullover and Press

Emphasis: This often overlooked exercise is an excellent all-around chest movement which hits virtually all sections of your pectorals. Significant stress is also placed on your deltoids and triceps.

Starting Position: Assume the same position with a barbell in your hands as for the start of a Bent-Arm Barbell Pullover movement.

Movement Performance: Allow the barbell to travel back over your face in a semicircular arc as for a Bent-Arm Pullover, then pull it back to your chest. Once the bar is on your chest, immediately push it to straight arms' length as when doing a Narrow-Grip Bench Press. Lower the weight back to your chest and repeat the exercise.

Exercise Variation: You can also effectively use two moderately heavy dumbbells for this exercise.

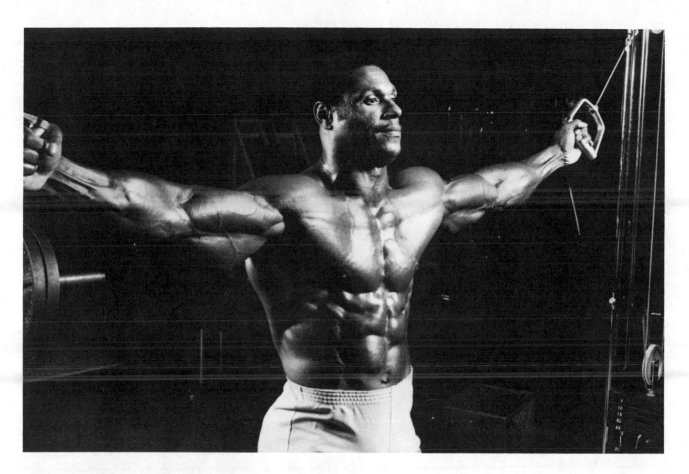

Cable Crossovers—start, above;
finish, below.

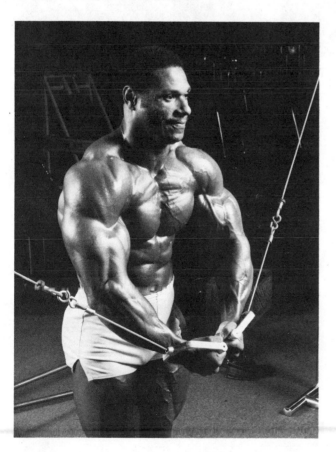

Cable Crossovers

Emphasis: Cable Crossovers stress primarily the lower, outer, and inner sections of the pectorals, plus the anterior delts. Most bodybuilders use Crossovers to etch deep grooves across the pectorals during a precontest cycle.

Starting Position: Attach loop handles to the cables running through two high pulleys. Stand between the pulleys with your feet set about shoulder-width apart and grasp the two pulley handles. With your palms down throughout the movement, extend your arms upward at 45-degree angles in relation to the floor. Bend your arms slightly during the exercise.

Movement Performance: Use pectoral strength to move your hands downward in semi-circular arcs and toward each other until they touch 6–8 inches in front of your hips. Hold this contracted position for two or three seconds, flexing your chest, shoulder, and arm muscles as hard as you can, somewhat like you were doing a most-muscular pose onstage at a competition.

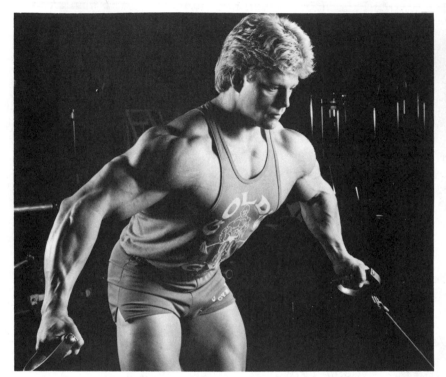
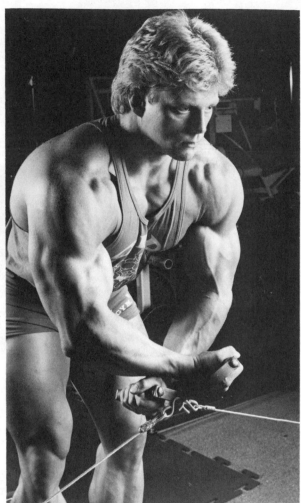

Low-Pulley Crossovers—start, left; finish, right.

Allow your hands to return slowly to the starting point and repeat the exercise for the suggested number of repetitions.

Training Tips: Normally, your torso will be either erect or inclined slightly forward during this exercise, but it can also be performed in a standing position with your torso parallel to the floor. This body position allows you to perform a movement very similar to Flat-Bench Pulley Flyes.

Exercise Variations: If you wish to isolate your legs from the movement, you can do Cable Crossovers in a kneeling position between the two pulleys. And both the standing and kneeling versions of the exercise can be performed with one arm at a time.

Low-Pulley Crossovers

Emphasis: This movement tends to isolate stress primarily in the inner edges of the pectorals.

Starting Position: Attach loop handles to cables running through two low pulleys. Stand directly between the two pulleys with your feet set about shoulder width apart and grasp the two handles. Bend over until your torso is parallel to the floor and extend your arms down toward the floor as illustrated.

Movement Performance: With your arms slightly bent during the movement, slowly move your hands toward each other in semicircular arcs until they meet each other directly below

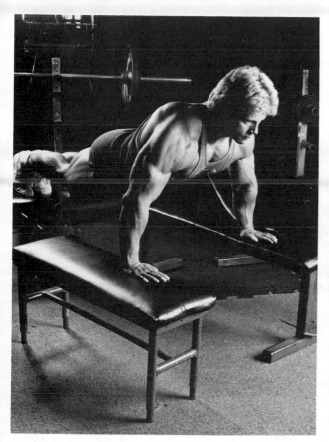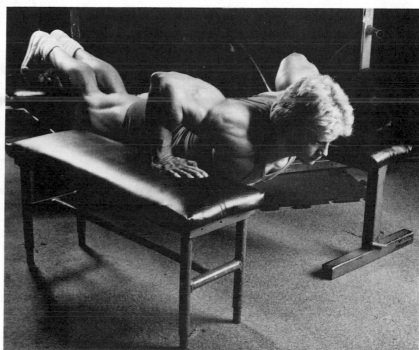

Push-Ups between Benches—start, left; finish, right.

your torso. Hold this position for two or three seconds, flexing your pectorals, deltoids, and arm muscles as intensely as you can. Allow the weights to pull your hands back to the starting position and repeat the movement for the desired number of repetitions.

Push-Ups between Benches

Emphasis: With this movement, you can adapt the old calisthenics Push-Up to become a resistance movement stressing your pecs, anterior deltoids, and triceps muscles.

Starting Position: Arrange three benches or stools so you can place your feet on one of them and one hand on each of the other two while in a supported position ready to do Push-Ups.

Movement Performance: Lower yourself down as far as possible between the benches by bending your arms, then push yourself back up to the starting position.

Training Tips: To add resistance to this movement, you can have a training partner either push down with appropriate force on your shoulders, or place a weight across your upper back.

Suggested Chest Routines

If you have less than a few weeks of training experience, the following routine can profitably be performed three nonconsecutive days per week:

Exercise	Sets	Reps
Barbell Bench Press	3	10-6*
Dumbbell Incline Press	3	10-6

* Pyramid weights and reps on exercises marked with an asterisk.

After 4–6 weeks of steady training on the foregoing program, you can use this chest routine three days per week:

Exercise	Sets	Reps
Incline Barbell Press	4	12-6*
Decline Dumbbell Press	3	10-6*
Flat-Bench Dumbbell Flyes	2	8-10

Following about three months of steady training, you should switch to a four-day split routine in which you train each major muscle group (including the chest) twice per week. This is typically how a lower-level competitive bodybuilder will work out in the off-season. Following is a sample chest-training program for off-season, competitive training:

Exercise	Sets	Reps
Incline Machine Press	4	12-6*
Parallel Bar Dips	4	12-6*
Pec Deck Flyes	3	10-6*
Cross-Bench Dumbbell Pullovers	3	10-15

Every bodybuilder trains differently from all others prior to a competition, as you will see in the following section listing the chest routines of a wide variety of men and women who have trained at Gold's Gym.

Chest Routines of the Champs

In this section, you will find a variety of chest training programs used by many of the Gold's Gym superstars who have won the sport's highest titles. Keep in mind as you examine these training programs that these men and women have been training for many years and have developed enormous recuperative powers. It is unlikely that you can make good gains using their full routines beginning from scratch, or even a year or two of experience. Instead, you should use these training programs as a guide to how you should work your own chest. In all likelihood, you can do the same exercises as your favorite champion, but scale down the number of sets he or she does of each movement to meet your own abilities.

CHARLES GLASS (MR. UNIVERSE)

Exercise	Sets	Reps
Barbell Bench Presses	4	12-15
Barbell Incline Presses	4	12-15
supersetted with		
Cross-Bench Dumbbell Pullovers	4	12-15
Decline Dumbbell Presses	4	12-15
supersetted with		
Pec Deck Flyes	4	12-15
Incline Dumbbell Flyes	4	12-15
supersetted with		
Pec Crunches	5	12-15

LOU FERRIGNO (MR. UNIVERSE)

Exercise	Sets	Reps
Bench Presses	5	6-10
Incline Presses	5	6-10
Decline Presses	5	6-10
Flat-Bench Flyes	4	10-12
Cross-Bench Pullovers	3	15
supersetted with		
Cable Crossovers	3	10-15

DR. FRANCO COLUMBU (MR. OLYMPIA)

Exercise	Sets	Reps
Bench Presses	7	12-6*
Barbell Incline Presses	4	10-6*
Flat-Bench Flyes	2-3	10-12
supersetted with		
Parallel Bar Dips	2-3	10-15

* All exercises marked with an asterisk should have the weights and reps pyramidded. With each succeeding set, the weight on the bar should be increased and the number of reps performed decreased.

CHRIS DICKERSON
(MR. OLYMPIA)

Exercise	Sets	Reps
Pec Deck Flyes	5	12
Incline Dumbbell Presses	5	12–8*
Dumbbell Bench Presses	5	6–8
Cable Crossovers	5	12

LISA ELLIOTT-KOLAKOWSKI
(GOLD'S CLASSIC CHAMP)

Exercise	Sets	Reps
Incline Machine Press	4	6–8
Barbell Bench Presses	4	6–8
Parallel Bar Dips	3–4	10–15
Pec Deck Flyes	3–4	8–10
Incline Cable Flyes	2–3	8–10
Cross-Bench Pullovers	2–3	10–15

CASEY VIATOR
(MR. AMERICA)

Exercise	Sets	Reps
Barbell Incline Presses	5–6	5–6
One-Arm Nautilus Flyes	4–5	6–8
Weighted Parallel Bar Dips	3–4	6–8
Incline Dumbbell Presses	3–4	5–6
Flat-Bench Flyes	3–4	6–8
Cable Crossovers	3–4	10–12

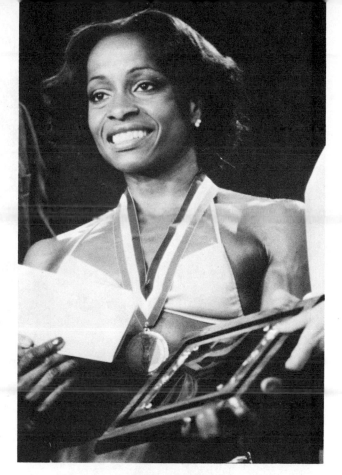

Carla Dunlap.

Lou Ferrigno.

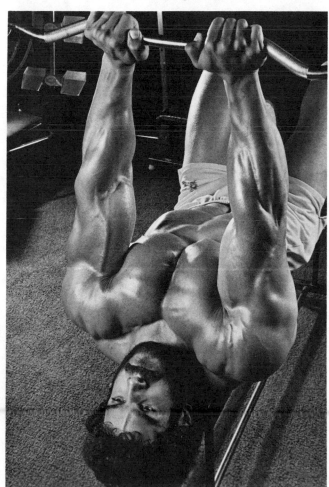

PATSY CHAPMAN
(BEST-IN-THE-WORLD CHAMP)

Exercise	Sets	Reps
Bench Presses	5	10
Flat-Bench Flyes	5	10
Incline Barbell Presses	5	10

ARNOLD SCHWARZENEGGER
(MR. OLYMPIA)

Exercise	Sets	Reps
Incline Barbell Presses	5	8–10
Bench Presses	5	8–10
Flat-Bench Flyes	5	8–10
Cable Crossovers	5	10–15

JUSUP WILKOSZ
(PRO MR. UNIVERSE)

Exercise	Sets	Reps
Incline Barbell Presses	5	10–12
Flat-Bench Flyes	5	10–12
Weighted Parallel Bar Dips	5	10–12
Cable Crossovers	5	10–12

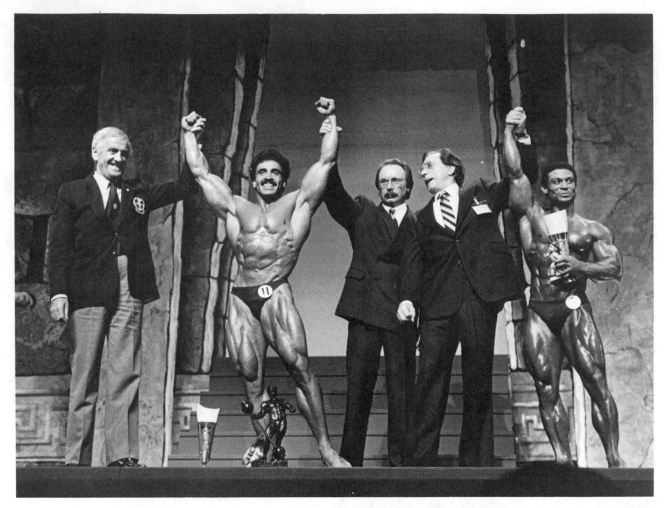

Ben Weider (at left) salutes Samir Bannout in triumph at the 1984 Olympia. At right, Joe Weider holds up runner-up Mohamed Makkawy's arm.

ROBBY ROBINSON
(MR. UNIVERSE)

Exercise	Sets	Reps
Incline Dumbbell Presses	4	8–10
Flat-Bench Flyes	4	8–10
Weighted Parallel Bar Dips	4	8–10
Cross-Bench Dumbbell Pullovers	2–3	10–15
supersetted with		
Cable Crossovers	2–3	10–15

LAURA COMBES
(MS. AMERICA)

Exercise	Sets	Reps
Bench Presses	5–7	12–4*
Incline Barbell Presses	4–5	10–5*
Incline Dumbbell Flyes	4–5	8–10
Pec Deck Flyes	3–4	8–10
Cross-Bench Dumbbell Pullovers	3–4	10–15

ANDREAS CAHLING
(MR. INTERNATIONAL)

Exercise	Sets	Reps
Incline Barbell Presses	2–3	8–12
Incline Flyes	2	10–12
Pec Deck Flyes	2	10–12
Parallel Bar Dips	2	10–15
Cross-Bench Dumbbell Pullovers	2	10–15
supersetted with		
Cable Crossovers	2	10–15

TOM PLATZ
(MR. UNIVERSE)

Exercise	Sets	Reps
Incline Dumbbell Presses	4–5	12–6*
Barbell Bench Presses	4–5	12–6*
Low Incline Flyes	3–4	10–12
Weighted Parallel Bar Dips	3–4	10–15
Cable Crossovers	3–4	10–15

CARLA DUNLAP
(MISS OLYMPIA)

Exercise	Sets	Reps
Incline Dumbbell Presses	4	8–10
Decline Dumbbell Presses	4	8–10
Decline Pullovers	4	8–10
Pec Deck Flyes	4	8–10

FRANK ZANE
(MR. OLYMPIA)

Exercise	Sets	Reps
Bench Presses	5	12–6*
Incline Dumbbell Presses	3	12–6*
Decline Flyes	3	10
Cross-Bench Dumbbell Pullovers	3	10

BERTIL FOX
(MR. UNIVERSE)

Exercise	Sets	Reps
Bench Presses	6–8	15–4*
Flat-Bench Flyes	6–8	6–8
Weighted Parallel Bar Dips	6–8	8–10
Incline Dumbbell Presses	6–8	6–8

SHELLEY GRUWELL
(WORLD GRAND PRIX CHAMPION)

Exercise	Sets	Reps
Flat-Bench Flyes	3	8–10
Dumbbell Bench Presses	3	8–10
Machine Bench Presses	3	8–10
Incline Barbell Presses	2–3	8–10
Cable Crossovers	2–3	10–15

SAMIR BANNOUT
(MR. OLYMPIA)

Exercise	Sets	Reps
Bench Presses	4–5	12–5*
Incline Dumbbell Presses	3–4	8–10
Flat-Bench Flyes	3–4	8–10
Parallel Bar Dips	3–4	10–15
supersetted with		
Cross-Bench Dumbbell Pullovers	3–4	10–15

SCOTT WILSON
(GRAND PRIX CHAMPION)

Exercise	Sets	Reps
Machine Incline Presses	4–5	8–5*
Dumbbell Incline Presses	4–5	8–5*
Incline Flyes	4–5	6–8
Barbell Bench Presses	4–5	8–5*
Flat-Bench Flyes	4–5	6–8
Weighted Parallel Bar Dips	4–5	8–10

DR. LYNNE PIRIE
(SOUTHWEST CHAMPION)

Exercise	Sets	Reps
Incline Dumbbell Presses	3–4	10–6*
Nautilus Flyes	2–3	8–10
Parallel Bar Dips	2–3	8–10
Flat-Bench Flyes	2–3	8–10

DANNY PADILLA
(MR. UNIVERSE)

Exercise	Sets	Reps
Bench Presses	5	10–12
Flat-Bench Flyes	5	10–12
Barbell Incline Presses	5	10–12
Barbell Decline Presses	5	10–12
Cross-Bench Dumbbell Pullovers	5	10–12
supersetted with		
Cable Crossovers	5	10–12

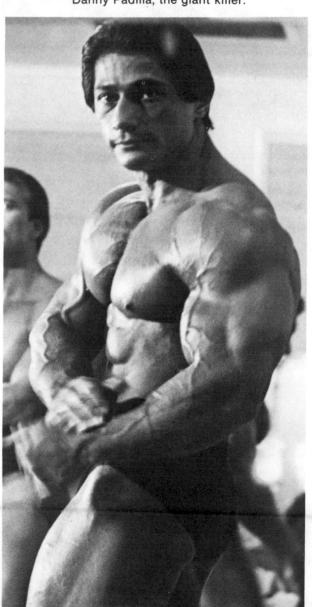

Danny Padilla, the giant killer.

RAY MENTZER
(MR. AMERICA)

Exercise	Sets	Reps
Barbell Incline Presses	2–3	8–3*
Pec Deck Flyes	2–3	6–8
Cable Crossovers (Kneeling)	2–3	6–8
Flat-Bench Flyes	2–3	6–8

RON TEUFEL
(MR. USA)

Exercise	Sets	Reps
Bench Presses	6–8	12–4*
supersetted with		
Cross-Bench Dumbbell Pullovers	6–8	10–15
Machine Incline Presses	5	8–10
supersetted with		
Dumbbell Decline Presses	5	8–10
Barbell Decline Presses	5	8–10
supersetted with		
Cable Crossovers	5	8–10

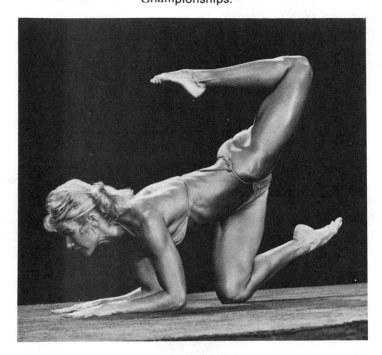

Shelley Gruwell poses at the 1983 Pro World Championships.

Looking Ahead

In Chapter 4, we will introduce you to all of the shoulder exercises that the superstar bodybuilders at Gold's Gym use in their workouts. And we will reveal many of these champs' actual shoulder-training programs.

4
SHOULDER TRAINING

Your shoulder muscular development is extremely important at a competition because it is impossible to hide poorly developed deltoids. Other weak muscle groups can be camouflaged in many poses, but your deltoids are visible in every pose that you throw at the judges and audience in your compulsory rounds and free-posing routine. Therefore, it's essential that you strive to develop massive, proportionate, and shredded delts.

The term *deltoid* derives from the Greek letter *delta,* which is shaped like a unilateral triangle. And when viewed from the side with your arm hanging down at your side, your deltoid muscle complex looks very much like an inverted letter delta.

Most champion bodybuilders have great deltoid development, but among men who have either trained at Gold's in the past or currently train there, the best delts belong to Chris Dickerson, Dr. Franco Columbu, Pete Grymkowski, Charles Glass, Andreas Cahling, Clint Beyerle, Mohamed Makkawy, and Samir Bannout. And among women, the best deltoid developments belong to Laura Combes, Kay Baxter, Carla Dunlap, Lisa Elliott-Kolakowski, Pillow, Dr. Lynne Pirie, Valerie Mayers, and Stella Martinez.

There are basically three types of deltoid movements that you will perform in your shoulder workouts—pushing exercises (e.g., Military Presses), leverage movements (e.g., Side Lateral Raises), and pulling exercises (e.g., Upright Rows). And if you faithfully and regularly perform all three types of movements with 100% intensity in all of your workouts, you will ultimately develop a set of broad, muscular, and fully developed shoulders that will be the envy of any man or woman.

Anatomy and Kinesiology

There are several small bundles of muscle fibers that make up the *rotator cuff* complex of the shoulder. This is the bundle of small muscles that many baseball pitchers rupture, have surgically repaired, and often fail to rehabilitate sufficiently to continue with their pitching careers. But as bodybuilders, we are concerned only with the large triangular-shaped deltoid muscle that forms a cap over the point of the shoulder.

The deltoid muscle has three distinct lobes called "heads" that contract either separately or in various combinations to move the humerus (upper arm bone) in a myriad of directions. The *anterior* (front) *head* of the deltoid primarily contracts to move the upper-arm bone forward and upward. The anterior deltoid head also comes powerfully into play in many chest exercises, such as Incline Presses, Bench Presses, Decline Presses, Parallel Bar Dips, and Flyes with both dumbbells and cables at a wide variety of bench angles.

The *medial* (side) *head* of the deltoid primarily contracts to move the humeris out to the side and upward. The medial deltoid head also comes peripherally into play in a large number of upper-body movements, particularly those for the chest and upper-back muscle groups.

The *posterior* (rear) *head* of the deltoid primarily contracts to move the upper-arm bone to the rear. The posterior deltoid head also comes strongly into play in many upper-back movements, such as Seated Pulley Rows, Barbell and Dumbbell Bent Rows, Upright Rows, Chins, and Lat Machine Pulldowns.

Shoulder Exercises

You will find 30 major shoulder movements in this section, each of which is fully described and depicted. Add in the numerous variations of each basic exercise, and you will have more than 60 shoulder movements in your basic pool of bodybuilding exercises. That should be a sufficient variety of deltoid exercises to satisfy any bodybuilder.

Military Presses

Emphasis: Sometimes referred to as Standing Presses or Barbell Overhead Presses, this movement strongly stresses the anterior delts and triceps. Secondary emphasis is placed on the medial deltoids, trapezius and other upper-back muscles, and the upper pectorals.

Starting Position: Place a moderately weighted barbell on the floor at your feet. Take an overgrip on the bar with your hands set 3–4 inches wider on each side than the width of your shoulders. Straighten your arms, straighten and

then arch your back, and bend your legs to dip your hips below the level of your shoulders. From this position, use a coordinated extension of your legs and torso, plus arm pull, to bring the barbell to your shoulders. Rotate your elbows directly beneath the bar. This complicated movement is called a Power Clean, and it is fully discussed and depicted in Chapter 5. It might be a good idea to refer to this exercise description (see pages 106–7) for a more precise elaboration of the correct method of cleaning a weight to your shoulders.

Movement Performance: Without allowing your torso to bend backward, slowly push the bar directly upward, close to your face until it is at straight arms' length directly above your head. If you happen to have a larger-than-average nose, you should take extra care as you press the weight upward. No joke, broken noses can happen with this exercise! Lower the weight slowly down to your shoulders, and without bouncing it at your shoulders, push it back to straight arms' length overhead.

Training Tips: Many bodybuilders prefer to avoid cleaning the weight to their shoulders by placing it on a weight-support rack, taking the correct grip on the bar, stepping back a pace or two, and pressing the weight. This movement is usually referred to as Presses Off the Rack.

Exercise Variations: When you do any type of Barbell Press—whether it be intended for shoulder or chest development—you can vary the width of the grip over quite a range. With Military Presses you can use a grip somewhat more narrow than the width of your shoulders, or you can use as wide a grip as the length of the bar will permit. Generally speaking, however, you will receive much more muscle-building benefit from using a medium-width grip. You can also do these Barbell Overhead Presses in a seated position, preferably on a bench with a back support.

Presses behind the Neck

Emphasis: Presses behind the Neck have a similar effect on the shoulder, arm, chest, and back muscles as do Military Presses, except that there is more involvement from the trapezius and posterior deltoids than in Militaries.

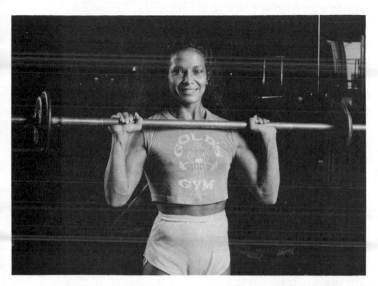

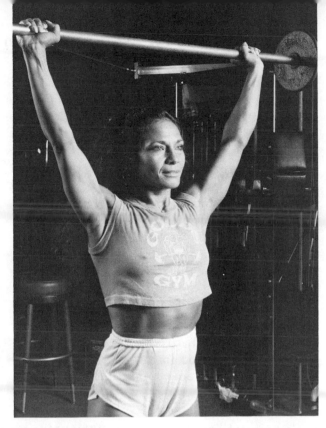

Military Press—start, left; finish, right.

Press behind the Neck—start, left; finish, right.

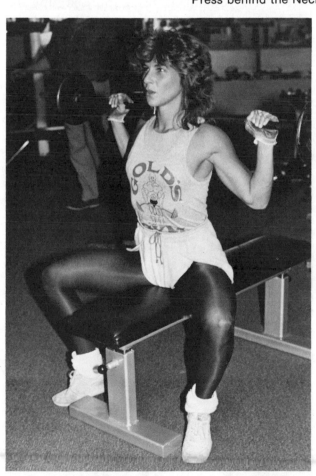

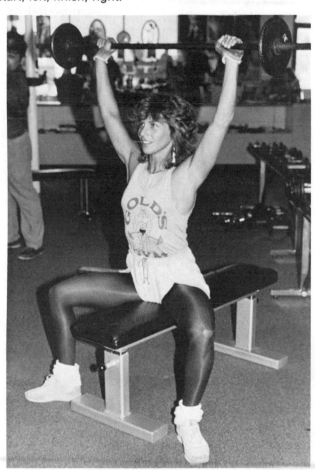

Starting Position: Take an overgrip on a barbell with your hands set 4–6 inches wider on each side than the width of your shoulders. Clean the bar to your shoulders and push it up over your head to a position resting across your trapezius muscles. Alternatively, you can rest the barbell on a weight-support rack and remove it from the rack after positioning it correctly behind your neck. Set your feet about shoulder-width apart and rotate your elbows beneath the bar.

Movement Performance: Keeping your elbows back during the movement, slowly press the weight directly upward until it is at straight arms' length over your head. Lower the bar back to the starting point and repeat the movement.

Exercise Variations: This movement is more frequently performed in a seated position than standing, and you can use all of the grip width variations outlined in the exercise description of Military Presses.

Comment: Some bodybuilders suffer neck vertebral injuries doing Presses behind the Neck, usually from a muscle spasm induced by the exercise. Frank Zane (three times Mr. Olympia) once had this problem, and he solved it with regular chiropractic care and a switch to Seated Dumbbell Presses done on a bench with a very high incline board attached to it.

Dumbbell Presses

Emphasis: This versatile deltoid movement primarily stresses the anterior and medial deltoid heads along with the triceps muscles. Secondary stress is placed on the posterior delts and the upper-back muscles.

Starting Position: Grasp two moderately weighted dumbbells and clean them to your shoulders. Rotate your palms so they are facing forward, and begin the movement with your upper arms pressed against the sides of your torso. Stand erect throughout the movement.

Movement Performance: Slowly push the dumbbells directly upward until they touch each other at straight arms' length directly above your head. Lower the weights slowly down to the starting point and repeat the movement.

Exercise Variations: For a slightly different feel in your anterior deltoids, you can press the dumbbells upward with your palms facing each other, rather than forward. With either hand position, you can press the dumbbells alternately, one dumbbell being pressed upward while the other is descending. And each of the foregoing variations of Dumbbell Presses can be performed while seated at the end of a flat exercise bench.

Dumbbell Press—start, left; finish, right.

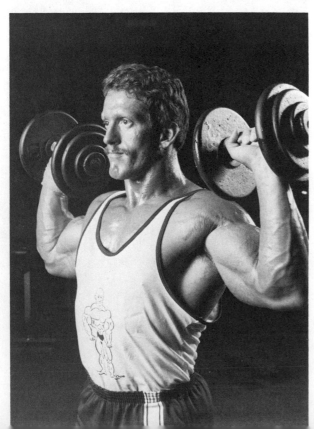
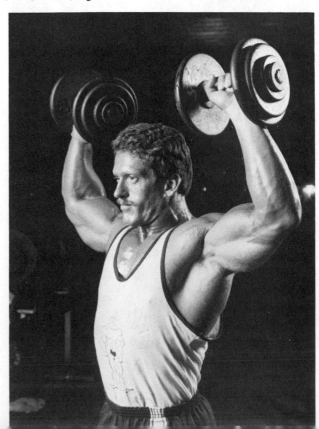

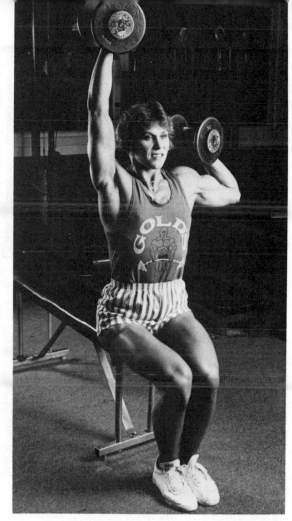

Alternate Dumbbell Press (seated with palms facing each other).

Comment: One of the most effective variations of Dumbbell Presses was originated at the original Gold's Gym on Pacific Avenue in Venice, California, by Arnold Schwarzenegger, and it became known as the Arnold Press. The Arnold Press starts with the hands in the same finish position as for a Dumbbell Curl. From there, the dumbbells are pressed upward and the hands simultaneously rotated 180 degrees so they are facing forward at the top point of the movement. And, to keep continuous tension on his deltoids, Arnold never locked out his elbows in this movement. If you give the Arnold Press a try, your deltoids will burn like never before.

Arnold Press—start, left; midpoint, center; finish, right.

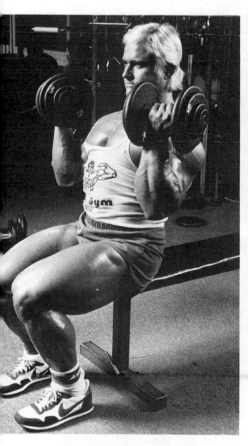
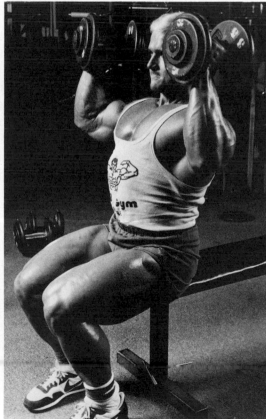
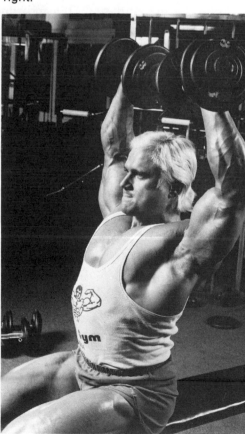

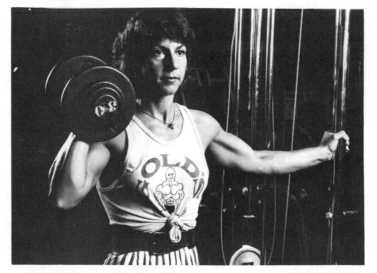

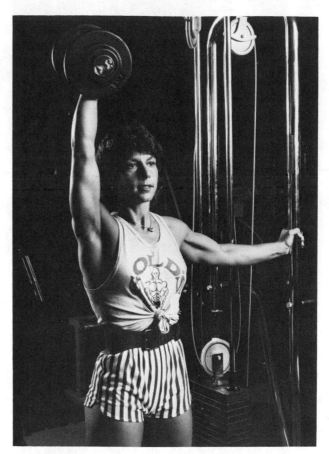

One-Arm Dumbbell Press—start, left; finish, right.

One-Arm Dumbbell Press

Emphasis: This movement stresses precisely the same muscles as all Dumbbell Presses, but whenever you perform a movement with one arm or one leg (versus two arms or two legs), you can invariably place greater mental concentration on the working muscles. Rather than splitting your focus on both shoulders as you do this exercise with two dumbbells, you can put all of your attention on one working deltoid.

Starting Position: Grasp a moderately heavy dumbbell in your right hand and clean it to your shoulder. Grasp a sturdy upright with your left hand to brace your body in a perfectly vertical position during the movement. If you allow your torso to bend to the left, you lose much of the range of motion in this exercise, so it must be supported vertically, or even in a position leaning slightly to the right. Rotate your wrist so your hand is facing forward.

Movement Performance: Slowly push the weight directly upward until your arm is completely straight. Lower the weight under full control back to the starting point and repeat the movement.

Training Tip: It will be tempting to use a bit of torso buck to get the dumbbell started from the bottom point of the movement, but this is best avoided. If you have to cheat the weight up in this manner, your dumbbell is probably too heavy.

Exercise Variations: You can also do One-Arm Dumbbell Presses with your palm facing inward toward the midline of your body. And you can even do the movement seated on a flat exercise bench placed an appropriate distance from the sturdy upright you are grasping as you do the exercise.

Universal Gym Overhead Press

Emphasis: This is a convenient machine movement with which you can directly stress your anterior delts and triceps, plus place secondary stress on your medial/posterior deltoid complex, upper-back muscles, and upper pectorals.

Starting Position: Place the stool that comes with a Universal Gym unit directly beneath the overhead pressing station handles of the machine. Sit on the seat facing the weight stack,

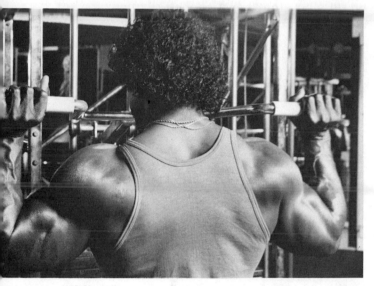
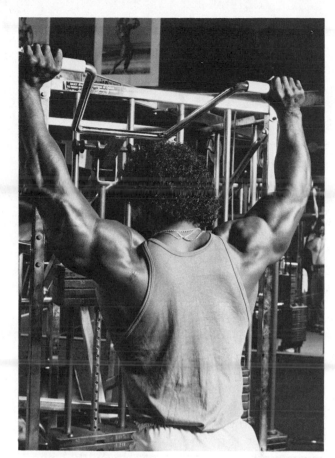

Universal Gym Overhead Press—start, left; finish, right.

grasp the handles with your palms facing away from your body, and entwine your legs around the legs of the stool to secure your body in position during the movement. Be sure to keep your torso in a totally upright position throughout the movement.

Movement Performance: Slowly straighten your arms completely, pause in the top position of the movement for a moment, return to the starting point, and repeat the movement.

Exercise Variations: You can also do this exercise facing away from the weight stack, which attacks your shoulders and arms from a slightly different angle. And, either facing toward or away from the weight stack, you can do the movement in a standing position. This latter variation was a favorite of Mike Mentzer (Mr. America, Mr. Universe), and Casey Viator.

Training Tips: A training partner can easily give you forced reps during this exercise in two ways. In the first method, he can cup his hands beneath your elbows and pull up with an appropriate degree of force. And in the second method, he can grasp one side of the fork that runs from the weight-stack lever arm out to the handles and pull upward with the right amount of force. In this same position, he can also pull downward and give you forced negative reps on your Universal Overhead Presses.

Smith Machine Overhead Presses

Emphasis: No hardcore bodybuilding gym is complete if it doesn't have a Smith machine, which is an apparatus consisting of two vertical runners on which a weight-loaded bar can slide. A Smith machine also has hooks that you can use to stop and secure a bar in any position if you fail to complete a rep. Overhead Presses for the shoulders and arms can easily be performed on a Smith machine.

Starting Position: Place a flat exercise bench in the middle of the machine parallel to the bar. Adjust the bar height so it is at shoulder level when you sit on the bench. Take a grip a bit wider than your shoulders on each side on the bar, sit on the bench with your feet in a comfortable position, and sit erect to bear the weight of the bar.

Movement Performance: Slowly push the bar

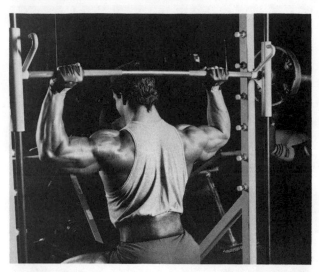

Smith Machine Overhead Press behind the Neck.

movements. Finally, you can do both Front Presses and Presses behind the Neck on a Smith machine while in a standing position.

Training Tip: The best way to do forced reps in this movement is to have your training partner cup your elbows with his or her hands and pull up on your elbows just enough to allow you to complete a forced rep that you wouldn't ordinarily have been able to finish on your own.

Nautilus Overhead Presses

Emphasis: With a Nautilus double-shoulder machine you can do Overhead Presses with your palms facing each other to strongly stress your anterior deltoids and triceps. Secondary stress in this movement is on the medial deltoids, upper-back and upper-chest muscles.

Starting Position: Adjust the height of the machine seat so the pressing handles of the machine are at the exact level of your shoulders when you sit on the seat. Sit in the machine, fasten the seat belt across your lap, and cross

to straight arms' length over your head, then lower it back to the starting point at your chest. Repeat the movement.

Exercise Variations: This movement can also be performed pressing the bar up from a position across your traps behind your shoulders, and you can use a wide variety of grip widths on both

Nautilus Overhead Press—start, left; finish, right.

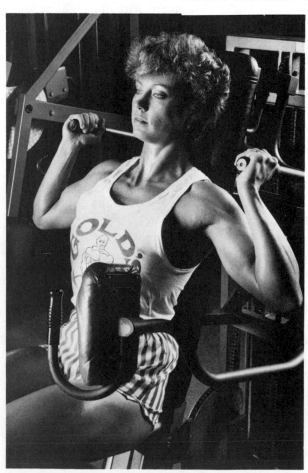

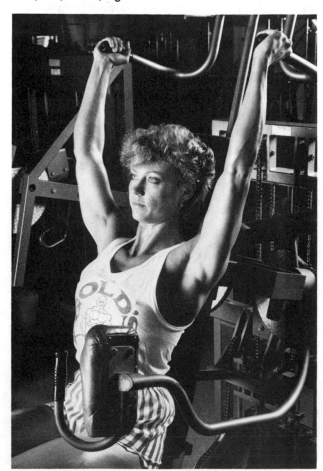

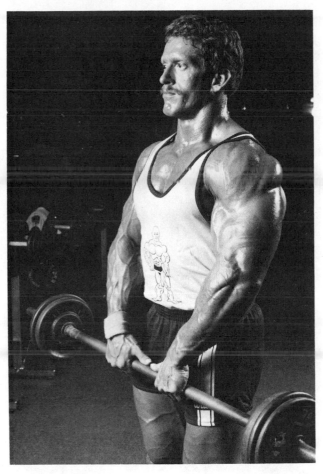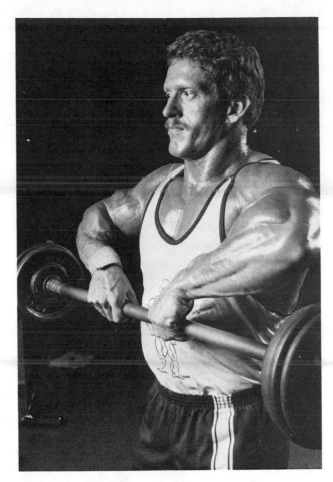

Barbell Upright Row—start, left; finish, right.

your ankles below the seat. Grasp the pressing handles of the machine with your palms facing toward each other. Place the back of your head against the padded back rest of the machine and keep it in that position throughout the movement.

Movement Performance: Slowly straighten your arms completely, hold the top position of the movement for a moment, lower back to the starting point, and repeat.

Training Tip: This is an excellent exercise in which you can use a technique called *negative emphasized* reps for your shoulders. This involves pressing the weight upward with both hands, shifting all the weight to your right hand and resisting the downward momentum of the weight with your right arm and shoulder muscles, pushing it back up with both hands, then lowering it with only your left hand. By alternating arms like this on the negative part of the movement, you can bomb your deltoids back to the Stone Age.

Barbell Upright Rows

Emphasis: Upright Rows place powerful stress on the entire shoulder girdle musculature, particularly the deltoids and trapezius muscles. Secondary emphasis is on the biceps, brachialis, and the gripping muscles of the forearms.

Starting Position: Take a narrow over-grip in the middle of a barbell handle, place your feet about shoulder-width apart, and stand erect with your arms running down the sides of your torso. Your hands and the barbell bar should rest across your upper thighs. Keep your torso erect and your legs straight throughout the movement.

Movement Performance: Being sure to keep your elbows above the level of your hands at all times, slowly pull the bar directly upward along the front of your body until your hands touch the underside of your chin. It's important that your elbows are in a high position, you roll your shoulders slightly backward, and you squeeze your shoulder blades together at the top position

of the movement. Slowly lower the barbell back
to the starting point and repeat the movement.

Training Tip: A common mistake when performing Upright Rows is to allow the bar to
drop from the top position back to the starting
point. If you don't lower it slowly and resist its
downward momentum, you will lose half the
value of the movement.

Exercise Variations: The main variations of
this movement are in the width of your grip. You
can use a very narrow grip with your index
fingers touching, a more normal grip with your
index fingers about six inches apart, or a wide
grip in which your hands are set at about
shoulder width. Each grip variation hits your
delts and traps differently.

Cable Upright Rows

Comment: This movement is precisely like
Barbell Upright Rows, except that it is performed with a floor pulley and a bar handle attached to the cable running through the pulley.
As you perform the movement, simply stand
about one foot back from the pulley and do the
exercise in precisely the same way as if you were
holding a barbell rather than the pulley handle.

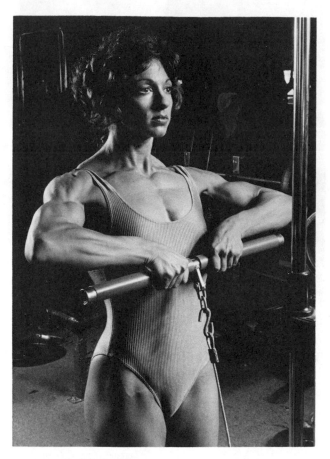

Cable Upright Row at midpoint.

Dumbbell Upright Row—start, left; finish, right.

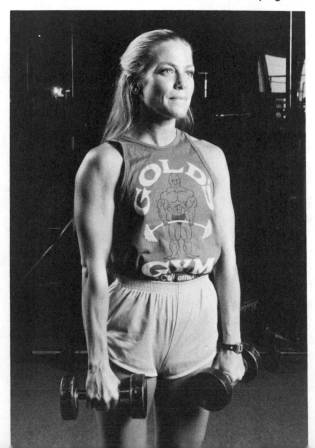
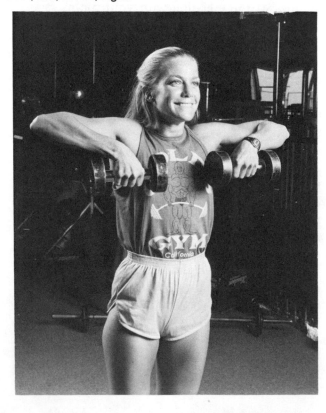

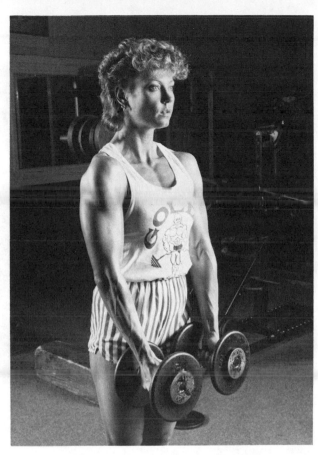
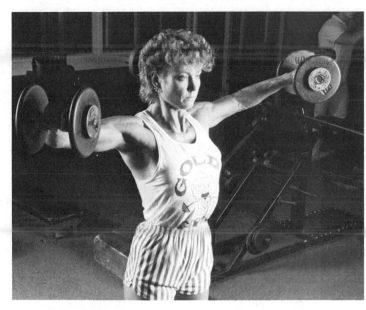

Standing Dumbbell Side Lateral—start, left; finish, right.

Dumbbell Upright Rows

Emphasis: Using two dumbbells, rather than a barbell or cable, gives you more freedom of movement when performing Upright Rows for your shoulder and trapezius muscles.

Starting Position: Grasp two moderately weighted dumbbells, set your feet about shoulder-width apart and stand erect. Your arms should be straight and running down the front of your body so the dumbbells touch each other while your palms are toward your body.

Movement Performance: Slowly pull the dumbbells directly upward an inch or two away from your torso until they reach shoulder level. As with Barbell Upright Rows, it is essential that you keep your elbows above the level of your hands throughout the movement. Lower the weights back to the starting point and repeat the movement.

Exercise Variations: Since your hands are restricted to a set distance apart as when you grasp a barbell bar, you can pull the dumbbells upward along a wide variety of movement arcs in Dumbbell Upright Rows.

Training Tip: You can ultimately use such heavy dumbbells in this movement that you will need to use straps to assist your grip on the dumbbell bars.

Standing Dumbbell Side Laterals

Emphasis: This movement is incorrectly performed more often than virtually all other exercises. Correctly executed, Dumbbell Side Laterals stress the medial heads of the deltoids in nearly total isolation from the rest of the body. Very minor secondary stress is placed on the anterior delts and the trapezius muscles.

Starting Position: Grasp two light dumbbells, place your feet about shoulder-width apart, and stand erect. Bend slightly forward at the waist and press the dumbbells together, palms facing each other, about six inches in front of your hips. Bend your arms slightly and keep them rounded like this throughout the movement.

Movement Performance: Using deltoid strength and keeping your palms toward the floor throughout the movement, raise the dumbbells in semicircular arcs out to the sides and slightly forward until they are above the level of your shoulders. At the top of the movement, it's essential that you rotate the front ends of the dumbbells below the level of the back ends for a moment to isolate stress on the medial deltoid heads. Lower the dumbbells slowly back along the same arc to the starting point and repeat the movement.

One-Arm Dumbbell Side Laterals

Comment: This movement is performed holding a sturdy upright post just the same as when performing One-Arm Dumbbell Presses. Leaning slightly away from the upright, raise the dumbbell in one hand up to shoulder level, pause for a second, lower it back to the starting point, and repeat the movement. Be sure to do the same number of sets and repetitions with each arm on all one-armed movements.

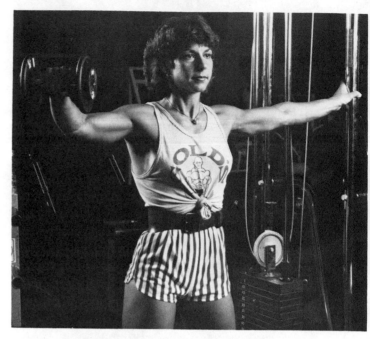

One-Arm Dumbbell Side Lateral.

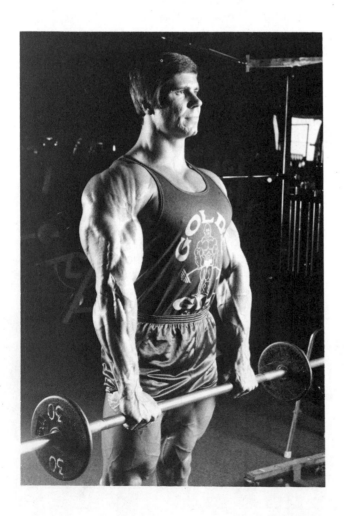

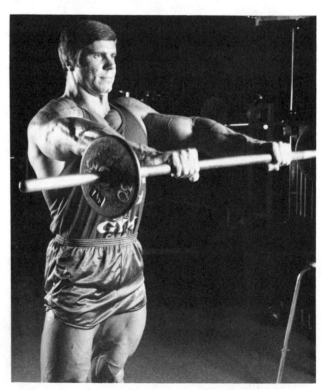

Standing Front Raise—start, left; finish, above.

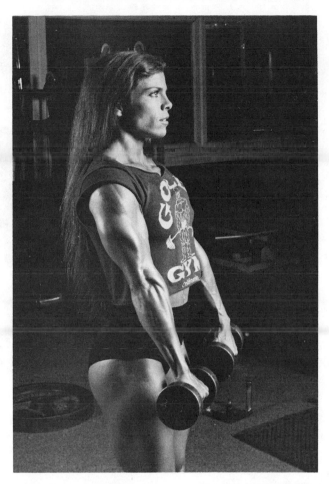 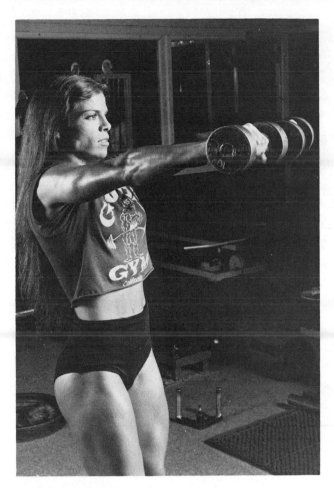

Dumbbell Front Raise—start, left; finish, right.

Standing Front Raises

Emphasis: This movement can be performed with a barbell, two dumbbells, or a single dumbbell held in both hands. Regardless of the variation used, Front Raises isolate stress on the anterior deltoid heads, with minor secondary stress placed on the medial delts and the trapezius muscles.

Starting Position: Take a shoulder-width over-grip on a light barbell. Set your feet a comfortable distance apart and stand erect with your arms straight down at your sides and the barbell resting across your upper thighs. Keep your torso motionless throughout the exercise.

Movement Performance: Moving just your arms, slowly raise the barbell in a semicircular arc from your thighs to the height of your shoulders. Or, for a more complete stress on your deltoids, you can raise the barbell all of the way to straight arms' length directly above your head. Lower the barbell back to the starting position and repeat the movement for the suggested number of repetitions.

Training Tip: A lot of very good bodybuilders like to flex their wrists so their hands hang downward during the movement.

Exercise Variations: This exercise is often performed with two dumbbells, either raising them both upward at the same time with your palms toward the floor, or lifting them in alternate fashion, one going upward as the other descends. In this case, the bells can be raised either to shoulder height in this fashion, or all the way to an overhead position. A second variation is performed with one dumbbell held in both hands—wrap a towel around the dumbbell handle and grasp the handle with both hands. In this case, the dumbbell can be raised up either to shoulder height, or completely overhead as well.

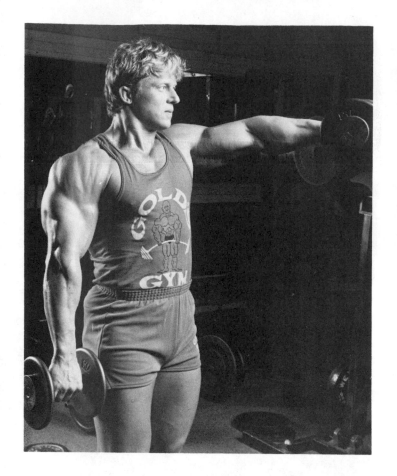

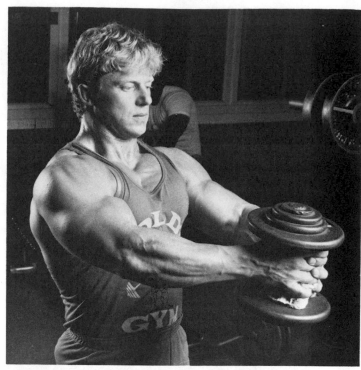

Front Raise variations—alternating arms, left; using both hands, above.

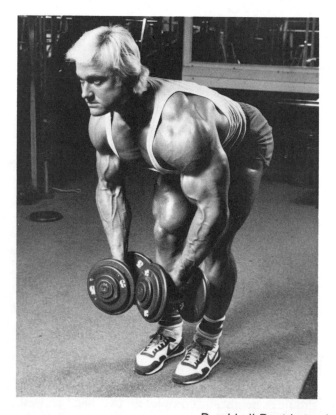

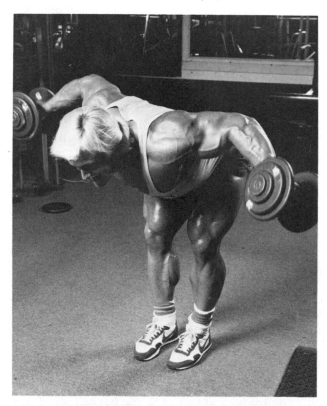

Dumbbell Bent Lateral—start, left; finish, right.

Dumbbell Bent Laterals

Emphasis: This movement is intended to isolate stress on the posterior heads of the deltoids, although it does so in combination with stressing the upper-back muscles and to some extent the medial deltoids.

Starting Position: Grasp two light dumbbells, set your feet about shoulder-width apart, and bend over until your torso is parallel to the floor. Hang your arms directly downward from your shoulders, your palms facing inward, and the dumbbells touching each other. You should bend your arms slightly and keep them rounded like this throughout the movement.

Movement Performance: Slowly raise the dumbbells in semicircular arcs directly out to the sides until they are slightly above shoulder level. Lower the weights back to the starting point and repeat the movement.

Training Tip: You will find that your lower back will take less stress if you keep your legs slightly bent during the movement.

One-Arm Dumbbell Bent Laterals

Comment: By bending over at the waist and grasping a sturdy upright with your free hand, you can easily perform Dumbbell Bent Laterals one arm at a time.

One-Arm Dumbbell Bent Lateral.

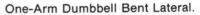

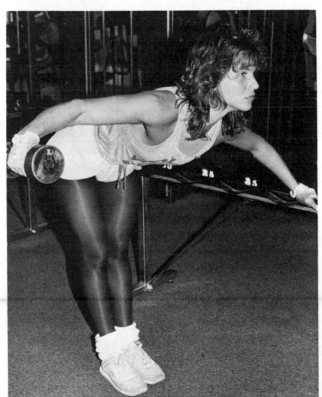

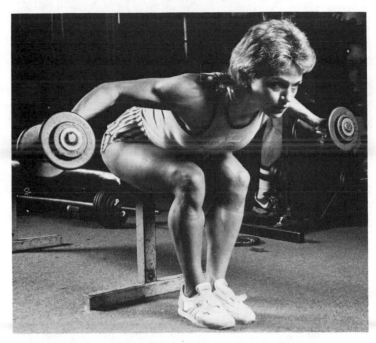

Seated Bent Lateral.

Seated Bent Laterals

Emphasis: As with the standing version of this movement, Seated Bent Laterals stress the posterior deltoids, upper-back muscles, and medial deltoids.

Starting Position: Grasp two light dumbbells and sit at the very end of a flat exercise bench, facing away from the length of the bench. Place your feet close to each other about two feet from the end of the bench. Bend over at the waist and rest your torso along your thighs. Hang your arms down as in Standing Bent Laterals, rounding them during the movement and turning your wrists so your palms face each other.

Movement Performance: Without moving your torso, slowly raise the dumbbells in semicircular arcs directly out to the sides until they are slightly above the level of your shoulders. Lower the weights slowly back to the starting point and repeat the movement.

Training Tip: The most common error when performing this exercise is to raise your torso from your thighs to help cheat up the dumbbells.

Exercise Variation: For a unique stress on your posterior and medial deltoids, you can raise the dumbbells slightly forward as you raise them out to the sides.

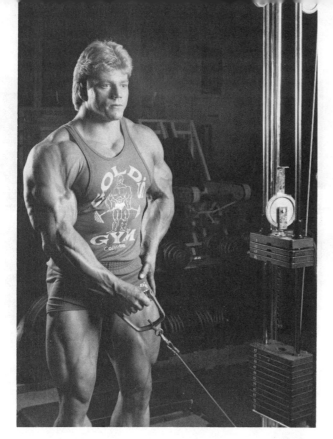 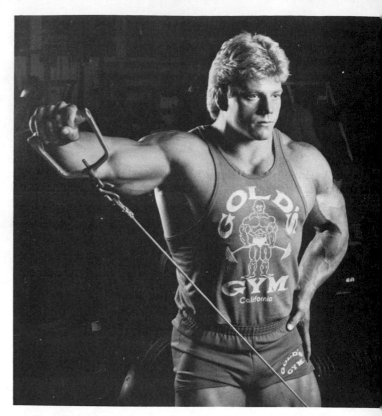

Cable Side Lateral—start, left; finish, right.

Cable Side Laterals

Emphasis: This Cable Side Lateral movement is one of the most effective exercises for isolating stress on the medial head of the deltoid. Only minor stress is placed on the anterior deltoid head and the trapezius muscles.

Starting Position: Attach a loop handle to the end of a cable passing through a floor pulley. Grasp the pulley handle in your left hand and stand with your right side about two feet away from the pulley. The cable should run diagonally across the front of your body as you perform the exercise. Bend your left arm slightly and keep it rounded like this throughout the movement. Place your right hand on your right hip.

Movement Performance: Slowly raise your left hand in a semicircular arc upward to the side and a bit forward until it is above the level of your shoulder. Slowly lower your hand back to the starting point and repeat the movement.

Exercise Variations: There are two other ways in which you can perform this exercise with one arm at a time and one way in which you can do it with both arms simultaneously. The first one-arm variation is performed with the cable running diagonally across your back rather than across the front of your body. And the second one-arm variation is performed with the arm toward the pulley raising the loop handle upward. The two-arm version of Cable Side Laterals is performed with the cables crossing each other in front of your body, your right hand raising the loop handle attached to the cable running through the pulley on the left side, and the left hand raising the pulley handle attached to the cable running through the pulley on the right side.

Cable Front Raises

Emphasis: By attaching a bar handle to a floor pulley, you can do a movement very similar to Barbell Front Raises to directly stress the anterior heads of your deltoids and place secondary stress on the medial delts and traps.

Starting Position: Attach a bar handle to a floor pulley and take an over-grip on the bar handle. Stand erect with your feet set about shoulder-width apart two feet back from the pulley. Straighten your arms and allow the pulley cable to pull them in a straight line toward the pulley.

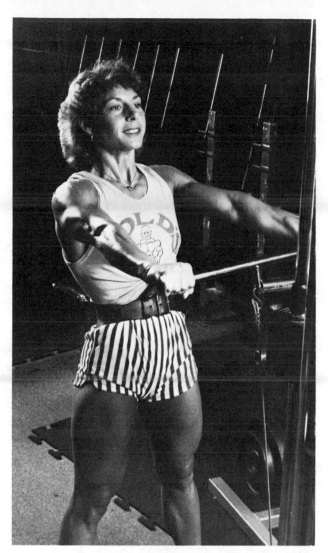

Cable Front Raise.

bench. If a seat is provided on the bench, you can sit on it as you do the movement. Otherwise, you can stand on the platforms attached to the foot end of the bench. Allow your arms to dangle downward from your shoulders and rotate your wrists so your palms face each other at the starting point of the movement. Bend your arms slightly and keep them rounded like this throughout the movement.

Movement Performance: Slowly raise the dumbbells in semicircular arcs directly out to the sides until they are slightly above shoulder level. Lower the dumbbells back to the starting point and repeat the movement.

Training Tip: The most common mistake when performing this exercise is moving the weights too much to the rear, rather than directly out to the sides. Raising the dumbbells to the rear removes stress from your deltoids and places them on your triceps.

Exercise Variation: For a very unique stress on your delts while lying in this position on an incline bench, you can raise the dumbbells directly to the front and upward to a point slightly above shoulder level, rather than out to the sides. Raising the dumbbells forward places more stress on the anterior deltoid heads than on the medial and side heads of your deltoids.

Movement Performance: Slowly raise the handle in a semicircular arc from the starting point up either to shoulder level or to a point directly above your head. Lower your hands and the handle back to the starting point and repeat the movement.

Exercise Variations: This movement can also be done with one arm at a time by attaching a loop handle to the cable.

Prone Incline Lateral Raises

Emphasis: Prone Incline Laterals stress the medial and posterior deltoid heads in concert. Strong secondary emphasis is on the trapezius and other upper-back muscles.

Starting Position: Grasp two light dumbbells and lie facedown on a 30–45-degree incline

Prone Incline Lateral Raise.

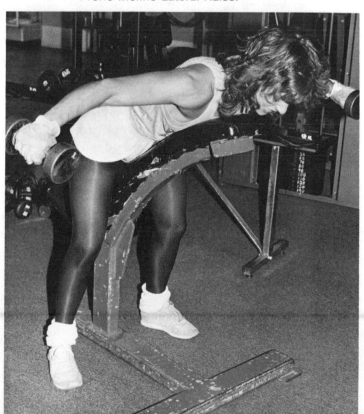

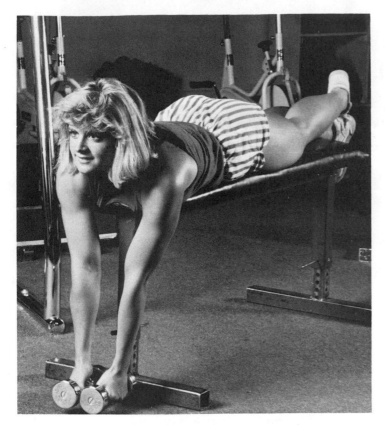

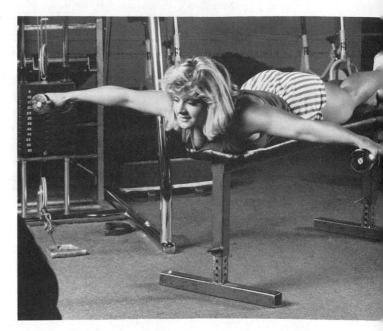

Prone Lateral Raise—start, left; finish, right.

Prone Lateral Raises

Comment: This movement is precisely the same as Prone Incline Laterals, except that they are performed while lying facedown on a flat exercise bench. You'll probably need to do this movement on a fairly high flat bench, since the dumbbells won't be clear of the floor in the bottom position of the movement if the bench is too low.

Incline Front Raises

Emphasis: Whether you perform this movement facedown as just described in the section on Prone Incline Laterals, or face up, this movement stresses the anterior heads of your deltoids quite intensely.

Starting Position: Grasp two light dumbbells and lie on your back on a 30–45-degree incline bench. You can sit on the bench seat if one is

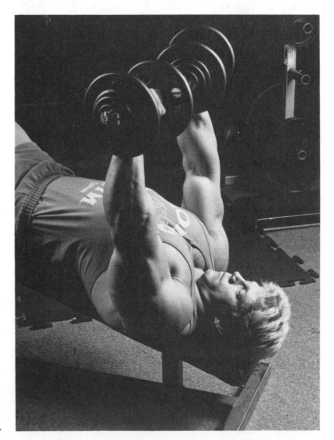

Incline Front Raise (face up) at finish.

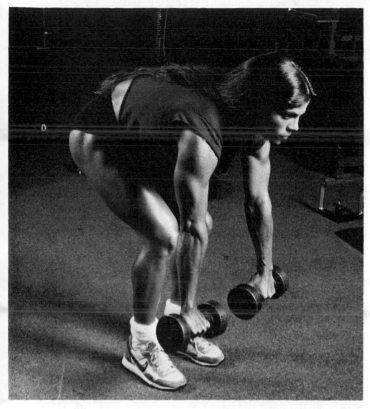

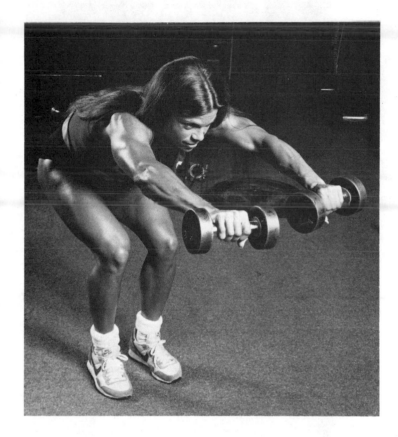

Bent-Over Front Raise—start, above; finish, right.

provided. Hang your arms straight down from your shoulders with your palms facing toward the rear.

Movement Performance: Keeping your arms straight, slowly raise the dumbbells directly forward and upward until they are directly above your shoulder joints. Lower the dumbbells back to the starting point and repeat the movement.

Exercise Variation: Rather than raising both dumbbells at once, you can do this exercise in alternate fashion, raising one dumbbell as the other is descending.

Bent-Over Front Raises

Emphasis: This unique movement strongly stresses the anterior and medial deltoid heads in concert. Secondary stress is placed on the poste-

rior deltoids, trapezius, and other upper-back muscles.

Starting Position: Take a shoulder-width over-grip on a light barbell, set your feet about shoulder-width apart, and bend over at the waist until your torso is parallel to the floor during the movement. Hang your arms directly down from your shoulders and keep your arms straight throughout the movement.

Movement Performance: Moving only your arms, slowly raise the barbell in a semicircular arc from the starting position to as high a point in front of, and above, your head as possible. Hold this top position for a moment, then return to the starting point to repeat the movement.

Exercise Variations: You can also do this movement with dumbbells, either raising them simultaneously or alternately.

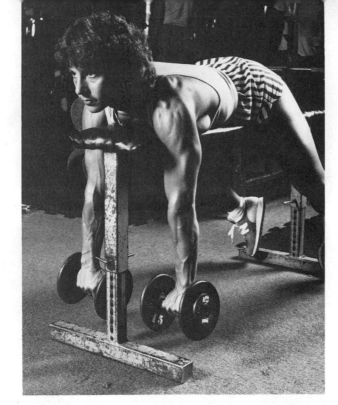 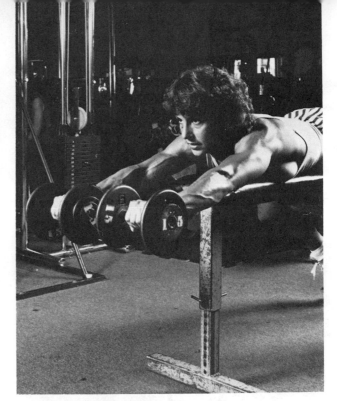

Prone Front Raise—start, left; finish, right.

Prone Front Raises

Comment: This movement is precisely the same as Bent Front Raises, except that it is performed lying facedown on a high, flat exercise bench with your head and shoulders positioned right at the end of the bench to allow freedom of arm and shoulder movement.

Incline Side Laterals

Emphasis: Incline Side Laterals place strong, direct stress on the medial deltoid head, with significant secondary stress on the anterior deltoid heads and trapezius.

Starting Position: Grasp a light dumbbell in your left hand and lie on your right side as illustrated on a 30–45-degree incline bench. Bend your arm slightly and keep it rounded like this throughout the movement. Allow the weight of the dumbbell to pull your left hand a few inches below the level of the incline bench.

Movement Performance: Slowly raise the

Incline Side Lateral—start, left; finish, right.

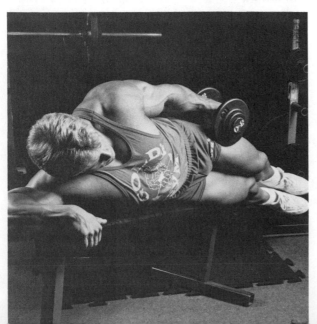 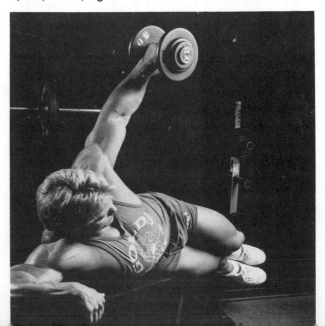

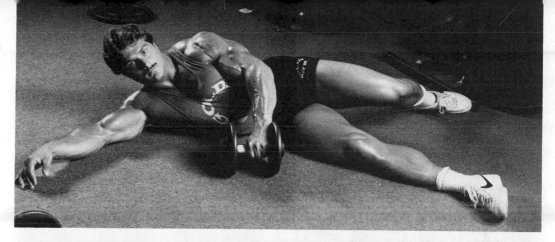

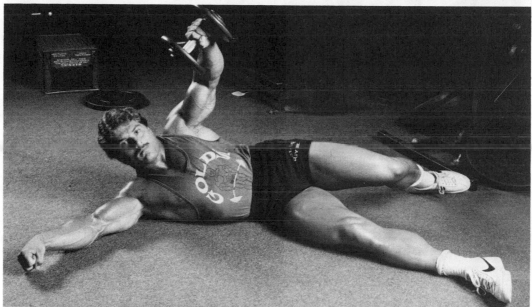

Floor Side Lateral—start, top; finish, bottom.

dumbbell directly out to the side and upward in a semicircular arc until it is directly above your left shoulder joint. Lower the weight back to the starting point and repeat the movement.

Exercise Variation: Rather than starting the movement with the dumbbell in front of your body, you can also begin the movement with the weight behind your butt.

Training Tip: Be sure to do the same number of sets and repetitions with each arm.

Floor Side Laterals

Emphasis: This movement, a favorite of the great French champion, Serge Nubret, is similar to Incline Side Laterals. Floor Side Laterals strongly stress the medial deltoid head, with significant secondary stress on the anterior delt and trapezius.

Starting Position: Lie on your right side on a mat placed on the floor and grasp a light dumbbell in your left hand. Balance your body in position during the movement by spreading your legs and using your right hand to push against the floor. Start with the dumbbell lying on the floor about six inches in front of your pelvis. Round your left arm and keep it slightly bent throughout the movement.

Movement Performance: Slowly raise the dumbbell from the starting point in a semicircular arc to a position directly above your shoulder joint. Lower the weight back to the starting point and repeat the movement.

Exercise Variation: Rather than starting the movement with the weight in front of your hips, you can begin with it behind your back.

Training Tip: Be sure to do the same number of sets and reps with each arm.

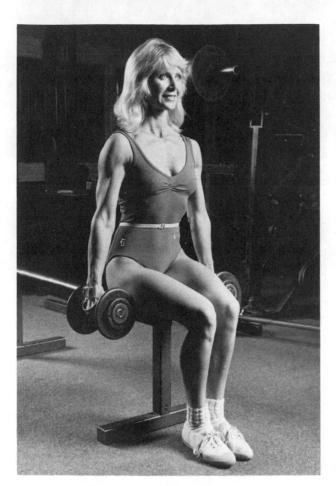

Seated Dumbbell Side Laterals

Emphasis: Seated Dumbbell Side Laterals primarily stress the medial deltoid heads and place secondary stress on the anterior deltoids and the upper-back muscles. This exercise is very similar to Standing Dumbbell Side Laterals, except that the legs are isolated from the movement.

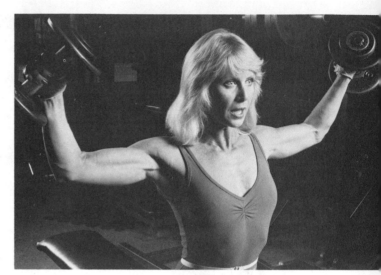

Seated Dumbbell Side Lateral—start, left; finish, right.

Palms-Up Dumbbell Side Laterals—start, left; finish, right.

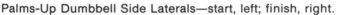

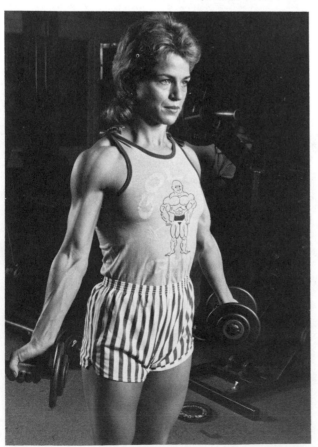

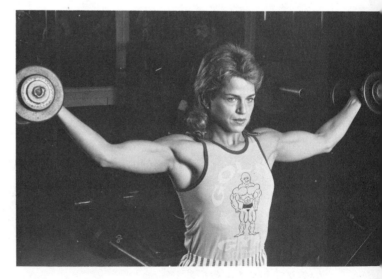

Starting Position: Grasp two light dumbbells and sit down at the end of a flat exercise bench. Place your feet in a comfortable position on the floor, or entwine your legs with the legs of the bench to brace your body in position during the movement. Hang your arms down at your sides

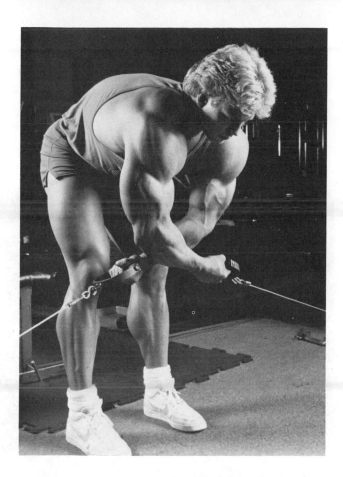

Cable Bent Lateral—start, left; finish, below.

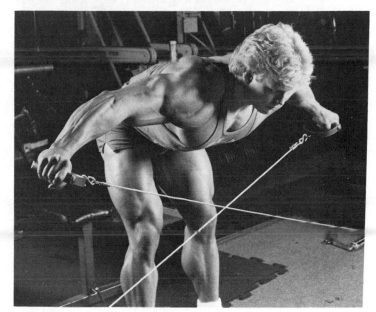

and keep your arms rounded during the movement.

Movement Performance: Slowly raise the dumbbells upward and slightly forward in semicircular arcs to a point just above shoulder level. Lower the weights back to the starting point and repeat the movement.

Exercise Variation: You can also perform Seated Dumbbell Front Raises in this position, raising the dumbbells forward and upward either simultaneously or alternately.

Palms-Up Dumbbell Side Laterals

Emphasis: To very directly stress the anterior heads of the deltoids in almost total isolation from the remainder of the body, you can do Palms-Up Dumbbell Side Laterals.

Starting Position: Grasp two light dumbbells in your hands, set your feet about shoulder-width apart, and stand erect with your arms hanging down at your sides. Rotate your wrists so your palms are facing away from your body. Bend your arms slightly and keep them rounded like this throughout the movement.

Movement Performance: Slowly raise the

dumbbells directly out to the sides in semicircular arcs until they are a bit above the level of your shoulders. Lower the dumbbells back to the starting point and repeat the movement.

Exercise Variation: You can perform this exercise with one arm at a time while grasping a sturdy upright with your free hand.

Cable Bent Laterals

Emphasis: Cable Bent Laterals place primary stress on the posterior deltoids, trapezius, and other upper-back muscles. Secondary stress is placed on the medial deltoids and triceps.

Starting Position: Attach loop handles to floor cables and stand between the two pulleys. Reach with your right hand to the left and grasp the loop handle attached to the cable running through the pulley on that side. Reach to the right with your left hand and grasp the loop handle on that side. Bend over at the waist until your torso is parallel to the floor and allow the weights on the ends of the cables to pull your arms across each other beneath your chest.

Movement Performance: From this position, slowly raise your hands in semicircular arcs

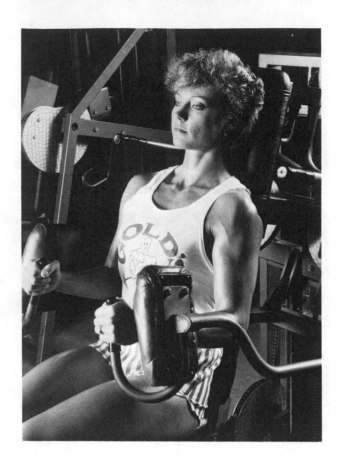

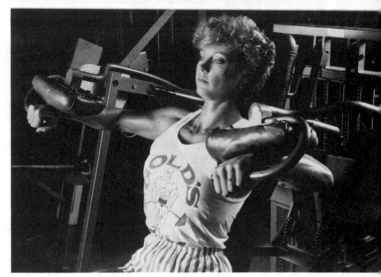

Nautilus Side Lateral—start, left; finish, below.

directly out to the sides and upward until they are slightly above the level of your shoulders. Pause at the top of the movement for a moment, and return to the starting point. Repeat the movement.

Exercise Variation: You can also do this exercise with one arm at a time by allowing the cable to pass beneath your torso as you move your hand upward. As you perform this movement, you can brace yourself with your torso parallel to the floor by placing your free hand on your knee.

Nautilus Side Laterals

Emphasis: Side Laterals performed on a Nautilus double-shoulder machine isolate stress primarily on the medial heads of the deltoids. Minor secondary stress is on the anterior deltoid heads and trapezius.

Starting Position: Adjust the height of the machine seat so, as you are sitting in the seat, your shoulder joints are at the level of the rotating cams of the machine. Sit in the machine, fasten the seat belt over your lap, and cross your ankles beneath the seat. Place the

backs of your wrists against the movement pads and grasp the handles attached to the pads.

Movement Performance: Using only deltoid strength, raise your elbows upward in semicircular arcs to as high a position as possible. Return to the starting point and repeat the movement.

Training Tip: The object in this exercise is to see how high you can raise your *elbows* in the movement, rather than how high you can raise your hands. So, it's essential that you keep your elbows above the level of your hands throughout the movement.

Exercise Variations: You can perform this exercise with one arm at a time. It is also possible to do the exercise in a standing position while facing the machine.

Pec Deck Rear Deltoid Movement

Emphasis: This exercise places direct stress on the posterior deltoids and upper-back muscles.

Starting Position: Sit backward in a pec deck machine (i.e., facing the upright padded board of the machine, rather than away from it). Push your elbows against the backs of the movement pads of the machine and allow the weights at-

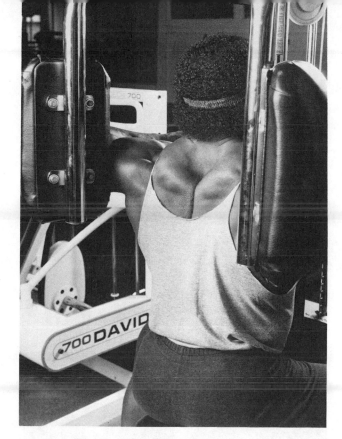

Pec Deck Rear Deltoid Movement.

tached to the pads to push your elbows as far away from the front of your body as possible.

Movement Performance: Using deltoid strength, push backward with your elbows against the pads as far as possible. Hold this fully contracted position for a moment, then return to the starting point. Repeat the movement.

Exercise Variations: You can do a very similar movement on the old Nautilus rowing machine.

Suggested Shoulder Routines

If you have less than a few weeks of training behind you, the following shoulder routine can profitably be performed three nonconsecutive days per week:

Exercise	Sets	Reps
Military Presses	3	12–8*
Upright Rows	2	8–12
Dumbbell Bent Laterals	2	8–12

* All exercises marked with an asterisk should have the weights and reps pyramidded. With each succeeding set, the weight on the bar should be increased and the number of reps performed decreased.

After 4–6 weeks of steady training on the foregoing program, you can use this routine three days per week:

Exercise	Sets	Reps
Military Presses (warmup)	1	15–20
Seated Presses Behind Neck	4	12–6*
Standing Side Laterals	3	8–10
Seated Dumbbell Bent Laterals	3	8–10
Barbell Upright Rows	3	12–8*

After about three months of training, you should switch to a four-day split routine in which you train each major muscle group (including the shoulders) twice per week. This is typically how a lower-level competitive bodybuilder will train in the off-season. Following is a sample shoulder training program for off-season competitive training:

Exercise	Sets	Reps
Smith Machine Front Presses	4	12–6*
One-Arm Dumbbell Press	4	12–6*
Seated Dumbbell Bent Laterals	3	8–12
Cable Bent Laterals	3	8–12
Barbell Upright Rows	4	12–6*
One-Arm Cable Side Laterals	3–4	10–15

Every advanced bodybuilder trains differently from all others prior to a competition, as you will see in the following section listing the shoulder routines of a wide variety of men and women who either train or have trained at Gold's Gym.

Shoulder Routines of the Gold's Champs

In this section, you will find a variety of shoulder training programs used by many of the Gold's Gym superstars who have won the sport's highest titles. Keep in mind as you examine these training programs that these men and women have been training for many years and have developed an enormous recuperative ability. It is unlikely that you can make good gains using their full routines without similar training experience. Instead, you should use these training programs as examples of how to work your own shoulders. In all likelihood, you can do the same exercises as your favorite champion, but scale down the number of sets that he or she does of each movement to meet your own abilities.

TIM BELKNAP
(MR. AMERICA)

Exercise	Sets	Reps
Seated Press behind the Neck	4	12-6*
Dumbbell Side Laterals	3	8-10
Cable Bent Laterals	3	8-10

TOM PLATZ
(MR. UNIVERSE)

Day 1 (with chest)

Exercise	Sets	Reps
Barbell Upright Rows	5-8	10-15
Barbell Front Raises	5-8	10-15
One-Arm Dumbbell Side Laterals	5-8	10-15
One-Arm Cable Side Laterals	5-8	10-15

Day 2 (with back)

Exercise	Sets	Reps
Smith Machine Press behind the Neck	5-8	10-15
Dumbbell Bent Laterals	5-8	10-15

SCOTT WILSON
(PORTLAND PRO GRAND PRIX CHAMP)

Exercise	Sets	Reps
Seated Press behind the Neck	5	6-10
Dumbbell Side Laterals	5	6-10
Dumbbell Bent Laterals	5	6-10

DR. LYNNE PIRIE
(HEAVYWEIGHT U.S.A. CHAMP)

Exercise	Sets	Reps
Nautilus Side Laterals	2-3	10-12
Nautilus Overhead Presses	2-3	10-12
Nautilus Rear Delt Rows	2-3	10-12

Note: All sets are done with forced reps, negatives, and forced negatives.

LARRY SCOTT
(MR. OLYMPIA)

Exercise	Sets	Reps
Dumbbell Presses	3-4	***
Side Laterals	3-4	***
Bent Laterals	3-4	***

Note: On all three exercises, Larry goes down the rack with several weight drops on each set, as marked by the asterisks.

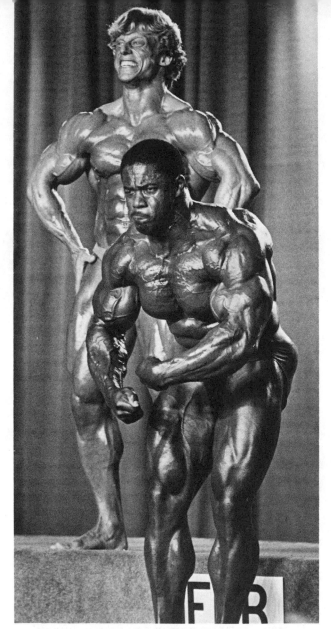

Andreas Cahling (elevated) and Bertil Fox.

RICHARD BALDWIN
(MR. AMERICA CLASS WINNER)

Exercise	Sets	Reps
Press behind the Neck	6	6-10
Dumbbell Bent Laterals	5	8-10
Cable Upright Rows	5	8-10
Dumbbell Presses	3	6-10
supersetted with		
Barbell Front Raises	3	8-10

CLINT BEYERLE
(MR. USA)

Exercise	Sets	Reps
Press behind the Neck	6-8	8-2*
Dumbbell Side Laterals	4-5	8-10
Dumbbell Presses	4-5	8-10
Cable Bent Laterals	5-6	8-10

JOHN BURKHOLDER
(MR. NORTH AMERICA)

Exercise	Sets	Reps
Military Press (warm-up)	1–2	10–15
Seated Press behind the Neck	4–5	6–8
Dumbbell Bent Laterals	3–4	8–10
Cable Side Laterals	3–4	8–10

ANDREAS CAHLING
(MR. INTERNATIONAL)

Exercise	Sets	Reps
Machine Press (warm-up)	2–3	10–15
Seated Press behind the Neck	3	6–8
Seated Bent Laterals	2	8–10
Standing Dumbbell Side Laterals	2	8–10
Cable Side Laterals	2	8–10
Cable Bent Laterals	2	8–10
Front Barbell Raises	2	8–10

LAURA COMBES
(MS. AMERICA)

Exercise	Sets	Reps
Dumbbell Presses (warm-up)	2–3	10–15
Military Presses	5	12–5*
Barbell Upright Rows	5	12–5*
Dumbbell Side Laterals	4	8–12
Seated Dumbbell Bent Laterals	4	8–12
Cable Side Laterals	1–2	10–15

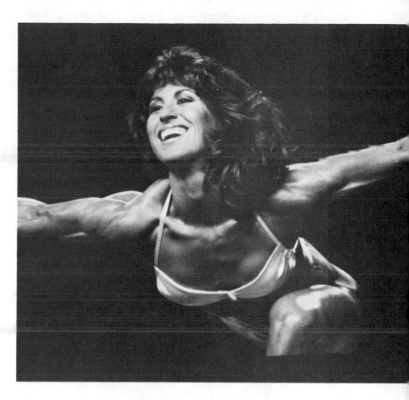

Rachel McLish.

STEVE DAVIS
(MR. WORLD)

Exercise	Sets	Reps
Dumbbell Presses	7	12–6*
Dumbbell Side Laterals	7	12–6*
Dumbbell Bent Laterals	7	12–6*

CHRIS DICKERSON
(MR. OLYMPIA)

Exercise	Sets	Reps
Seated Press behind the Neck	6	12–8*
Standing Dumbbell Side Laterals	6	8–10
Seated Dumbbell Presses	6	8
Seated Bent Laterals	6	12–15
Upright Rows	4	10–12

Lisa Elliott-Kolakowski.

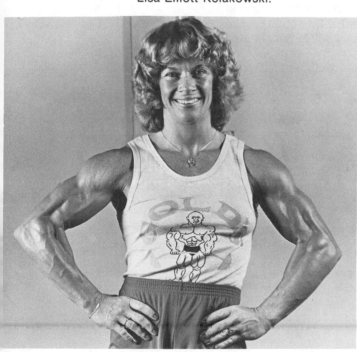

LISA ELLIOTT-KOLAKOWSKI
(GOLD'S CLASS CHAMP)

Exercise	Sets	Reps
Arnold Dumbbell Presses	4	6
Machine Press behind the Neck	4	6
Dumbbell Side Laterals	4	6
Seated Bent Laterals	4	6
Upright Rows	4	6
Cable Side Laterals	4	6–8

CHARLES GLASS
(AMATEUR WORLD CHAMP)

Exercise	Sets	Reps
Dumbbell Presses (warm-up)	2-3	10-15
Machine Press behind the Neck	6	12-2*
Seated Dumbbell Presses	4	10-6*
Seated Bent Laterals	5	8-10
supersetted with		
Standing Dumbbell Side Laterals	5	8-10
Barbell Upright Rows	5	8-10

ROD KOONTZ
(NATURAL MR. AMERICA)

Exercise	Sets	Reps
Dumbbell Side Laterals	4	10-12
Heavy Partial Side Laterals	4	12-15
Press behind the Neck	4	8-10
Note: Above exercises are performed as a triset		
Dumbbell Shrugs	4	12-15
supersetted with		
Partial Front Raises	4	8-10

1983 Lightweight World Champion Erica Mes.

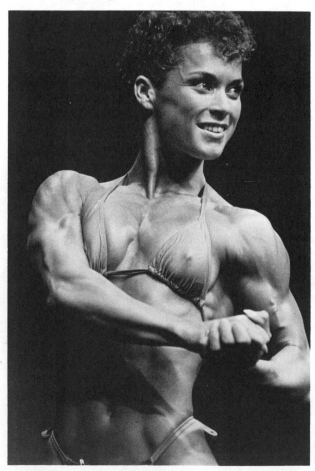

RACHEL McLISH
(MISS OLYMPIA)

Exercise	Sets	Reps
Machine Side Laterals	3	6-8
Machine Overhead Presses	3	6-8
supersetted with		
Dumbbell Bent Laterals	3	6-8

JOE NAZARIO
(MR. INTERNATIONAL)

Exercise	Sets	Reps
Seated Press behind the Neck	5	8-10
supersetted with		
Dumbbell Side Laterals	5	8-10
Dumbbell Presses	5	8-10
supersetted with		
Front Raises	5	8-10
Nautilus Side Laterals	5	8-10
supersetted with		
Dumbbell Bent Laterals	5	8-10

JACQUES NEUVILLE
(WORLD CHAMPION)

Exercise	Sets	Reps
Seated Press behind the Neck	5	10-12
Seated Bent Laterals	5	10-12
Cable Side Laterals	5	10-12
Upright Rows	5	10-12

CARLOS RODRIGUEZ
(MR. UNIVERSE)

Exercise	Sets	Reps
Military Presses (warm-up)	1-2	15-20
Seated Machine Presses	4-5	6-8
Seated Dumbbell Presses	4-5	6-8
Dumbbell Side Laterals	4-5	8-10
Cable Side Laterals	4-5	8-10
Dumbbell Bent Laterals	4-5	8-10

DON ROSS
(PRO MR. AMERICA)

Exercise	Sets	Reps
Dumbbell Side Laterals	8	8
Dumbbell Front Raises	8	8
Dumbbell Bent Laterals	6	8

PAT STEWART
(MR. NORTH AMERICA)

Exercise	Sets	Reps
Press behind the Neck	4	12-6*
Alternate Dumbbell Presses	3	8-12
Dumbbell Side Laterals	2	8-12
Cable Bent Laterals	2	10-12
Upright Rows	3	8-10

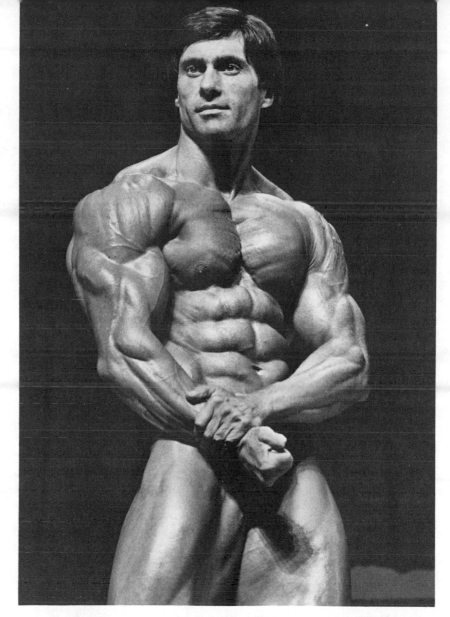

Jacques Neuville.

DENNIS TINERINO
(PRO MR. UNIVERSE)

Exercise	Sets	Reps
Machine Front Presses	6	6
Seated Dumbbell Presses	4	6–8
Dumbbell Bent Laterals	4	8–10
Dumbbell Side Laterals	4	8–10
Cable Side Laterals	4	8–10

CASEY VIATOR
(PRO GRAND PRIX CHAMP)

Exercise	Sets	Reps
One-Arm Nautilus Side Laterals	3–5	15–20
Seated Press behind the Neck	5–6	10–12
Dumbbell Side Laterals	4–5	10–12
Dumbbell Bent Laterals	4–5	10–12
Barbell Upright Rows	4–5	10–15

JUSUP WILKOSZ
(PRO MR. UNIVERSE)

Exercise	Sets	Reps
Alternate Dumbbell Front Raises	5	10–12
supersetted with		
Dumbbell Side Laterals	5	10–12
Seated Bent Laterals	5	10–12
Seated Military Presses	5	10 12
Cable Side Laterals	5	10–12

ARNOLD SCHWARZENEGGER
(MR. OLYMPIA)

Exercise	Sets	Reps
Seated Press behind the Neck	4–5	8–10
Arnold Dumbbell Presses	4–5	8–10
Dumbbell Side Laterals	4–5	8–10
Seated Dumbbell Bent Laterals	4–5	8–10
Cable Side Laterals	4–5	8–10

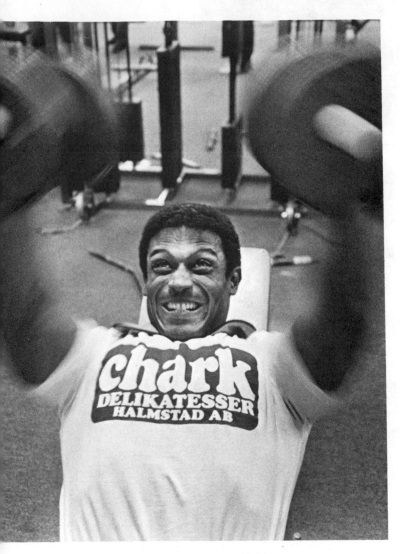

Mohamed Makkawy.

ALBERT BECKLES
(MR. UNIVERSE)

Exercise	Sets	Reps
Seated Dumbbell Presses	4	10–12
Seated Press behind the Neck	4	10–12
Dumbbell Side Laterals	4	10–12
Dumbbell Bent Laterals	4	10–12
Barbell Upright Rows	4	10–12

* All exercises marked with an asterisk should have the weights and reps pyramidded. With each succeeding set, the weight on the bar should be increased and the number of reps performed decreased.

SAMIR BANNOUT
(MR. OLYMPIA)

Exercise	Sets	Reps
Seated Machine Press behind the Neck	4–5	6–8
supersetted with		
Seated Bent Laterals	4–5	8–10
Seated Dumbbell Presses	4–5	6–8
supersetted with		
Standing Dumbbell Side Laterals	4–5	8–10
One-Arm Cable Side Laterals	4–5	8–10

DANNY PADILLA
(MR. UNIVERSE)

Exercise	Sets	Reps
Seated Barbell Front Presses	4	6–10
Seated Machine Presses behind the Neck	4	6–10
Dumbbell Side Laterals	4	8–12
One-Arm Cable Side Laterals	4	8–12
Seated Dumbbell Bent Laterals	4	8–12
Cable Bent Laterals	4	8–12

LOU FERRIGNO
(MR. INTERNATIONAL)

Exercise	Sets	Reps
Seated Press behind the Neck	5	6–10
Seated Machine Front Presses	5	10–12
Dumbbell Side Laterals	5	10–12
Dumbbell Bent Laterals	5	10–12
Dumbbell Alternate Front Raises	5	10–12

DR. FRANCO COLUMBU
(MR. OLYMPIA)

Exercise	Sets	Reps
Dumbbell Side Laterals	4	10
Dumbbell Bent Laterals	6	10
Seated Press behind the Neck	4	8
Dumbbell Alternate Front Raises	3	8
One-Arm Cable Side Laterals	3	10

Looking Ahead

In Chapter 5, we will introduce you to all the back exercises that the superstar bodybuilders at Gold's Gym use in their workouts. And we will reveal many of these champions' actual back training routines.

5
BACK TRAINING

The back is a very complex body part that, when fully developed, is nearly as large in muscle mass as the thighs and hips. Like leg training, back workouts are extremely fatiguing. A rapid build-up of fatigue toxins invariably occurs when you work your back that makes the pain barrier a very real enemy in back training. As a result, many otherwise great bodybuilders have failed to carry their back development to the level necessary to move them from the ordinary to the superstar class.

Back training can also be a problem for individuals (usually those who have an inherent structural weakness in their spines) who have suffered from lower-back injuries. While it's possible to train around a lower-back injury by avoiding those movements that aggravate the injury, it is much more difficult to achieve maximum back development when you have a chronic spinal problem.

Among male bodybuilders, Samir Bannout, Dr. Franco Columbu, and Sergio Oliva probably have the best all-around back development. Closely following these great athletes are a number of other champions such as Casey Viator, Frank Zane, Tony Pearson, Tom Platz, Arnold Schwarzenegger, Andreas Cahling,

Larry Jackson, Danny Padilla, Chris Dickerson, Albert Beckles, Roy Callender and Greg De-Ferro.

Interestingly, women seem to achieve comparably outstanding leg and back development in comparison to men, so a great number of women bodybuilders have achieved super back musculature. Still, it's difficult to conceive of back development better than that of Carla Dunlap, Laura Combes, and Sue Ann McKean. Other women with very good back development are Lisa Elliott-Kolakowski, Candy Csencsits, Kay Baxter, Claudia Wilborn, and Stella Martinez.

Anatomy and Kinesiology

Most champion bodybuilders treat their backs as three separate muscle groups—upper back (primarily the *trapezius* muscle complex), the middle back (primarily the *latissimus dorsi* group), and the lower back (primarily the *erector spinae* muscles). So they don't necessarily train all three areas in the same workout. Many bodybuilders do their trap work with deltoids and/or lower-back training with hip and thigh work.

The trapezius is a large kite-shaped muscle

that covers the upper back, giving a sloping look to the shoulders of a powerfully developed bodybuilder. The top and bottom points of the kite originate at about the base of the skull and insert on the spinal column near the middle of your thorax. The traps contract to pull your shoulders upward and backward.

The latissimus dorsi muscles give a wedge-like shape to the torso when viewed from the front or back. In a front or back lat spread pose, they look almost like wings. The lats originate from the sides of the spinal column and attach via thick tendons to the upper arm bones. They contract to pull the upper arms downward and backward. Crucially, you can't fully contract your latissimus dorsi muscles unless you arch your back during the movement, so you should keep this fact in mind as you train lats.

Your erector spinae muscle group lies like two thick columns of muscle on either side of the spine along your lower back. The spinal erectors contract primarily to straighten the spine from a bent-over position in relation to your legs and to bring your back into an arched position.

Back Exercises

There are nearly 40 major back exercises included in this section, each fully described and depicted. Add in the numerous variations of each basic exercise, and you will add more than 60 back movements to your basic pool of bodybuilding exercises.

Barbell Power Clean

Emphasis: This complex movement ultimately stresses most of the major muscle groups of the body, so it is often used as a general body warm-up prior to a workout. Primary stress is on the spinal erectors and trapezius muscles, and secondary emphasis is on the hip, thigh, biceps, and forearm muscles.

Starting Position: It might help you to visualize this exercise better if you understand that it is the basic movement that you use to bring a barbell to your shoulders when preparing to do Military Presses. Stand up to a barbell resting on the floor and place your feet about shoulder-width apart, your toes pointed directly forward.

Bend over and take an over-grip on the bar with your hands set two or three inches wider than your shoulders on each side. Straighten your arms, flatten and slightly arch your back, and bend your legs so your hips are lower than your shoulders and your knees are lower than your hips. *This is the best mechanical position in which to pull any heavy weight from the floor,* so be especially careful to analyze the photo of it that accompanies this exercise description.

Movement Performance: Start the movement by first straightening your legs to start the bar moving upward off the floor. As your legs begin to come to a straight position, begin to straighten your back as well. And when your legs and back are both in one long line, quickly rise up on your toes and pull hard on the bar with your arms. To fix the bar at your shoulders, you should quickly dip your legs and whip your elbows beneath the bar to catch the bar across your shoulders at the base of your neck. Lower the bar back to the floor and repeat the movement for the number of repetitions suggested in your training program.

Training Tips: We feel that you should always wear a weightlifting belt cinched tightly around your waist as you perform this movement. And if you don't want to wear your hands out doing this exercise, you should learn to use weightlifting straps to fix your hands more securely on the bar.

Exercise Variations: This movement can be done precisely the same way while holding two dumbbells in your hands. And with both barbell and dumbbell variations of Power Cleans, you can pull each rep past the first one "from the hang," or from a position just above your knees, rather than from the floor.

High Pulls

Emphasis: This movement is often used by competitive weightlifters to improve their explosive pulling power. Primary emphasis in High Pulls is on the spinal erectors and trapezius muscles; secondary stress is on the hip, thigh, biceps, and forearm muscles.

Starting Position: This movement is the first three-fourths of a Power Clean, with only the fixation of the bar at your shoulders deleted.

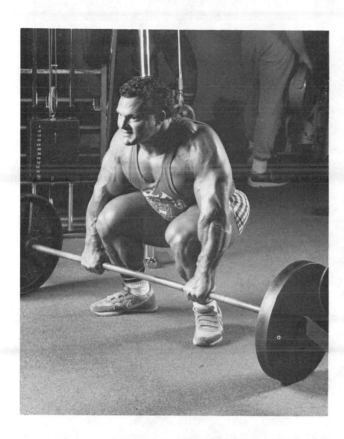
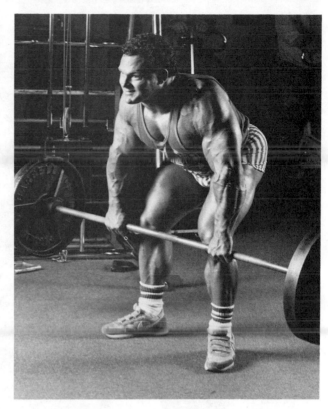

Barbell Power Clean—start, above left; midpoint, above right; near finish, below left; finish, below right.

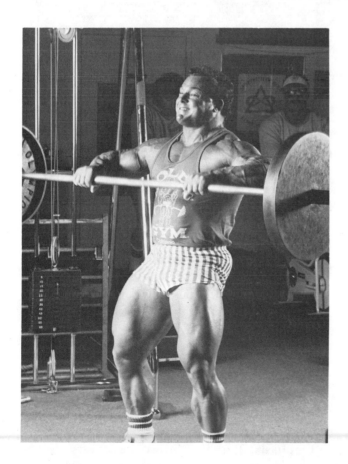
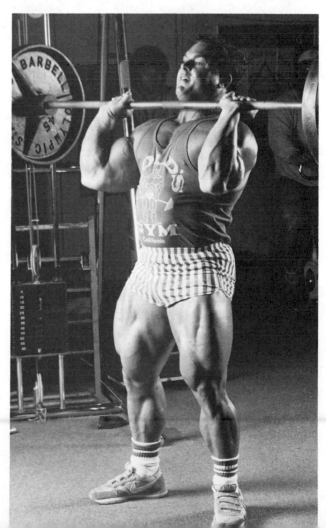

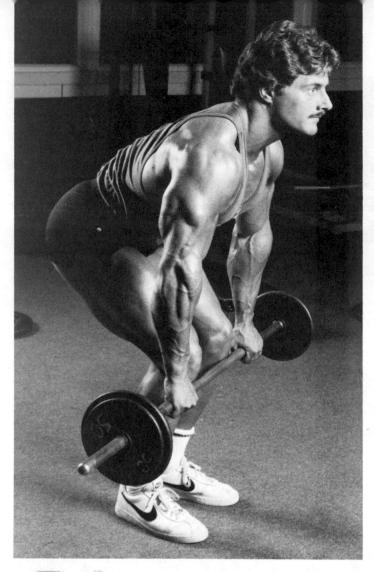

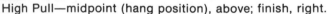

High Pull—midpoint (hang position), above; finish, right.

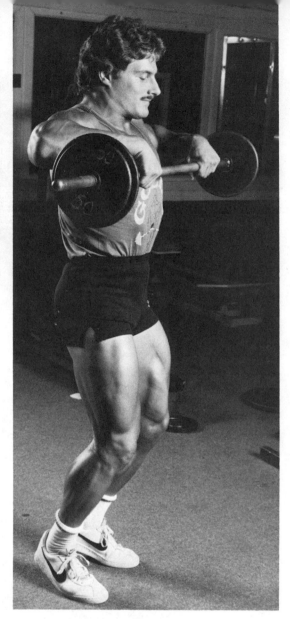

Stand up to a barbell resting on the floor and place your feet about shoulder-width apart, and your toes pointed directly forward. Bend over and take an over-grip on the bar with your hands set two or three inches wider than your shoulders on each side. Straighten your arms, flatten and slightly arch your back, and bend your legs so your hips are lower than your shoulders and your knees are lower than your hips.

Movement Performance: Initiate the movement by first straightening your legs to start the bar moving upward from the floor. As your legs begin to come to a straight position, begin to straighten your back as well. And when your legs and back are both in one long line, quickly rise up on your toes and pull hard on the bar with your arms. Your elbows should be held out to the sides in the top position of the movement and you should lean forward to touch your chest to

the bar. Lower the weight back to the floor and perform an appropriate number of repetitions.

Training Tips: You should always wear a lifting belt when you do High Pulls in your back workouts. And it's usually a good idea to use only an Olympic bar for this exercise and utilize straps to reinforce your grip on the bar.

Exercise Variations: *Don't use dumbbells in this exercise,* since you will be using a much heavier weight for High Pulls than for Power Cleans and the dumbbells are so unwieldly that you could injure yourself using them. As with Power Cleans, you can do some of your High Pulls from a hang position.

Barbell Shrugs

Emphasis: Barbell Shrugs are a very direct movement for stressing the trapezius and other

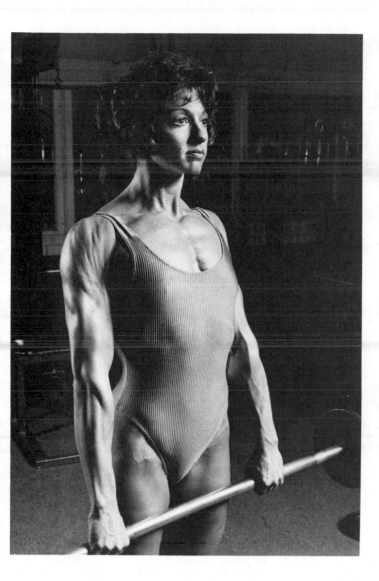

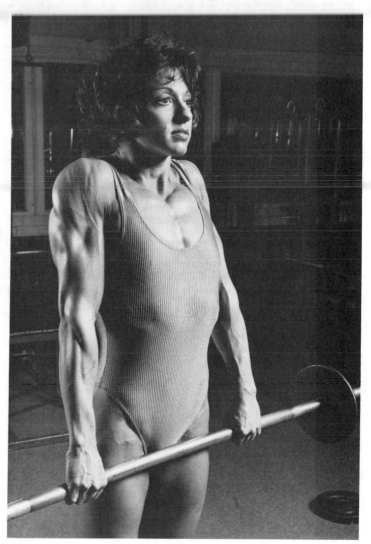

Barbell Shrug—start, left; finish, right.

upper back muscles. Secondary stress is on the gripping muscles of your forearms.

Starting Position: Assume the same starting position as for a Power Clean or a High Pull movement, but pull the barbell upward only until it is resting across your upper thighs when your arms are straight down at your sides and your torso is erect. Sag your shoulders forward and downward as far as comfortably possible. Be sure *not* to sag your torso forward at the waist or bend your arms as you do Shrugs.

Movement Performance: Slowly shrug your shoulders upward and backward as high and as far back as possible. Hold this peak-contracted, top position for a moment, return the barbell to the starting point, and repeat the movement for an appropriate number of repetitions.

Training Tips: With very heavy weights, you will definitely need to wear a weightlifting belt

and use straps to reinforce your grip. Bodybuilders frequently perform this exercise standing in a power rack with the pins set so the barbell is a little above knee height; this procedure keeps you from having to use up valuable energy lifting the bar up to the starting position in the first place.

Exercise Variations: The main variation in this movement consists of using a grip wider or more narrow than the recommended shoulder-width grip.

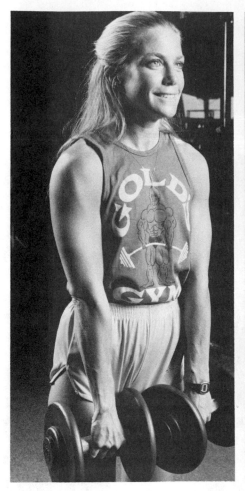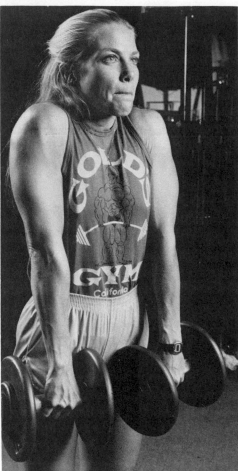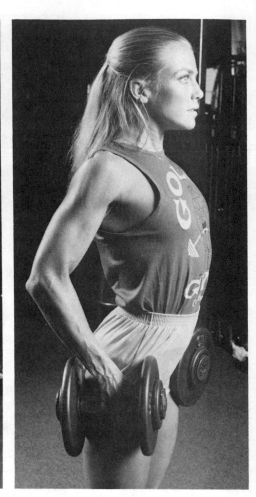

Dumbbell Shrug—start, left; midpoint of rotation forward, center; midpoint of rotation backward, right.

Dumbbell Shrugs

Emphasis: Dumbbell Shrugs are also a very direct movement for stressing the trapezius and other upper-back muscles. Secondary stress is on the gripping muscles of your forearms. You will have more mobility in your shoulders when using a pair of dumbbells, so in many ways Dumbbell Shrugs are superior to Barbell Shrugs.

Starting Position: Grasp two heavy dumbbells, assume the basic pulling position, and lift the weights up to your thighs; your arms should be held straight and your torso erect throughout the movement. Sag your shoulders forward and downward as far as comfortably possible.

Movement Performance: Slowly shrug your shoulders upward and backward as high and as far as possible. Hold this peak-contracted, top

position for a moment, then lower the dumbbells back to the starting point, and repeat the movement for the required number of reps.

Training Tips: You can wear a weightlifting belt and use straps to reinforce your grip when doing Dumbbell Shrugs.

Exercise Variations: When using dumbbells, you can do Rotating Shrugs, a far superior movement to Barbell Shrugs. In this exercise, you actually rotate your shoulders forward and/ or backward as you shrug the dumbbells upward.

Universal Shrugs

Emphasis: As with all Shrug movements, Universal Shrugs place primary stress on the traps and secondary emphasis on the gripping muscles of the forearms.

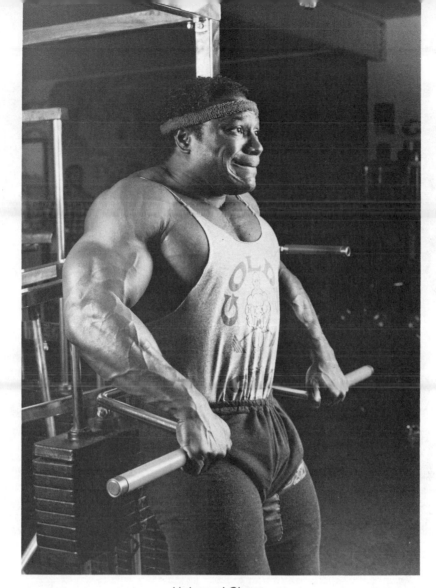

Universal Shrug.

Starting Position: This exercise is performed at the Bench Press station of a Universal Gym machine. Stand facing the weight stack and take an over-grip in the middle of the machine handles. Stand erect and keep your arms straight during the movement. Sag your shoulders forward and downward.

Movement Performance: Slowly shrug your shoulders upward and backward as high and as far as possible. Hold this peak-contracted, top position for a moment, then lower the handles back to the starting position, and repeat the exercise.

Training Tips: You should wear a weightlifting belt and use straps to reinforce your grip as you do Universal Shrugs. If you are less than about 5′6″ tall, you will probably need to stand on a thick block of wood to position your shoulders high enough to have resistance on your traps in the low position of the movement.

Exercise Variations: This exercise is also frequently performed facing away from the weight stack.

Barbell Upright Rows

Emphasis: All variations of the Upright Rows exercise strongly stress both the trapezius and deltoid muscle groups. Secondary emphasis is on the biceps, brachialis, and forearm muscles.

Starting Position: Take a narrow over-grip in the middle of a barbell handle, about six inches between your index fingers. Stand erect with your arms straight down at your sides and your fists resting on your upper thighs.

Movement Performance: Being sure to keep

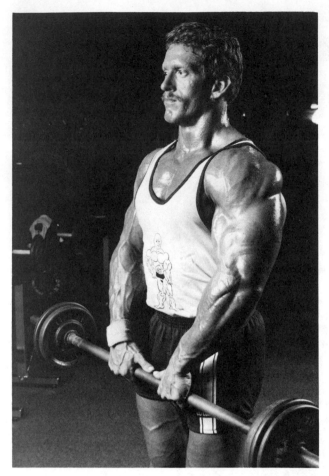 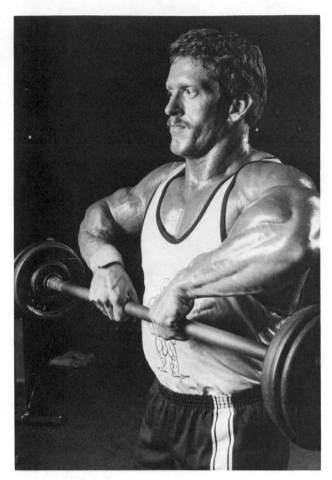

Barbell Upright Row—start, left; finish, right.

your elbows well above the level of your grip on the bar at all times, slowly pull the barbell directly upward close to your body until the backs of your hands contact the underside of your chin. In the top position of the movement, you should roll your shoulders backward and squeeze your shoulder blades together. Lower the weight slowly back to the starting point and repeat the movement for an appropriate number of repetitions.

Training Tips: Be very careful to lower the weight slowly back to the starting point. There is a natural tendency in this exercise to drop the weight from the top point of the movement back to the starting position. Since you receive almost half of the benefit of an exercise during the lowering phase of the movement, you should lower the bar slowly and emphasize the negative half of the exercise.

Exercise Variations: You can vary the width of

your grip on the bar inward until your hands are touching and outward to about shoulder width. However, the wider your grip when performing Upright Rows, the more the exercise stresses your deltoid muscles at the expense of your trapezius group.

Dumbbell Upright Rows

Emphasis: Dumbbells give you somewhat more freedom of movement when you perform Upright Rows to strongly stress your deltoids and trapezius muscles. Secondary emphasis is on your biceps, brachialis, and forearm flexors.

Starting Point: Grasp two moderately heavy dumbbells and stand erect with your arms hanging straight down, your palms facing the front of your body, and the dumbbells resting across your upper thighs.

Movement Performance: Being sure to keep

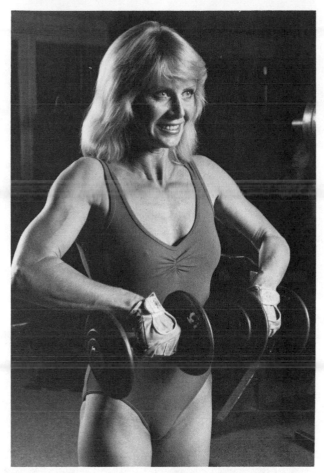

Dumbbell Upright Row at midpoint.

Cable Upright Row—start, left; finish, below right.

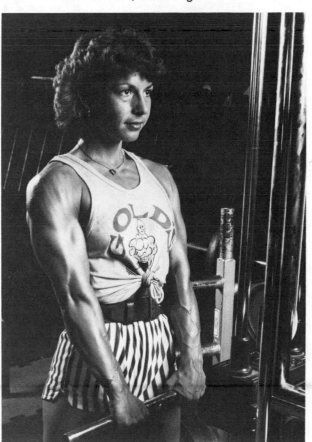

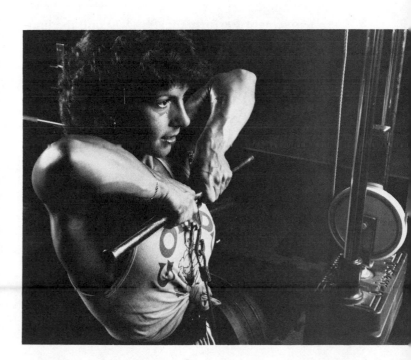

your elbows well above the level of your hands, slowly pull the dumbbells directly upward along the front of your body until they are above the level of your lower pectorals. Lower the weights slowly and deliberately back to the starting point, and continue the movement until you have done a full set.

Training Tips: You'll ultimately need to use straps to reinforce your grip when you are doing heavy Dumbbell Upright Rows. And with all variations of the movement, you might wish to wear a weightlifting belt around your waist to protect your lower back from injury.

Exercise Variations: Rather than shifting your grip width on a barbell, you can pull the dumbbells upward in Dumbbell Bent Rows along different paths—closer together, farther apart, and perhaps a little farther away from your body than under normal circumstances.

Cable Upright Rows

Emphasis: Cable Upright Rows stress primarily the traps and delts, while placing secondary stress on the biceps, brachialis, and forearm flexors. Cable Upright Rows place a somewhat more continuous form of resistance on the working muscles than either the barbell or dumbbell variations.

Starting Position: Attach a bar handle to the pulley leading through a floor pulley. Grasp the handle with a narrow over-grip (about six inches

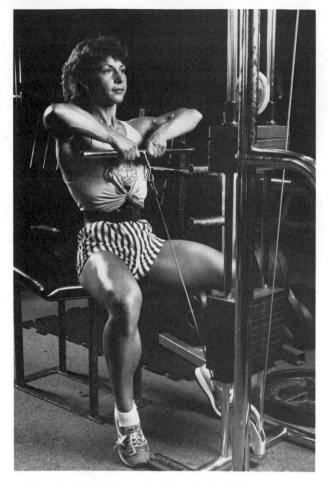

Seated version of Cable Upright Row.

stabilizing muscles as the abdominals. The Dead-lift is such a good test of basic body strength that it is one of the three lifts contested in powerlifting championships.

Starting Position: Load a relatively heavy weight on a barbell, and take the same starting position with it as for a Power Clean movement.

Movement Performance: Slowly lift the bar with straight arms from the floor up to a position with your torso erect and the bar resting across your upper thighs. Start the movement by beginning to straigthen your legs. Follow through by straightening your spine as your legs come straight, and pull your shoulders back at the end of the movement. Reverse the procedure by first bending your back and then your legs to return the weight to the floor. Repeat the movement for an appropriate number of repetitions.

Training Tips: To achieve a longer range of movement, you can stand on a thick block of wood while performing the exercise. You should wear a weightlifting belt and use straps to reinforce your grip with the heaviest weights.

Exercise Variations: The powerlifting version

Deadlift at midpoint.

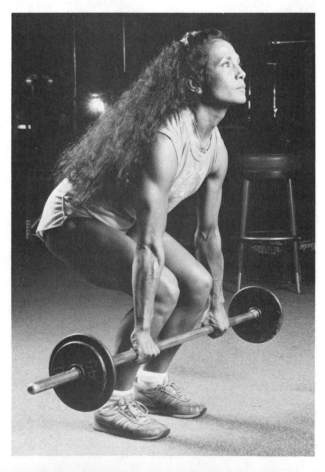

between your index fingers). Stand erect with your feet set about shoulder-width apart one or two feet back from the pulley and facing toward the pulley. Extend your arms straight down at your sides with your hands resting across your upper thighs.

Movement Performance: Slowly pull the handle directly upward along your body, emphasizing a high elbow position, until your hands touch the underside of your chin. Lower your hands slowly back to the starting position and repeat the movement.

Exercise Variations: You can vary the width of your grip on the bar handle. You can also attach two loop handles that attach via their own short individual cables to the main cable; with this handle, the movement is somewhat similar to Dumbbell Upright Rows.

Deadlifts

Emphasis: This is a very good, basic exercise for building power in your back, thigh, hip, and buttock muscles. Secondary stress is on the gripping muscles of your forearms and such

of this exercise is usually performed with a reversed grip, that is with one hand facing forward and the other to the rear. A reversed grip makes it easier to hold a heavy weight when you aren't using straps.

Stiff-Leg Deadlifts

Emphasis: This movement places very strong stress on both the lumbar muscles of your lower back and your hamstrings. Secondary emphasis is on your upper-back muscles and the gripping muscles of your forearms.

Starting Position: You must always perform your Stiff-Leg Deadlifts while standing on a thick block of wood or a flat exercise bench, or you won't be able to achieve a full range of motion in the exercise. Take a shoulder-width over-grip on the barbell and stand erect with it on the block or bench, your arms straight and the barbell resting across your upper thighs. Straighten your thighs and keep them straight throughout the movement.

Movement Performance: Slowly and deliberately bend forward at the waist and lower the barbell downward until it touches your toes or the bench/block you are standing on. Reverse the procedure to return to the starting point of the exercise. Repeat it for the required number of reps.

Training Tips: You can use straps to reinforce your grip, but you will probably find a weightlifting belt restrictive when you perform Stiff-Leg Deadlifts. It's absolutely essential that you do this movement slowly and deliberately, since your lower back is in a weak mechanical position when your legs are held straight. And if the exercise causes any pain in your lower spine, it should be entirely avoided.

Exercise Variations: Another way to increase the range of motion when performing Stiff-Leg Deadlifts is to use plates of a small diameter. You can also do Stiff-Leg Deadlifts while holding two heavy dumbbells in your hands, a variation that uniquely stresses your hamstrings and lower-back muscles.

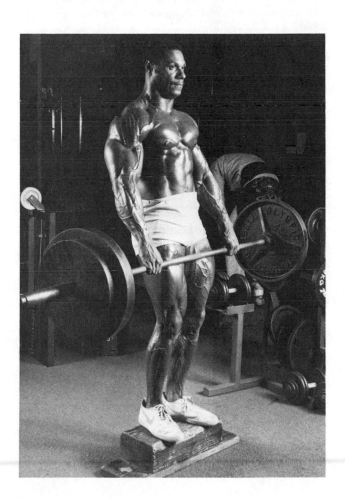

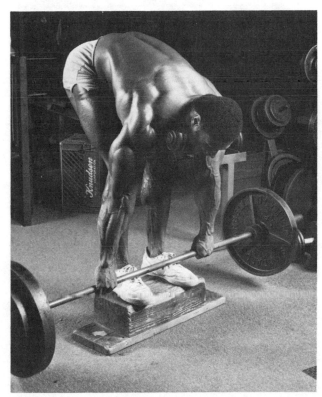

Stiff-Leg Deadlift—start, left; finish, above.

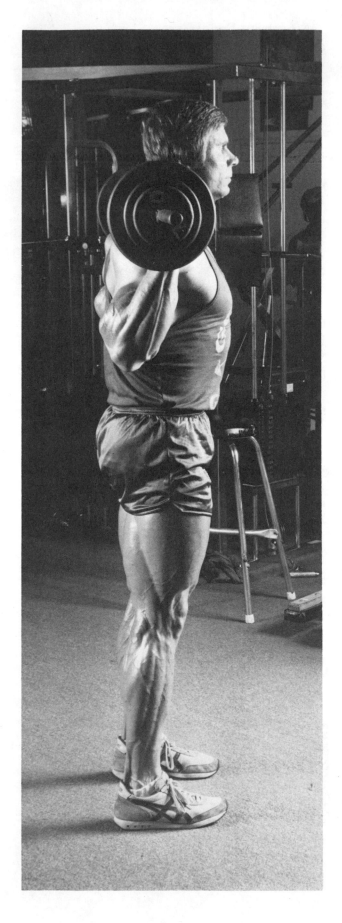

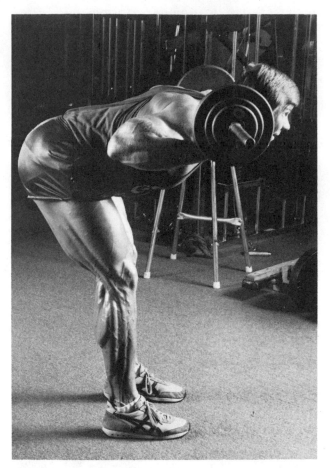

Good Mornings—start, left; finish, above.

Good Mornings

Emphasis: This oddly named exercise directly stresses the erector spinae and hamstring muscles. Secondary stress is on the upper-back muscles.

Starting Position: Lift a light barbell to a position across your shoulders behind your head. Balance the bar in this position during the movement by holding on to the bar out near the plates. Place your feet about shoulder-width apart and point your toes directly forward. Stand erect and hold your legs straight throughout the movement.

Movement Performance: Slowly bend forward at the waist, keeping your upper back as flat as possible as you do so. As soon as your torso has descended past a position parallel to the floor, reverse the movement, and return to the starting point. Repeat the exercise for the suggested number of repetitions.

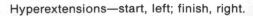

Hyperextensions—start, left; finish, right.

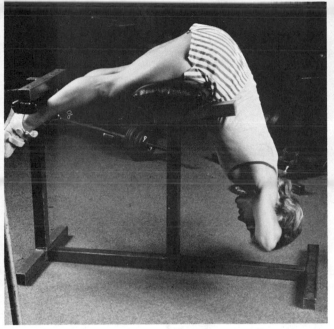

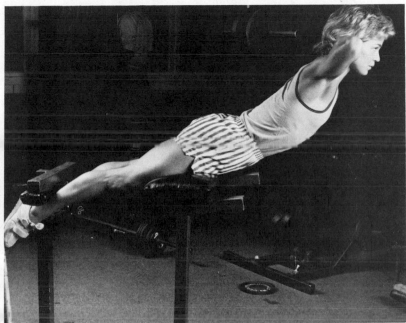

Training Tips: If you find that the bar cuts painfully into your neck vertebrae, you should pad the bar by wrapping a towel around it.

Exercise Variations: With your legs held slightly bent, you can use much heavier weights in this exercise. However, the heavier poundages can place a potentially harmful stress on your lower back.

Hyperextensions

Emphasis: This excellent movement effectively isolates stress on the spinal erector, buttock, and hamstring muscles.

Starting Position: Usually, this exercise is performed on a special bench constructed specifically for it. Stand facing the larger pad. Lean forward and grasp the handles in front of the pad to lever your body into a position with your hips across the large pad and the backs of your ankles resting beneath the smaller pads at the back of the apparatus. Be sure to hold your legs straight throughout the movement. Place your hands behind your head and neck as you do the exercise. Flex forward at the waist until your torso is in a position vertical to the floor.

Movement Performance: Arch upward and backward until your torso is above a position parallel to the floor. You should not arch upward excessively, however, because such a movement can compress your spinal vertebrae. Return to the starting position and repeat the movement.

Training Tips: You can add resistance to this exercise by holding a light barbell or loose barbell plate against the back of your head and neck. You can almost always do Hyperextensions for your erectors, even with a sore back, because the movement places a type of stress on the spine that fails to compress your vertebrae. In contrast, all Deadlift movements do compress the spinal vertebrae.

Exercise Variations: If you don't have a bench specifically constructed for use in Hyperextensions, you can still do the movement by resting your legs across a high table or exercise bench and having a training partner lie across them to restrain your legs in position as you perform the exercise.

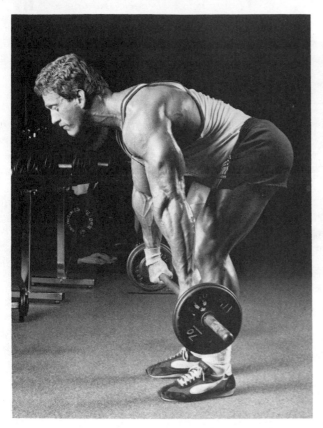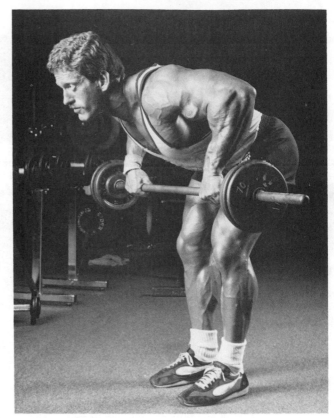

Barbell Bent Row—start, left; near finish, right.

Barbell Bent Rows

Emphasis: This is an excellent upper-back movement that places major stress on the latissimus dorsi, biceps, brachialis, and forearm flexor muscles. Secondary emphasis in the exercise is on the trapezius, posterior deltoid, and erector spinae muscles. As you perhaps know, all rowing-type lat movements primarily build thickness in the latissimus dorsi muscle group, while chinning- and pulldown-type lat exercises primarily build width in the latissimus dorsi muscles.

Starting Position: Stand about one-and-a-half feet back from a moderately heavy barbell lying on the floor. Bend over and take a shoulder-width over-grip on the barbell. Straighten your arms completely, keep your legs slightly bent to relieve strain from your lower back, and bring your torso into a position parallel to the floor. In this correct starting position, the barbell should be just clear of the floor.

Movement Performance: Moving just your arms, slowly pull the barbell directly upward to touch lightly against the lower part of your ribcage. As you pull the weight upward, your upper arms should travel out away from your torso at approximate 45-degree angles. Lower the weight slowly back to the starting point and repeat the movement.

Training Tips: With large diameter plates on the bar, you must stand on a thick block of wood or a flat exercise bench as you do the movement. This will allow you to completely straighten your arms and stretch your lats in the bottom position of the movement without the plates contacting the floor and terminating the movement. You should wear a weightlifting belt when you do Barbell Rows, and you can use straps to reinforce your grip as you do the movement.

Exercise Variations: You can use a wide variety of grip widths as you perform your Barbell Bent Rows. Your grip can be as narrow as one with your hands touching each other in the middle of the bar, to as wide as the length of the bar will permit. You can also do Barbell Rows with an under-grip on the bar, a grip which places your biceps in a more powerful pulling position than does the over-grip. If you have a sore lower back, you can comfortably do this movement with your forehead resting on a padded exercise bench supporting your torso parallel to the floor.

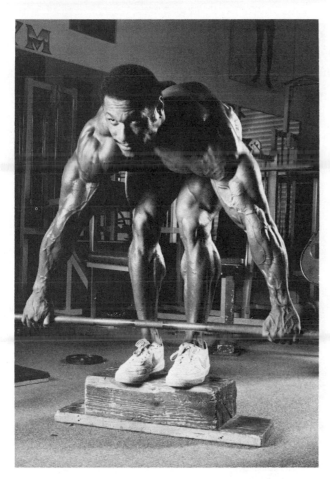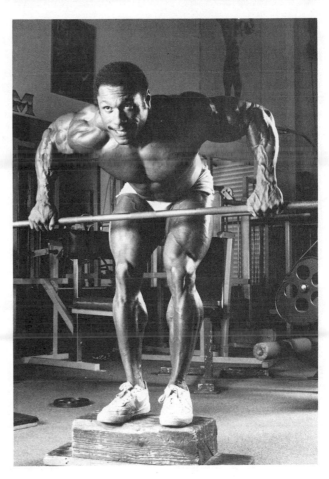

Barbell Bent Row (on block)—start, left; finish, right.

Barbell Bent Row (using head for support)—start, left; finish, right.

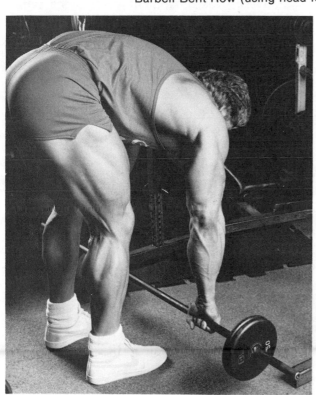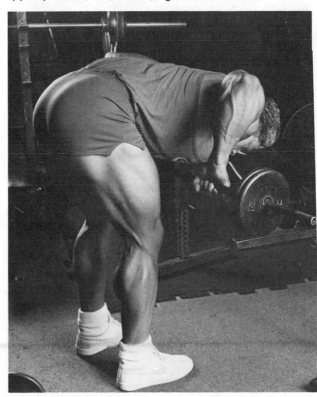

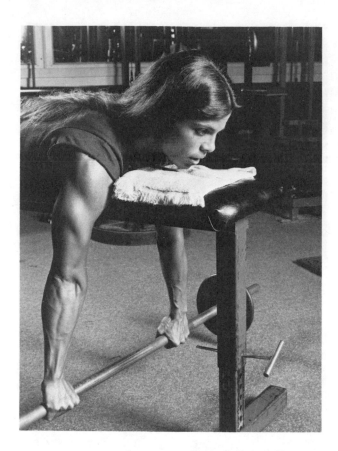

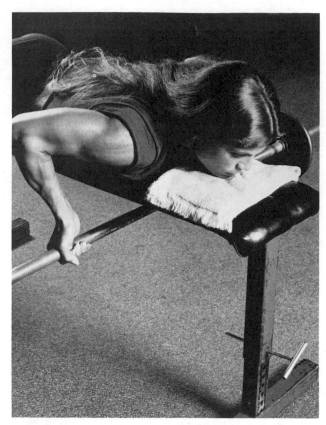

Barbell Bench Row—start, above; midpoint, below;
finish (with reversed grip), above right.

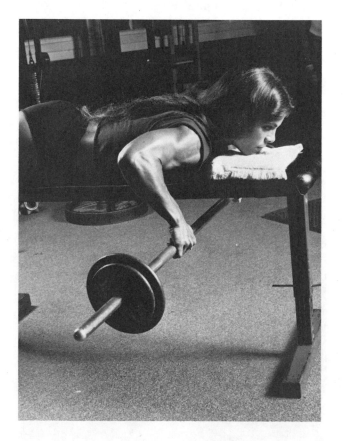

Barbell Bench Rows

Emphasis: This movement stresses the same back and arm muscles as Barbell Bent Rows, except that the erectors are isolated from the movement. Therefore, this is a great way to thicken your upper and middle back muscles when you have a sore lower back.

Starting Position: Adjust a flat exercise bench to a level that allows you to straighten your arms at the bottom point of the movement without the plates touching the floor. Lie facedown on the bench and have two training partners lift a barbell up to where you can take a shoulder-width overgrip on the bar. Fully straighten your arms.

Movement Performance: Being sure that your upper arms travel outward at approximate 45-degree angles from your torso, slowly pull the barbell directly upward until it touches the underside of the bench directly beneath your lower ribcage. Hold this peak-contracted, top position of the exercise for a moment, lower the barbell

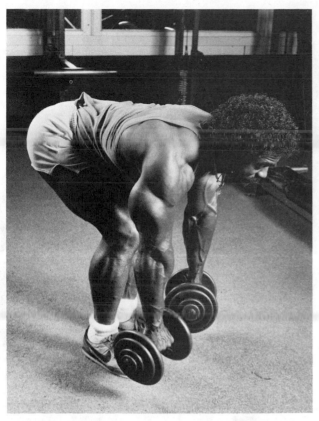 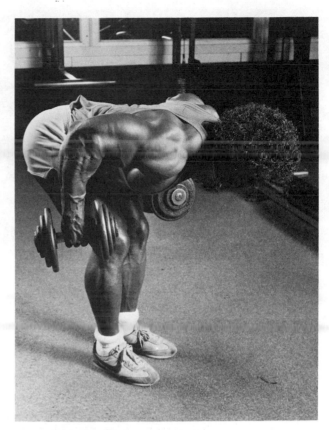

Dumbbell Bent Row—start, left; finish, right.

back to straight arms' length below your chest, and repeat the movement for the required number of repetitions.

Exercise Variations: You can shift major stress in this exercise to your trapezius muscles by placing a 4 × 4-inch block of wood under the legs of the head end of the bench. And by placing the block of wood beneath the legs at the other end of the bench, you can intensify the effect that the movement has on your lower lats. You can also vary the movement by performing it with two dumbbells rather than a barbell. You should also occasionally vary the width of your grip on the barbell that you use, or even change your hands to an under-grip position on the bar.

Dumbbell Bent Rows

Emphasis: Performing Bent Rows with two dumbbells in place of a barbell allows you more freedom of movement with your hands as you stress your lats, biceps, brachialis, and forearm flexor muscles. Secondary stress in this move-

ment is on the trapezius, posterior deltoid, and erector spinae muscles.

Starting Position: Place two moderately heavy dumbbells on the floor in front of you. Set your feet about shoulder-width apart with your toes angled slightly outward. Unlock your legs throughout your set and bend over to grasp the weights. Straighten your arms fully and bring your torso up to a position parallel to the floor. You should keep your back slightly arched during this and all rowing exercises.

Movement Performance: Keeping your elbows near the sides of your torso, slowly pull the dumbbells directly upward until they touch the sides of your chest. Lower the weights slowly back to the starting position and repeat the movement.

Exercise Variations: You can do this movement with the palms of your hands either both facing your legs, or facing toward each other. You can also pull the dumbbells upward close together, or outward away from each other, as you do the exercise.

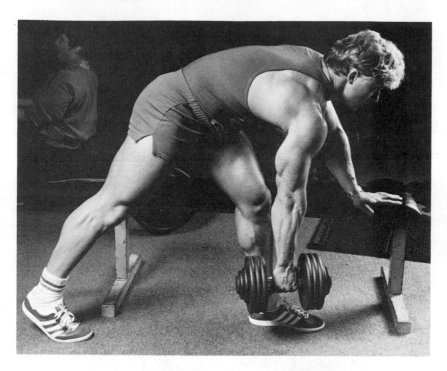

One-Arm Dumbbell Bent Row—start (both feet on floor), above; finish (knee on bench), right.

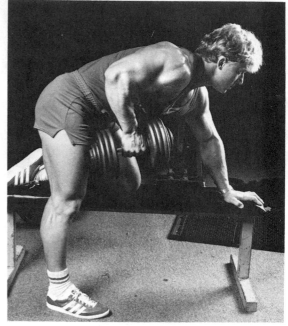

One-Arm Dumbbell Bent Rows

Emphasis: As in the previous movement, One-Arm Dumbbell Bent Rows strongly stress the latissimus dorsi, biceps, brachialis, and forearm flexor muscles. Lesser stress is on the trapezius and posterior deltoids.

Starting Position: Place a dumbbell on the floor at one side of a flat exercise bench. Kneel with your right knee and lower leg on the bench and place your right hand on the bench about two feet ahead of your knee. Reach down and grasp the dumbbell in your left hand. Completely straighten your left arm and slightly rotate your left shoulder downward toward the dumbbell in order to fully stretch your left lat muscle group.

Movement Performance: Keeping your elbow in at your side, slowly pull the dumbbell directly upward and roll your left shoulder slightly upward as the dumbbell touches the side of your ribcage. Lower the weight back to the starting point and repeat the movement. Be sure to do an equal number of sets and repetitions for each side of your body.

Training Tip: It's good to do one-arm and one-leg movements from time to time, because you can put more mental concentration into the movement performed with one limb than into the same exercise done with two arms or two legs. On the other side of the coin, however, some one-arm movements can put a twisting strain on the spine, so they should be used with discretion.

Exercise Variations: The version of this exercise performed with your knee on the bench has

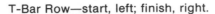
T-Bar Row—start, left; finish, right.

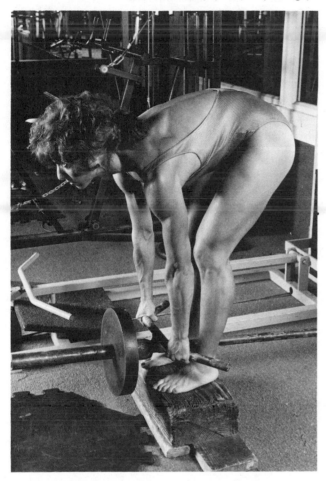

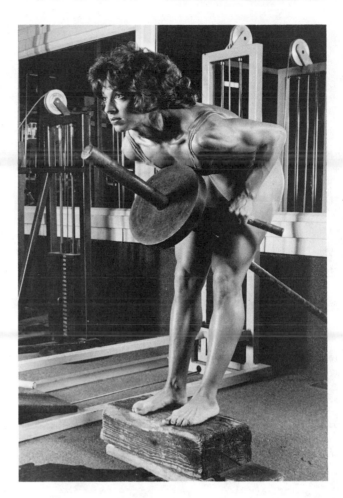

become popular in recent years. In the older variation of the movement, both feet are kept on the floor. When using a dumbbell in your left hand, your right hand should remain on the bench, your right leg should be placed forward and slightly bent, and your left leg must be placed to the rear and held relatively straight.

T-Bar Rows

Emphasis: T-Bar Rows place very strong stress on the latissimus dorsi, erector spinae, biceps, brachialis, and forearm flexor muscles. Less intense stress is on the posterior deltoids and the traps.

Starting Position: Load up the T-bar apparatus and place your feet on the platforms provided with it. Bend over and grasp the handles of the machine, unlock your legs a couple of degrees, straighten your arms, and raise your torso up to a position parallel to the floor.

Movement Performance: Without moving your torso upward and downward more than three or four inches each rep, slowly pull the handle of the machine upward until either the plates or the handle itself touches your chest. Lower your hands back to the starting position and repeat the movement.

Exercise Variations: The plate-loading T-bar apparatus has limitations in its range of motion due to the diameter of the plates. A better form of T-bar machine utilizes a plate stack attached to the end of the lever arm with a pulley, since this variation of T-bar apparatus does not use large-diameter barbell plates to provide resistance against your working muscles.

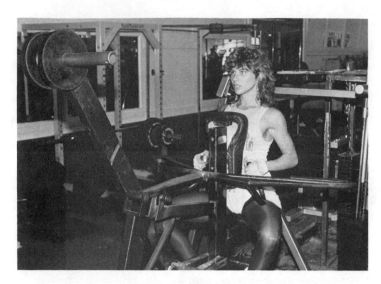

Corbin-Pacific Row at finish.

Corbin-Pacific Rows

Emphasis: This machine allows you to isolate stress on your latissimus dorsi, biceps, brachialis, and forearm flexor muscle groups, while placing secondary resistance on the posterior deltoids and trapezius muscles.

Starting Position: Sit in the machine facing the upright pad and place your chest firmly against this pad. Reach forward and grasp the handles of the machine. Lift up slightly to release the weight for use and allow the weight on the machine to pull your arms straight.

Movement Performance: Keeping your elbows down below shoulder level, slowly bend your arms and pull the handles of the machine as far toward your torso as comfortably possible. Return to the starting point and repeat the exercise. At the end of your set, you can pull the handles halfway toward you and lower them a bit to lock the weight in position prior to exiting the machine.

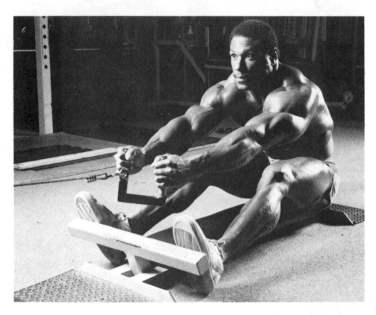

Seated Pulley Row—start, left; finish, below.

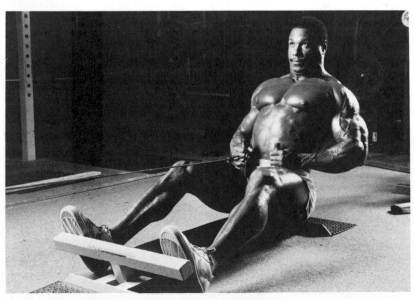

Seated Pulley Rows

Emphasis: This is an excellent movement for developing all of the back muscles: trapezius, latissimus dorsi, and erector spinae. Strong stress is also placed on the posterior deltoids, biceps, brachialis, and forearm flexor muscles.

Starting Position: Most commonly this exercise is performed with a handle that allows you to take a narrow grip with your palms facing inward toward each other. Grasp the handle in this manner, place your feet against the foot bars at the front end of the apparatus seat, straighten your arms, and sit down on the seat with your legs slightly bent throughout the movement. Lean forward toward the pulley and lower your head between your arms to completely stretch your lats at the beginning of the movement.

Movement Performance: Keeping your elbows in tight against your sides, simultaneously sit erect and pull in the handle to touch your upper abdominals. Be sure to arch your back in this position, and don't sit back past a position in which your torso is perpendicular to the floor.

Return to the starting point of the exercise and repeat the movement for the suggested number of repetitions.

Training Tip: You will probably find it unnecessary to wear a weightlifting belt when you perform Seated Pulley Rows.

Exercise Variations: You will most frequently do this exercise with a pulley set near the floor, but it can also be done with a high pulley set 3–5 feet above floor level. On either version of the movement, there are several different types of handles that you can use. Most commonly, you will probably use a type of handle that gives you a shoulder-width parallel grip (one in which your palms face inward toward each other as you do the exercise). A straight-bar handle can also be used with either an over-grip or an under-grip set at a variety of widths. You can also use the type of arrangement that attaches two loop handles to the main cable via smaller individual cables. And while you could perform this exercise with one hand at a time, it will place potentially harmful stress on your back and for that reason should be avoided.

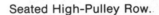

Seated High-Pulley Row.

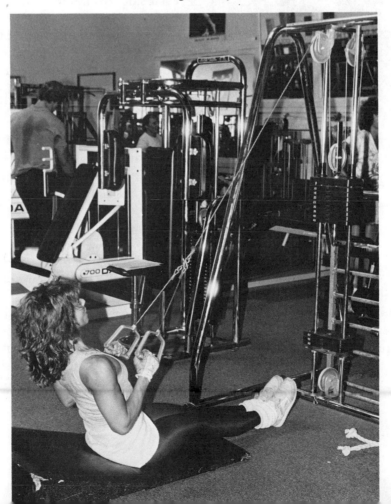

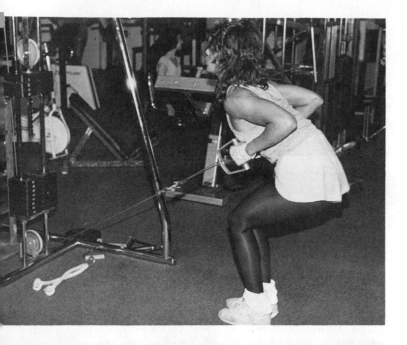

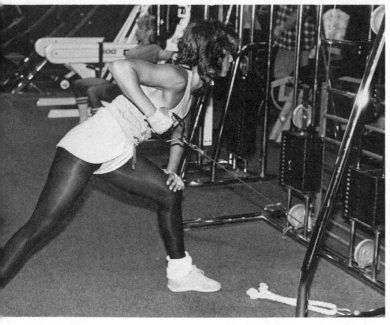

Standing Low-Pulley Row, top; Standing One-Arm, Low-Pulley Row, bottom.

Standing Pulley Rows

Emphasis: While the biceps, brachialis, posterior deltoid, and forearm flexor muscle groups are involved in this version of the movement, you can isolate more of the stress on your lats doing the exercise standing with either two hands or one hand.

Starting Position: Attach your choice of handle to the cable running through a floor pulley, place your feet about shoulder-width apart, and assume a crouching position with your arms held straight at the beginning of the movement.

Movement Performance: Slowly pull the handle in to touch the lower part of your ribcage. Be sure to keep your elbows in at the sides of your torso as you pull against the weight. Return to the starting point and repeat the exercise for the desired number of repetitions.

Exercise Variations: You can also perform this exercise with one arm at a time. Both the one-armed and two-armed versions of the exercise can be done with a high pulley.

Chins

Emphasis: The wide variety of Chins that you can perform all place very strong stress on the lats, biceps, and brachialis muscles. Keep in mind that rowing movements build primarily latissimus dorsi thickness, while Chins and Pulldowns develop lat width.

Starting Position: Jump up to grasp a chinning bar with an over-grip, your hands set two or three inches wider than your shoulders on each side. Straighten your arms completely and curl your legs up behind you.

Movement Performance: Concentrate on pulling your elbows downward and backward as you pull your body up to the bar and touch the upper part of your chest on the chinning bar. Arch your back at the top point of the movement. Slowly lower yourself back to the starting position, stretching your lats in the process. Repeat the movement.

Training Tips: If you are too weak to perform more than four or five reps of Chins, you should continue working with Lat Machine Pulldowns until you have developed enough strength to do Chins. And when Chins become easy to perform, you can add resistance to the movement by strapping a light dumbbell or loose barbell plate around your waist.

Exercise Variations: You can also perform this exercise with any width of under-grip on the bar; an under-grip actually puts your biceps in a more powerful pulling position than the more commonly used 'over-grip. You can also vary the

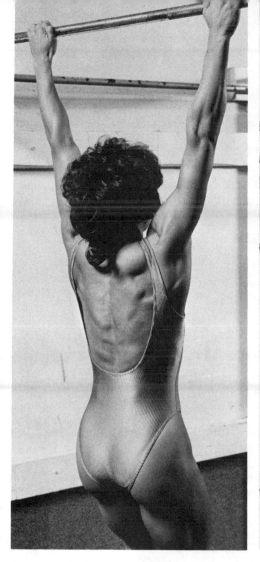
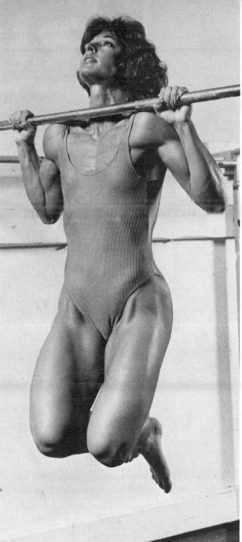
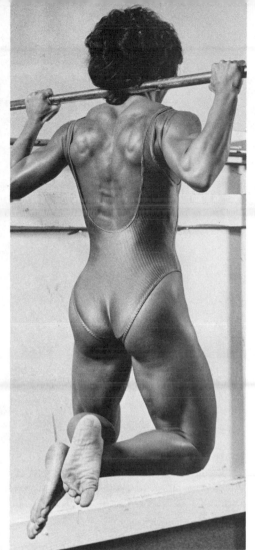

Chins—start, left; finish (in front of neck), center; finish (behind neck), right.

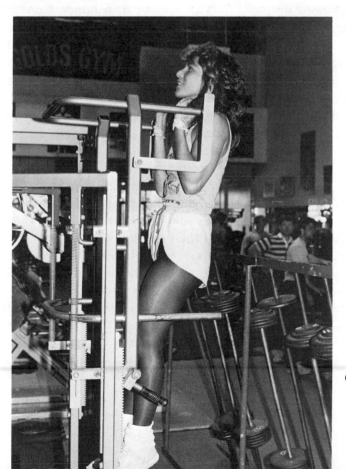

Chins on Nautilus Multi Machine.

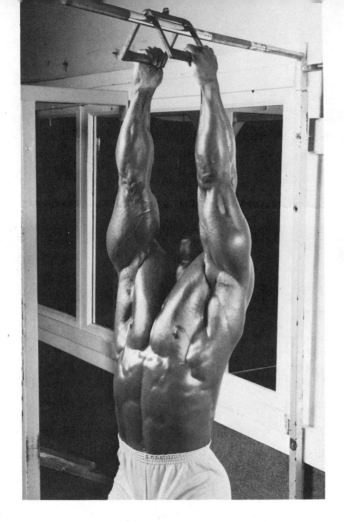

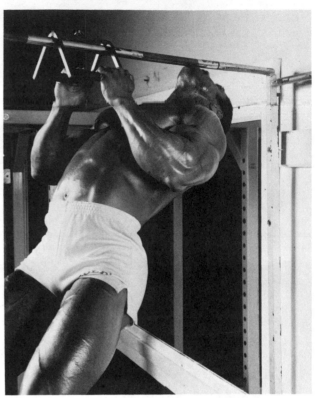

V-Bar Chins—start, left; finish, below.

width of your over-grip on the bar to as narrow as having your hands touching, to as wide as you can grasp the bar and still pull your body up to it. With any width over-grip wider than your shoulders, you can also do Chins behind the Neck by pulling your body up so you touch the bar on your trapezius muscles behind your neck. There is also a special attachment that fits over a chinning bar that allows you to use a narrow parallel grip as you do your Chins. The movement done with this V-bar attachment is called V-Bar Chins.

Lat Machine Pulldowns

Emphasis: Lat Pulldowns directly stress the lats, posterior delts, biceps, brachialis muscles, and forearm flexors.

Starting Position: Take an over-grip on the lat machine handle with your hands set two or three inches wider on each side than the width of your shoulders. Straighten your arms and sit on the seat provided with the machine, wedging your knees beneath the restraint bar to keep your body from moving as you do the exercise. Arch

your back and keep it slightly arched throughout the exercise.

Movement Performance: Concentrate on pulling your elbows downward and backward as you pull the bar down in front of your neck to touch the upper part of your chest. Slowly return to the starting position and repeat the movement.

Training Tips: Some lat machines don't have a seat and restraint bar. So, if your lat machine doesn't have a set, you should either sit or kneel on the floor directly beneath the pulley as you do the exercise. And with very heavy weights, you should have a training partner push down with his hands on either side of your shoulders to keep your body from coming off the floor as you pull the bar downward.

Exercise Variations: You can vary the width of your grip on the bar, or use an under-grip. You can pull the bar down in front of your neck, or alternate repetitions to both the front and back of your neck within a single set. You can also use both the narrow- and medium-width, parallel-grip handles to do this exercise. And, you can do a special type of Pulldown movement on the Nautilus torso-arm machine.

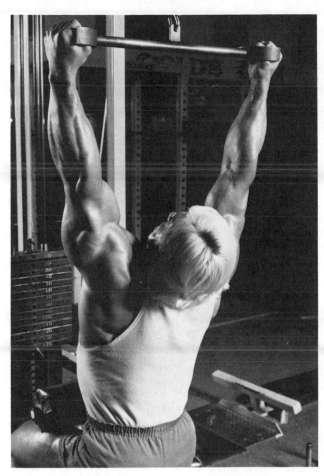
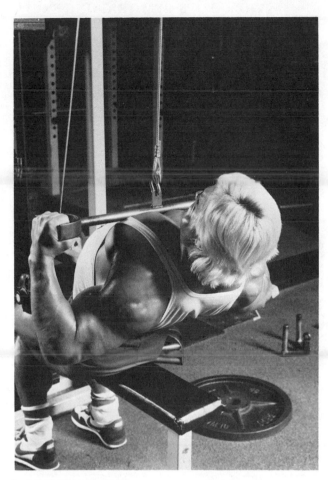

Lat Machine Pulldown—start, left; finish, right.

Lat Machine Pulldown—wide grip, left; narrow grip, right.

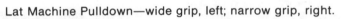
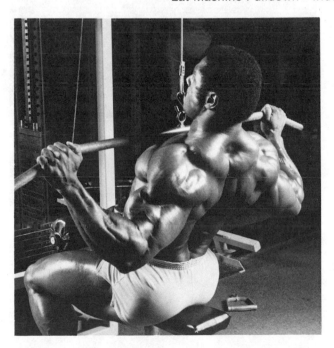
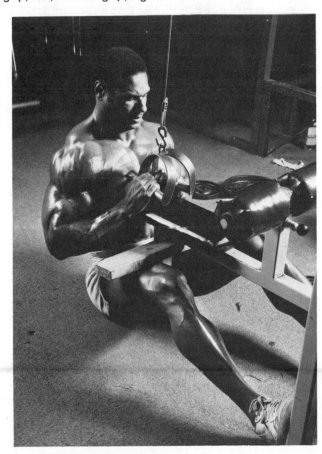

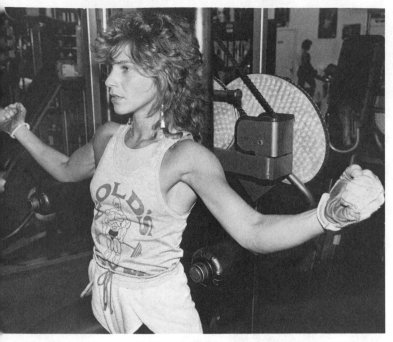

Nautilus behind the Neck Movement.

Nautilus behind the Neck Movement

Emphasis: This excellent machine is becoming obsolete, but if you have access to one you can effectively isolate your lats from the rest of your body by making use of it.

Starting Position: Adjust the height of the machine's seat to a position that puts your shoulder joints at the level of the pivot points on the cams when you sit down. Sit in the seat and secure the seat belt over your lap to keep you from coming out of the seat as you do the exercise. With your palms facing forward, force your elbows against the inner sides of the machine's roller pads.

Movement Performance: Use lat strength to force the pads downward in semicircular arcs to as low a position as possible. Return to the starting point and repeat the exercise.

Nautilus Rows

Emphasis: This machine allows you to isolate stress in your upper-back muscles and posterior deltoids.

Starting Position: Sit in the machine facing the two vertical roller pads. With your palms

toward the floor, slip your arms between the pads and position your elbows against those pads.

Movement Performance: Slowly move your elbows directly to the rear, holding the finish position for a moment, return to the starting point, and repeat the movement for the desired number of repetitions.

Exercise Variations: You can do a very similar movement, Pec Deck Rows, sitting backward in a pec deck machine and positioning your elbows against the movement pads of the apparatus.

Nautilus Pullovers

Emphasis: Nautilus Pullovers isolate stress on the lats and other middle- and upper-back muscles. Secondary stress is on the abdominal muscles and pectorals.

Starting Position: Sit in the machine on enough pads to place your shoulder joints at the same level as the pivot point of the machine. Push down on the foot pedal with your feet to bring the movement pads of the machine in a

Nautilus Row.

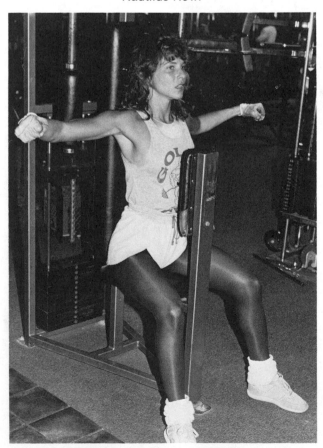

position where you can place your elbows against the pads and grasp the cross bar lightly. Release the foot pedal and allow the weight on the machine to pull your elbows upward and backward as far as is comfortably possible.

Movement Performance: Push on the pads with your elbows to move them forward and downward as far as possible. Hold this finish position for a moment to achieve a good peak contraction effect in your muscles. Return to the starting point and repeat the movement for the suggested number of repetitions.

Bent-Arm Pullovers

Emphasis: This free-weight movement essentially stresses the same muscles (upper back and pectorals) as the Nautilus Pullovers, although in a slightly less intense manner.

Starting Position: Take a narrow over-grip on a barbell (there should be about six inches of space between your index fingers) and lie on your back on a flat exercise bench with your head off the end of the bench. You should have your arms fully bent and the weight resting on your chest.

Movement Performance: Keeping your arms

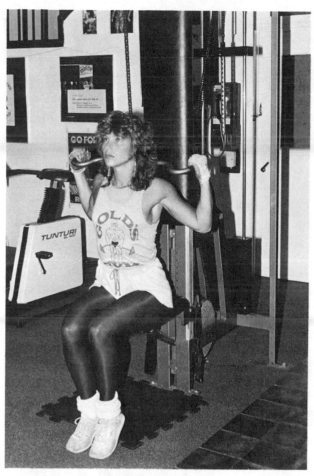
Nautilus Pulldown.

Bent-Arm Pullovers—start/finish, left; midpoint, right.

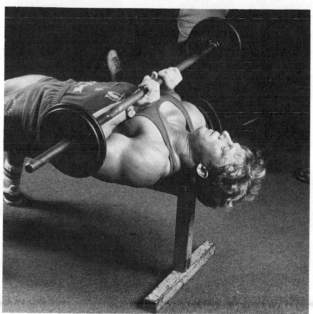
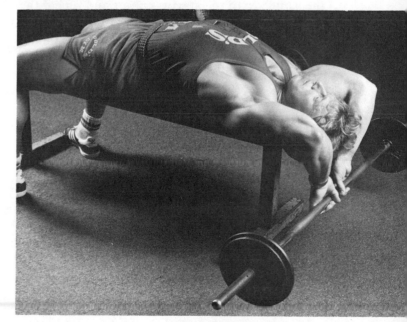

bent and your elbows as close together as possible, slowly lower the barbell past your face and down behind your head to as low a position as comfortably possible. Pull the weight back along the same arc to the starting point and repeat the movement for the required number of repetitions.

Training Tips: It's absolutely essential that you keep your elbows pulled toward the centerline of your body as you perform Bent-Arm Pullovers. Allowing your elbows to travel out away from each other can put your shoulders in a position in which they are vulnerable to injury.

Stiff-Arm Lat Pulldowns

Emphasis: You can do a movement similar to Bent-Arm Pullovers on a lat machine to stress your lats, serratus muscles, and pectorals.

Starting Position: Place your feet slightly wider than shoulder-width about two feet back from a lat machine pulley. Lean forward and take a narrow over-grip on the lat machine bar, your arms slightly bent. With your torso inclined forward at approximately a 45-degree angle with the floor, allow the weight on the machine to pull your hands upward and bring your arms in line with your torso.

Movement Performance: Slowly move your hands in semicircular arcs from the starting point downward until the lat bar rests across your upper thighs. Return the weight back along the same arc to the starting point and repeat the exercise.

Training Tip: You can also use a rope handle or two loops of nylon webbing to secure your grip to the lat pulley cable.

Pulley Crunches

Emphasis: This movement is primarily intended to stress the *rectus abdominis* muscles, but it also places strong stress on the serratus and lower latissimus dorsi muscles.

Starting Position: Attach a rope or webbing handle to the end of a lat machine cable and kneel down on the floor about two feet back from the pulley. Extend your arms above your head and bend your arms slightly throughout the movement.

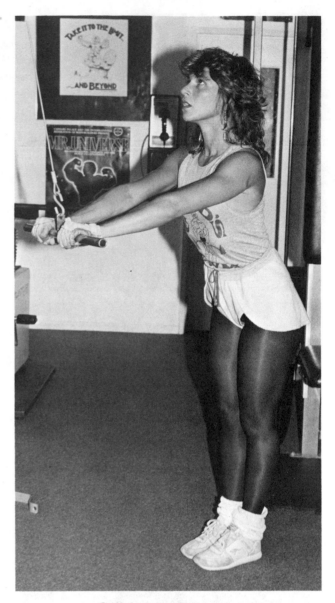

Stiff-Arm Lat Pulldown.

Movement Performance: Simultaneously flex your torso forward at the waist to bring your forehead to the floor, do a sort of pullover motion with your hands to bring them to the floor directly in front of your head, and briskly exhale. When you do this correctly, you will feel a strong contraction in your abdominal, serratus, and latissimus dorsi muscles.

Exercise Variations: To place more intense stress on your lats, you can do this movement with one arm at a time, but be sure to do an equal number of sets and repetitions for each side of your body.

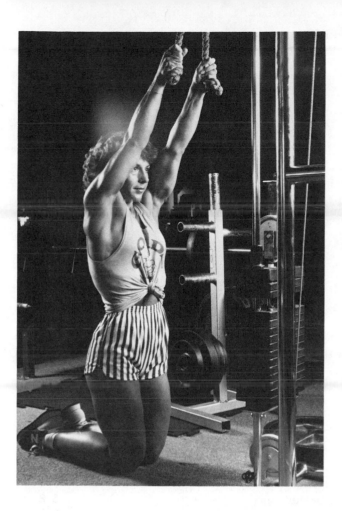

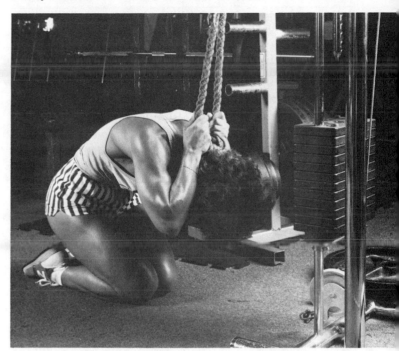

Pulley Crunches—start, left; finish, below.

Suggested Back Routines

If you have less than a few weeks of training behind you, the following back routine can profitably be performed three nonconsecutive days per week:

Exercise	Sets	Reps
Barbell Bent Rows	3	8–12
Barbell Upright Rows	2	8–12

After 4–6 weeks of steady and progressive training on the foregoing program, you can use this more intense back routine three days per week:

Exercise	Sets	Reps
Hyperextensions	2–3	10–15
Barbell Shrugs	3	10–15
Seated Pulley Rows	3	12–8*
Front Lat Machine Pulldowns	2	8–12

* All exercises marked with an asterisk should have the weights and reps pyramidded. With each succeeding set, the weight on the bar should be increased and the number of reps performed decreased.

After about three months of steady training, you should switch to a four-day split routine in which you train each major muscle group (including the back) twice per week. This is typically how a lower-level competitive bodybuilder will work out in the off-season. Following is a sample back-training program for off-season, competition-level training:

Exercise	Sets	Reps
Good Mornings	4	10–15
Upright Rows	3	8–12
Rotating Dumbbell Shrugs	2	10–15
Barbell Bent Rows	4	12–6*
Lat Pulldowns behind the Neck	4	12–6*
Seated Pulley Rowing	4	12–6*
Pulley Crunches	2–3	10–15

Every advanced bodybuilder trains differently from all others prior to a competition, as you will see in the following section listing the back routines of a wide variety of men and women who either train or have trained at Gold's Gym.

Back Routines of the Gold's Champs

In this section, you will find a variety of back training programs used by many of the Gold's Gym superstars who have won the sport's highest titles. Keep in mind as you examine these training programs that these men and women have been training for many years and have developed enormous recuperative abilities. It is highly unlikely that you would make good gains using their full routines without similar experience. Instead, you should use these training programs as examples of how to work your own back. In all likelihood, you can do the same exercises as your favorite champion, but scale down the number of sets that he or she does of each movement to meet your own abilities.

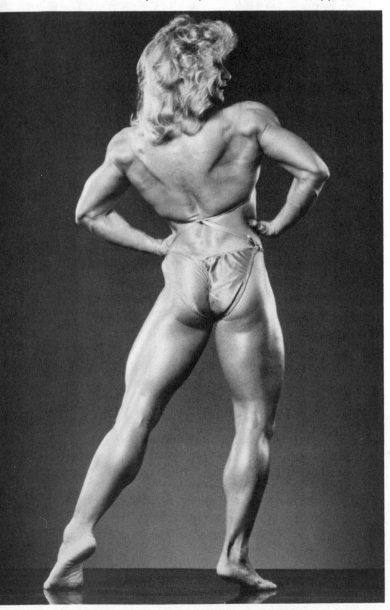

Kay Baxter (Gold's Classic Champ).

GREG DeFERRO
(MR. INTERNATIONAL)

Exercise	Sets	Reps
Wide-Grip Front Lat Pulldowns	3	8–12
supersetted with		
Bench Rows	3	8–12
Medium-Grip Front Lat Pulldowns	3	10
supersetted with		
T-Bar Rows	3	10
Low Pulley Rows	3	10
High Pulley Rows	3	10
Hyperextensions	4	10–12

COREY EVERSON
(NORTH AMERICAN CHAMPION)

Exercise	Sets	Reps
Lat Pulldowns behind the Neck	5	10–15
Close-Grip Pulldowns	5	10–15
Hyperextensions	5	15–20

BRONSTON AUSTIN, JR.
(MR. WESTERN AMERICA)

Exercise	Sets	Reps
Seated Pulley Rows	5–8	5–8
T-Bar Rows	5–8	5–8
Barbell Bent Rows	5–8	5–8
One-Arm Dumbbell Bent Rows	5–8	5–8
Nautilus Pullovers	5–8	5–8
Front Lat Pulldowns	5–8	8–10

LAURA COMBES
(AMERICAN CHAMPION)

Exercise	Sets	Reps
Barbell Shrugs	4–5	10–15
Stiff-Leg Deadlifts	4–5	10–15
Barbell Bent Rows	5	8–10
Front Chins	5	8–10
Seated Pulley Rows	3–4	8–10
Lat Pulldowns behind the Neck	3–4	8–10

SAMIR BANNOUT
(MR. OLYMPIA)

Exercise	Sets	Reps
Wide-Grip Front Chins	4–5	10–12
Lat Pulldowns behind the Neck	4–5	10–12
Seated Pulley Rows	4–5	8–10
One-Arm Dumbbell Bent Rows	4–5	8–10
Nautilus Pullovers	4–5	10–15

CANDY CSENCSITS
(MS. EASTERN AMERICA)

Exercise	Sets	Reps
Dumbbell Bent Rows	3	8–10
Lat Pulldowns behind the Neck	3	8–10
Seated Pulley Rows	3	8–10
Upright Rows	3	8–10
Hyperextensions	3	12–15

ANDREAS CAHLING
(MR. INTERNATIONAL)

Exercise	Sets	Reps
Front Chins	2–3	10–15
Reverse-Grip Lat Pulldowns	2	8–12
Medium-Grip Front Pulldowns	2	8–12
Wide-Grip Front Pulldowns	2	8–12
Wide-Grip Pulldowns behind the Neck	2	8–12
One-Arm Dumbbell Bent Rows	2	8–12
Hyperextensions	2–3	8–12

CHRIS DICKERSON
(MR. OLYMPIA)

Exercise	Sets	Reps
Front Chins	4–5	10–15
One-Arm Dumbbell Bent Rows	4–6	8–10
Lat Pulldowns behind the Neck	4	8–10
One-Arm Pulley Rows	4	8–10
Seated Pulley Rows	4	8–10

VALERIE MAYERS
(MS. EASTERN SEABOARD)

Exercise	Sets	Reps
Wide-Grip Chins	4–5	Max
One-Arm Dumbbell Bent Rows	4–5	10–6*
Lat Pulldowns behind the Neck	4–5	8–10
Narrow-Grip High Pulley Rows	4–5	8–10
Bent-Arm Pullovers	3–4	8–10

CASEY VIATOR
(PRO GRAND PRIX CHAMP)

Exercise	Sets	Reps
Deadlifts	4–6	8–5*
Nautilus Pullovers	4–6	10–15
Lat Pulldowns behind the Neck	4–6	10–15
One-Arm Dumbbell Bent Rows	4–6	10–12
Chins behind the Neck	6–8	10–15
Front Chins	6–8	10–15
Barbell Shrugs	6–8	15–20

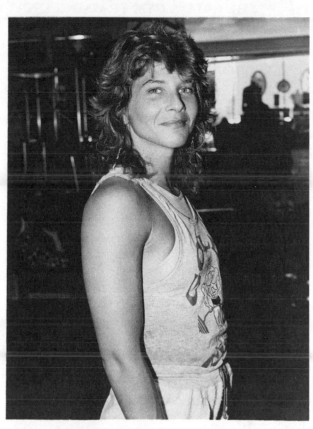

Nautilus exercise model, Cindy Lee.

CLAUDIA WILBOURN
(MS. CALIFORNIA)

Exercise	Sets	Reps
Lat Pulldowns	3	6–10
Seated Pulley Rows	3	6–10
One-Arm Dumbbell Bent Rows	3	6–10
Barbell Shrugs	3	8
One-Arm Low Pulley Rows	2	8

TONY PEARSON
(MR. UNIVERSE)

Exercise	Sets	Reps
Front Chins/Chins behind the Neck	8	10–12
T-Bar Rows	5	8–10
Barbell Bent Rows	5	8–10
Hyperextensions	3–5	10–15

SUE ANN McKEAN
(SUPERBOWL BODYBUILDING CHAMP)

Exercise	Sets	Reps
Pulley Upright Rows	5	10–12
Dumbbell Stiff-Leg Deadlifts	5–8	10–15
Front Chins	5–8	10–12
Dumbbell Bent Rows	4–5	8–10
Lat Pulldowns behind the Neck	4–5	8–10
Stiff-Arm Pulldowns	2–3	10–15

SCOTT WILSON
(PRO MR. AMERICA)

Exercise	Sets	Reps
Deadlifts	5	5
Barbell Bent Rows	5	6–8
T-Bar Rows	5	6–8
Front Lat Pulldowns	5	8
One-Arm Dumbbell Bent Rows	5	8
Barbell Shrugs	5	8
Upright Rows	5	8

ARNOLD SCHWARZENEGGER
(MR. OLYMPIA)

Exercise	Sets	Reps
Wide-Grip Front Chins	4–5	8–10
Lat Pulldowns behind the Neck	4–5	8–10
Barbell Bent Rows	4–5	8–10
T-Bar Rows	4–5	8–10
Seated Pulley Rows	4–5	8–10

STACEY BENTLEY
(ZANE PRO INVITATIONAL CHAMPION)

Exercise	Sets	Reps
Deadlifts	5	12–12
Dumbbell Bent Rows	5	12–15
Hyperextensions	5	12–15
Front Lat Pulldowns	3	6–8
Seated Pulley Rows	3–5	8–12

DR. FRANCO COLUMBU
(MR. OLYMPIA)

Exercise	Sets	Reps
Wide-Grip Front Chins	6	10–15
T-Bar Rows	4	10
Seated Pulley Rows	4	10
One-Arm Dumbbell Bent Rows supersetted with	3	10
Close-Grip Chins	3	10

BERTIL FOX
(MR. UNIVERSE)

Exercise	Sets	Reps
Lat Pulldowns behind the Neck	5	8–10
Front Lat Pulldowns	5	8–10
One-Arm Dumbbell Bent Rows	6	8–10
Chins (various types) supersetted with	6	8–10
Cross-Bench Dumbbell Pullovers	6	8–10
Seated Pulley Rows	6	8–10

TIM BELKNAP
(MR. AMERICA)

Exercise	Sets	Reps
Wide-Grip Front Chins	2–3	10–15
Wide-Grip Front Lat Pulldowns	3	12–15
Wide-Grip Seated Pulley Rows	3	12–15
Narrow-Grip Seated Pulley Rows	3	12–15
Nautilus Pullovers	3	10–12
Stiff-Leg Deadlifts	3	10–12
Hyperextensions	3	20–30

* All exercises marked with an asterisk should have the weights and reps pyramidded. With each succeeding set, the weight on the bar should be increased and the number of reps performed decreased.

Looking Ahead

In Chapter 6, we'll discuss how to train your thighs, including descriptions and photographs of almost 30 exercises, plus more routines of the top men and women who train at the Hall of Champions, Gold's Gym!

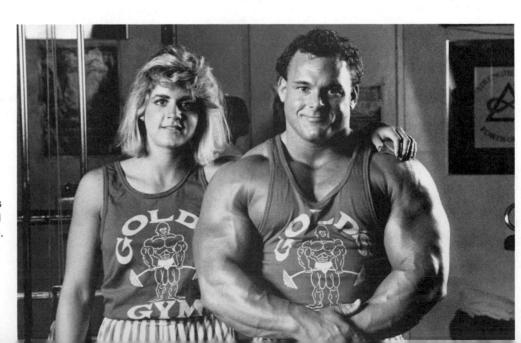

Exercise models Vickie Schiff and Tim Belknap.

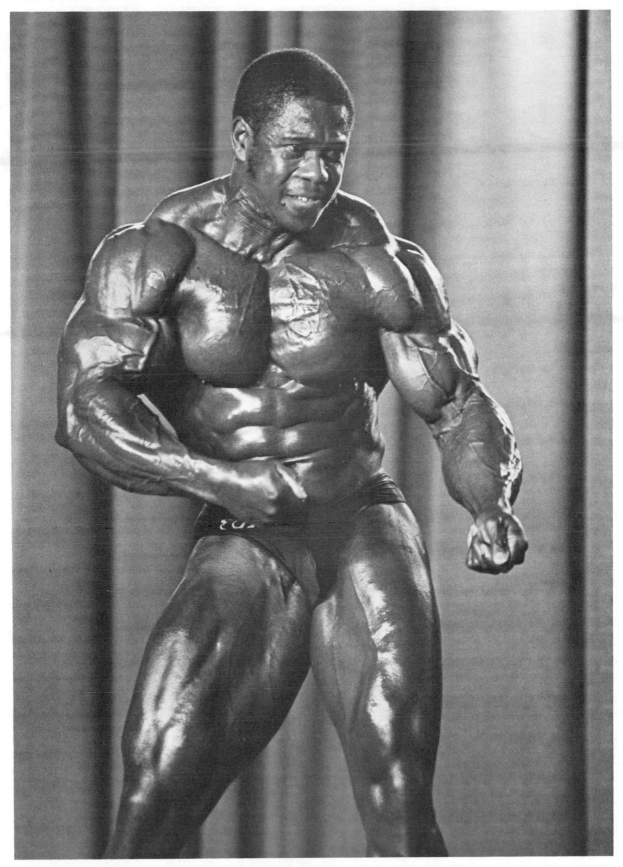

Bertil Fox.

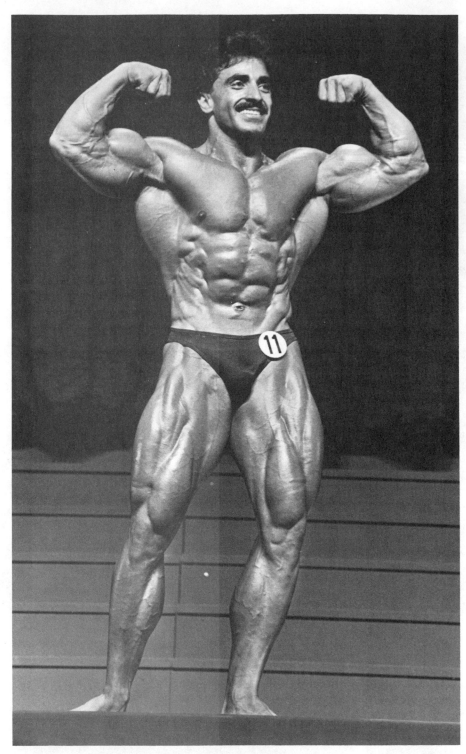

Samir Bannout.

6
THIGH AND HIP TRAINING

The thigh and hip muscles are among the largest and strongest in the human body. Because your leg muscles are so large, you must expend a great deal of energy when training them. There is such a heavy build-up of fatigue toxins when you work your legs to the limit that it is quite painful to bomb your thighs and hips. And this pain deters many bodybuilders from developing their thigh and hip muscle groups to the limit.

Among male bodybuilders, Tom Platz is acknowledged as having the best thigh development of all time. Other men with incredible leg and hip development are Tim Belknap, Sergio Oliva, Mike Mentzer, Jeff King, and Lee Haney. And three female bodybuilders with awesome leg and hip development are Kay Baxter, Sue Ann McKean, and Rachel McLish.

Within certain genetic limitations, any man or woman with full use of his or her legs can develop incredible leg mass, shape, and muscularity. It merely requires a willingness to bear the moderate pain of consistently hard and heavy workouts featuring plenty of Squats, Leg Presses, and other thigh and hip exercises. Those bodybuilders with underdeveloped legs are invariably men and women who are unwilling to pay the price of achieving optimum thigh and hip muscularity.

Anatomy and Kinesiology

The largest muscle group of the thigh is the *quadriceps,* which consist of four individual muscles. The quads contract to straighten the leg from a bent position, plus, to an extent, to pull the knees toward each other.

On the back of the thigh is the *biceps femoris* muscle group, which is frequently referred to as the *hamstrings* or *leg biceps.* The leg biceps muscles contract to bend the leg from a straight position.

There are also *adductor muscles* on the inner side of each thigh that contract to pull your thighs toward each other. And there are *abductor muscles* on the outsides of your thigh and hips that serve to move your thighs apart from each other.

Finally, there is the *buttocks* muscle group, primarily consisting of the *gluteus maximus,* which contract to move a straight leg to the rear. The buttocks also contract to move your body to an erect position when you are flexed forward at the waist.

Thigh and Hip Exercises

You will find nearly 30 major thigh and hip

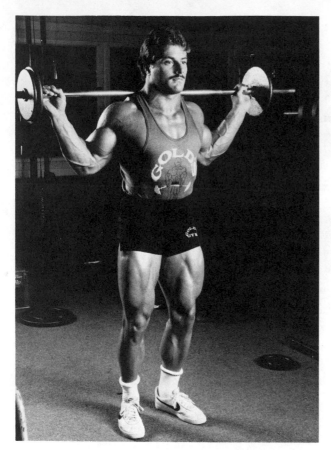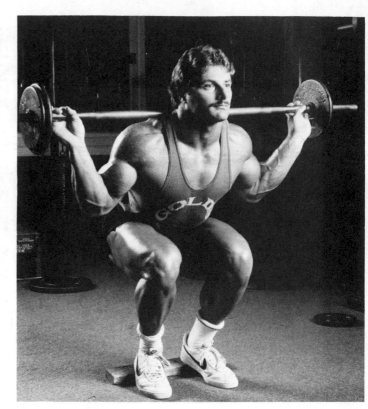

Squat—start, left; finish, right.

movements in this section, each fully described and depicted. Add in the numerous variations of each basic exercise, and you will have more than 50 leg and hip movements in your basic pool of bodybuilding exercises.

Squats

Emphasis: Squats are considered to be the best single lower body exercise, as well as a valuable movement for stimulating a full-body, anabolic metabolism. Squats strongly stress the quadriceps, buttocks, and lower-back muscles. Significant secondary stress is placed on the hamstrings, upper back, and abdominal muscles.

Starting Position: Place a barbell on a squat rack and load it with enough plates to allow you to perform at least 8–10 repetitions of Squats. Bend your legs and position the bar across your trapezius muscles and shoulders as illustrated. Grasp the bar with your hands out near the plates on each side to balance it across your upper back. If you find that the bar presses painfully against your neck vertebrae, you can pad the barbell bar by wrapping a thick towel around it. Straighten your legs to lift the bar from the rack and step backward one or two paces. Set your feet with your heels about shoulder-width apart, your toes angled slightly outward. Tense your back muscles throughout the movement to keep your torso upright during the exercise. As another way of keeping your torso upright during the movement, you should also pick a point on the wall in front of you at eye level and focus your eyes on that point throughout each repetition.

Movement Performance: Keeping your torso erect, slowly bend your legs and lower yourself into a full squatting position. As you bend your legs, your knees should travel slightly outward directly over your toes. Without bouncing in the bottom position of the movement, slowly straighten your legs and return to the starting position.

Training Tips: If you have inflexible ankles, you will find it difficult to squat flat-footed. In this case, you should elevate your heels during the movement by resting them on a 2 × 4-inch

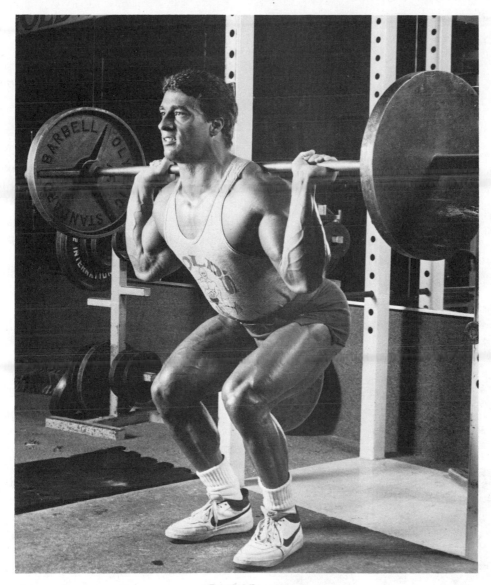

Partial Squat.

board or two thick barbell plates. To maximize stability throughout your midsection as you squat, you should wear a weightlifting belt tightly cinched around your waist. And if you have ever injured one or both of your knees, you should use elastic gauze bandages wrapped around them as you do your Squats.

Exercise Variations: For varying types of stress on your thigh muscles, you can squat with your feet either closer to each other, or with them spread wider than shoulder-width. You can also do your Squats with your toes pointed directly forward, or with them angled slightly inward.

Partial Squats

Comment: Partial Squats affect the same mus-cle groups as full Squats, but they can be performed with much heavier weights. Partial Squats are done the same as full Squats, except that you go down either a quarter of the way to a full squatting position (Quarter Squat), half of the way down (Half Squat), three quarters of the way (Three-Quarters Squat), or only until your thigh bones reach a position parallel to the floor (Parallel Squat).

Bench Squats

Comment: Bench Squats are a form of Partial Squat in which you straddle a low, flat exercise bench and squat down until your buttocks lightly touch the bench, then recover to the starting position. Alternatively, you squat down to a low stool set directly behind your heels. In

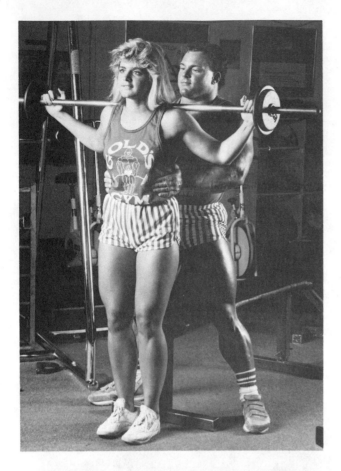

either case, it is essential that you refrain from bouncing off the bench, since bouncing can cause a lower-back injury.

Jump Squats

Emphasis: Jump Squats are an excellent way to build explosive power into your thigh and calf muscles.

Starting Position: Place a light barbell across your shoulders and balance it in place as you would for a full Squat movement.

Movement Performance: Squat slowly down, then come upward as explosively as possible, attempting to actually leap into the air. As soon as you land back on the floor, squat downward again and repeat the movement.

Dumbbell Squats

Emphasis: When you perform Squats holding two dumbbells, you strongly stress your quadriceps and buttocks, as well as the gripping muscles of your forearms. Secondary stress is placed on your hamstrings, lower back, and abdominal muscles.

Starting Position: Grasp a pair of moderately heavy dumbbells in your hands and stand erect with your arms hanging directly down at your sides. Place your feet about shoulder-width apart and angle your toes slightly outward. Be sure to keep your arms straight throughout the movement, and maintain an upright position of your torso.

Movement Performance: Slowly bend your legs and sink into a full squatting position. Without bouncing in the bottom position of the movement, immediately return to the starting position.

Comment: It is very difficult to hold dumbbells heavy enough to tax the thigh muscles of a very strong bodybuilder, so most superstars avoid this exercise in favor of Squats performed with a barbell. Alternatively, you can use straps to reinforce your grip on the dumbbells.

Exercise Variations: You can do Jumping Squats while holding two dumbbells.

Training Tip: If you discover that the dumbbells come in contact with the floor before you reach a full squatting position, you should do Dumbbell Squats while standing on a thick block of wood.

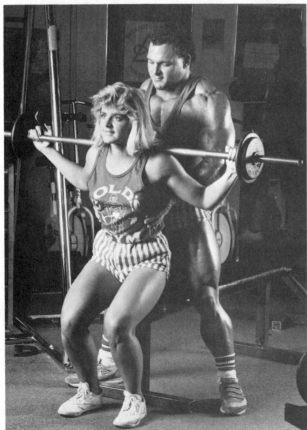

Bench Squat—start, top; finish, bottom. Note position of spotter steadying lifter with hand pressure on sides of waist.

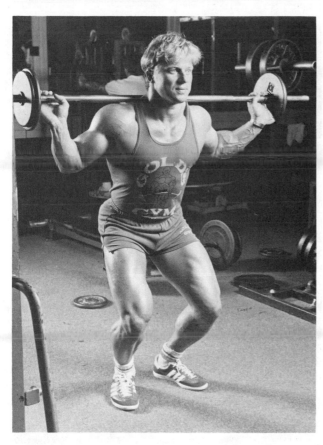 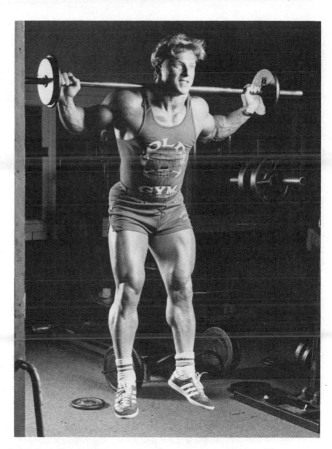

Jump Squat—start, left; finish, right.

Dumbbell Squat—start, left; finish, right.

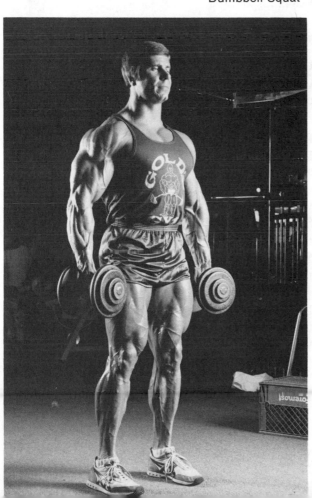 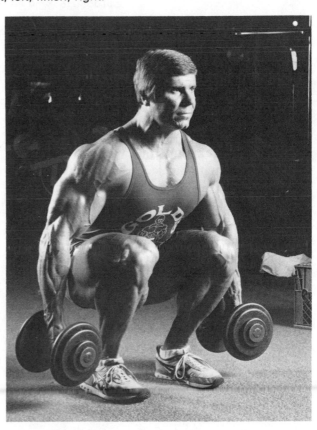

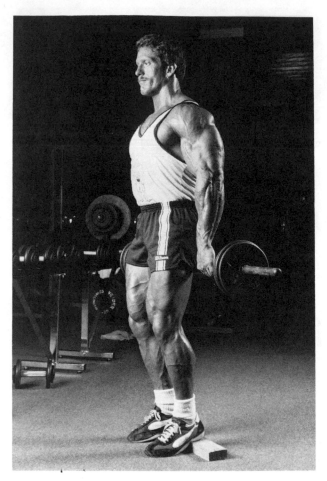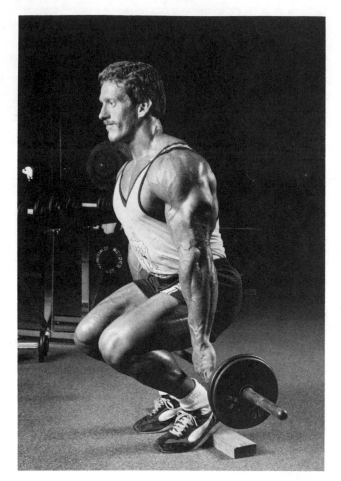

Barbell Hack Squat—start, left; finish, right.

Barbell Hack Squats

Emphasis: Hack Squats performed either with a barbell or on one of the various types of hack machines stress the quadriceps in relative isolation from the remainder of your body. Moreover, Hack Squats particularly stress the quads just above the knees and add sweep to the quads on the outer sides of your thighs.

Starting Position: Place a barbell on the floor so the handle rests above a thick block of wood. Place your heels on the block of wood with your feet set slightly narrower than shoulder-width. Bend your legs and grasp the bar with your hands set at shoulder-width and your palms toward the rear. Straighten your arms and hold them straight throughout the movement. Keeping your torso upright, straighten your legs and stand with your body erect, the bar resting across your upper thighs just beneath your but-

tocks. You must hold the bar tightly against your upper thighs in this position until you have completed your set.

Movement Performance: Keeping your torso perfectly erect, squat slowly down as far as possible, then recover to the starting position by straightening your legs.

Training Tips: Some bodybuilders wear a weightlifting belt while doing Barbell Hack Squats and rest the bar against the upper edge of the belt, a method popularized by the great Steve Reeves (winner of the 1947 Mr. America title and star of numerous muscle flicks). You will find it difficult at first to maintain your balance when doing Hack Squats with a barbell, but within two or three workouts your balance will improve until you can do the movement flawlessly.

Comment: Most bodybuilders are in favor of Hack Squats performed on a machine, so the

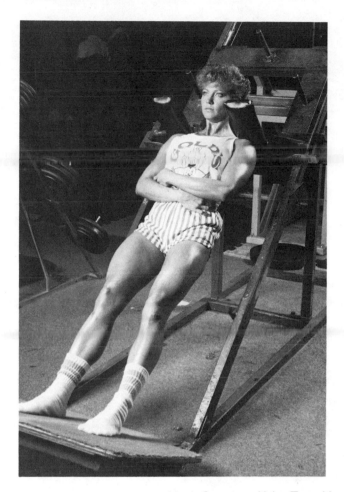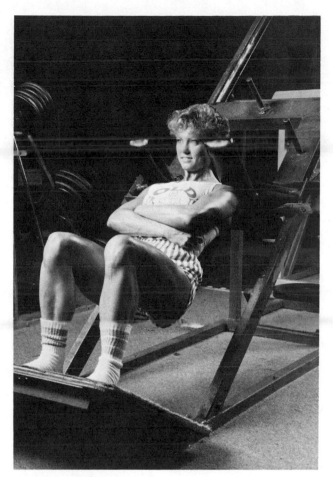

Hack Squat on Yoke-Type Machine—start, left; finish, right.

barbell version is probably most appropriate for use in a home gym setting.

Machine Hack Squats

Emphasis: Machine Hack Squats also stress the quadriceps in relative isolation from the remainder of your body, with particular emphasis placed on the quads just above the knees and on the outer sides of your thighs.

Starting Position (Yoke-Type Machine): Place your feet on the angled foot rest with your heels about eight inches apart and your toes angled outward. Bend your legs so you can position your shoulders beneath the yokes attached to the sliding platform of the machine. Straighten your legs completely and rotate the stop bars near your shoulders to a position that releases the weight for Hack Squats.

Starting Position (Sliding Platform-Type Ma-

chine): Place your feet on the angled foot rest with your heels about eight inches apart and your toes angled outward. Place your back against the sliding platform of the machine and bend your legs to slip your body down the platform until you can grasp the handles at the lower edge of the platform. Keep your arms straight throughout the movement. Straighten your legs fully.

Movement Performance: Slowly bend your legs and sink down into as low a squatting position as possible, being sure that your knees travel out over your feet as you do the movement. Slowly straighten your legs to return to the starting position.

Comment: With the yoke-type machine, be sure to rotate the stop bars to the locking position at the end of your set before stepping from the machine. With the platform-type machine, you can simply lower the slide down until

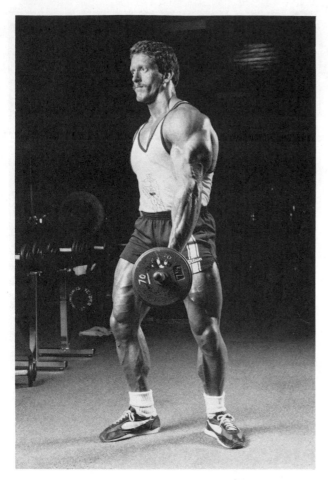
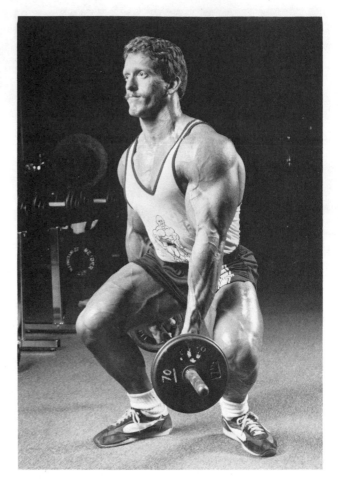

Jefferson Lift Squat—start, left; finish, right.

it comes to rest against its stops, then exit the machine.

Exercise Variations: For a super-intense contraction in your quads, you should try to rise up with your hips thrust forward as far as possible. This type of movement is analogous to Sissy Squats, which will be described and illustrated a bit later in this chapter.

Jefferson Lift Squats

Emphasis: This is a relatively classic leg and hip movement that packs plenty of power and muscle mass into the quadriceps and buttocks, as well as into the trapezius and the gripping muscles of the forearms.

Starting Position: Straddle a moderately heavy barbell as illustrated, your feet set about shoulder-width apart and your toes pointed di-

rectly forward. Bend your legs completely enough so you can reach to the rear with one hand and grasp the bar, your palm facing the midline of your body, then reach to the front with your other hand and grasp the bar in front of your body in the same manner. You should hold your arms completely straight and keep your torso erect throughout the movement.

Movement Performance: Slowly straighten your legs until you are standing erect with the barbell resting directly beneath your groin. Return to the full squatting position and repeat the movement for an appropriate number of repetitions.

Training Tips: For a longer range of motion, you can perform Jefferson Lift Squats while standing on a thick block of wood. And if you experience any difficulty in grasping the bar, you can use straps to strengthen your grip.

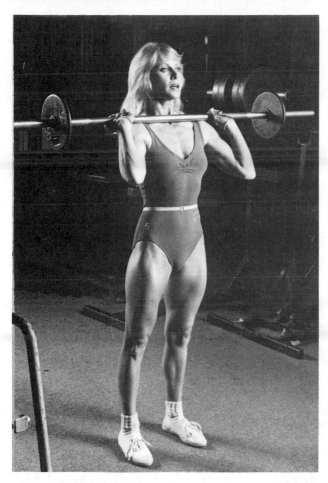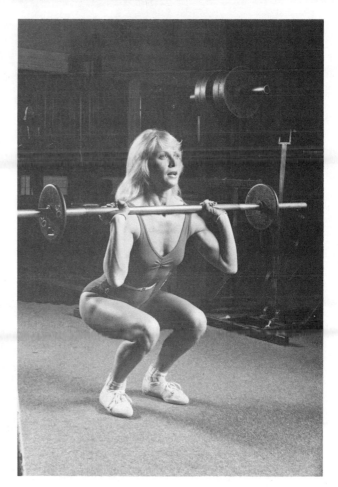

Front Squat—start, left; finish, right.

Front Squats

Emphasis: Front Squats are similar to normal Squats, except that the bar is held across the shoulders and upper chest in front of the neck. Primary emphasis in this movement is on the quadriceps, particularly the lower part of the quads just above the knees. Secondary emphasis is on the buttocks, abdomen, and back muscles.

Starting Position: Place a barbell on a pair of squat stands and load it up with a moderate weight. Position your feet about shoulder width apart, toes angled slightly outward, directly beneath the bar. Bend your legs and extend your arms directly forward, parallel to the floor, so you can position the bar across your deltoids and upper chest at the base of your neck. Keeping your elbows up, cross your arms over the bar. As long as you don't allow your elbows to drop, the bar will remain securely placed in this position.

Straighten your legs, step back, and position your feet for your Front Squats.

Movement Performance: Keeping your torso perfectly erect, bend your legs and slowly lower yourself into a full squatting position. Without bouncing at the bottom of the movement, slowly return to the starting point.

Training Tip: It's essential that you wear a weightlifting belt when you do Front Squats. And most bodybuilders find that they must stand with their heels on a block of wood when they perform the movement.

Exercise Variations: You can also hold the bar without your arms crossed over it. Simply set your grip on the bar with your hands about six inches wider on each side than shoulder-width. Maintaining this grip on the bar, move your elbows forward and upward as you position the bar across your upper chest and deltoids. As

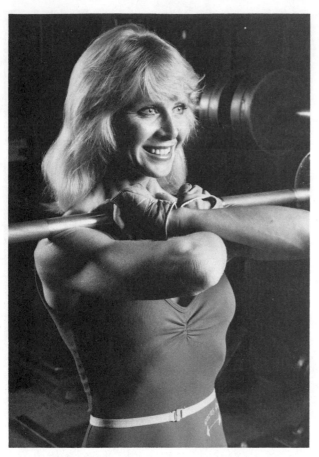

Front Squat with crossed-arm alternate position.

long as you keep your elbows held high in this position, the bar will remain securely in position. Regardless of the grip position, you can do Front Squats to various partial-squat depths if you prefer.

Sissy Squats

Emphasis: This movement is often performed during a peaking cycle because it is good for carving deep cuts in the quadriceps group. You will also find Sissy Squats to be one of the best ways of strongly stretching your quads.

Starting Position: You will find it easier to balance your body during Sissy Squats if you stand between a set of parallel bars and lightly grasp the uprights attached to the bars as you perform the movement. Your feet should be set about shoulder-width apart, your toes pointed directly forward. You probably won't need to add resistance to the movement.

Movement Performance: You must simultaneously do four movements in order to reach the correct bottom position of the exercise: rise up on your toes, bend your legs to at least a 90-degree angle, thrust your knees as far forward as possible, and incline your torso backward until

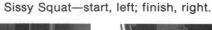

Sissy Squat—start, left; finish, right.

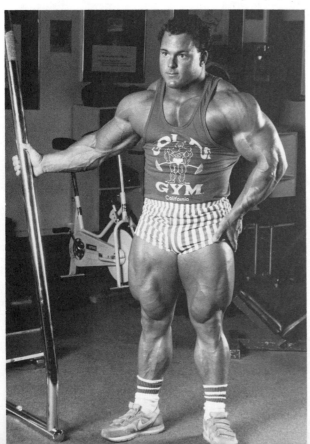

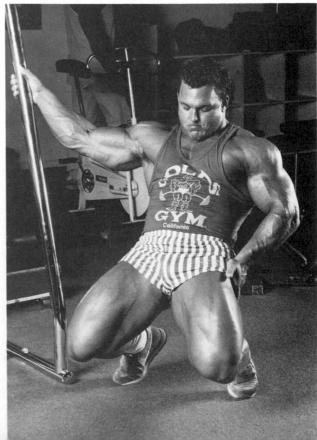

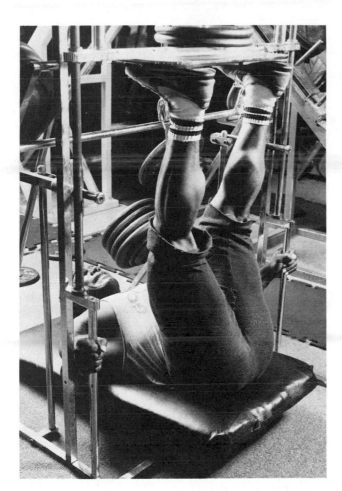 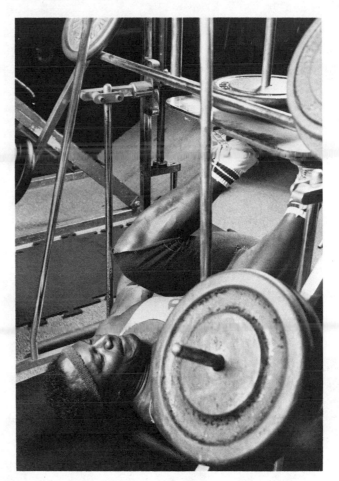

Vertical Leg-Press Machine—start, left; finish, right.

it is approximately parallel to the floor. If you correctly perform these movements, you will feel a very strong stretching sensation in your quads. Slowly reverse the procedure to return to the starting point, then repeat the movement.

Training Tip: If you eventually require added resistance for Sissy Squats, you should securely belt a loose barbell plate against your waist.

Exercise Variations: While it is more difficult to balance your body, you can do Sissy Squats while holding on to a single upright with one hand. And to keep continuous tension on your quads, you can come only about three-quarters of the way up in the movement before descending again into the full squatting position.

Leg Presses

Emphasis: At the present time, there are five distinctly different types of leg-press machines,

each of which places direct stress on the quadriceps and buttocks, with secondary emphasis on the hamstrings.

Starting Position (Vertical Leg-Press Machine): You will find a pad beneath this machine that has one end higher than the other. Position this pad so you can lie on your back with your hips at the high end of the pad and directly beneath the sliding platform of the machine. Place your feet on the sliding platform a little wider than shoulder-width, your toes angled slightly outward. Keeping your feet flat on the platform at all times, straighten your legs and rotate the stop bars to the sides to release the platform for use in the exercise. (Of course, you must rotate the stop bars to the locked position when you are finished with your set.)

Starting Position (45-Degree-Angled Leg-Press Machine): Lie back on the angled backboard of the machine and grasp the handles

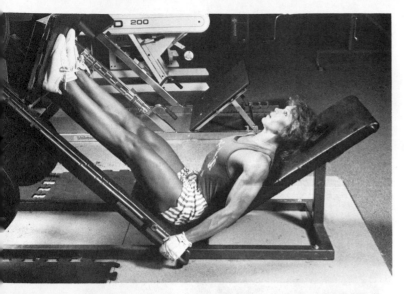

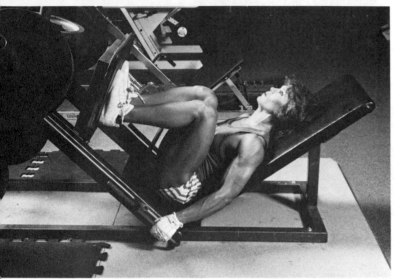

45-Degree-Angled Leg-Press Machine—start, top; finish, bottom.

provided to steady your body in position during your set. Place your feet on the sliding platform at about shoulder-width, your toes angled slightly outward. Straighten your legs and release the stop bars. (Be sure to move these stop bars to a locked position when you finish your set.)

Starting Position (Universal Gym Leg-Press Machine): The seat of this leg-press machine is adjustable. You need merely pull up on the knob at the front of the seat to release the seat. Then move the seat as close to the machine's pedals as possible; the closer it is to the pedals, the longer will be your range of motion in the exercise. Sit in the seat, bend your legs, and place your feet on the pedals attached to the movement arm of the machine. If there are two sets of pedals, be sure to use the lower set because it stresses the thigh muscles more directly than the upper pair of pedals. Grasp the handles provided at the sides of the seat to maintain your body position during the movement. And be sure that you keep your torso held perfectly upright throughout the set. Slumping forward can place a harmful strain on your upper spine as you do Leg Presses on a Universal Gym machine. Finally, straighten your legs.

Starting Position (Nautilus Leg-Press Machine): This machine is somewhat similar to the Universal Gym apparatus. The seat can be ad-

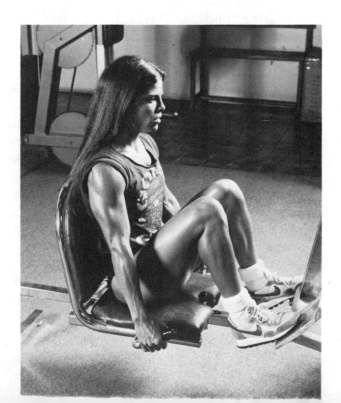

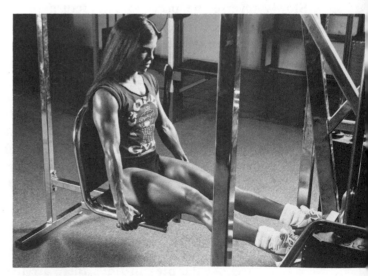

Universal Gym Leg-Press Machine—start, left; finish, above.

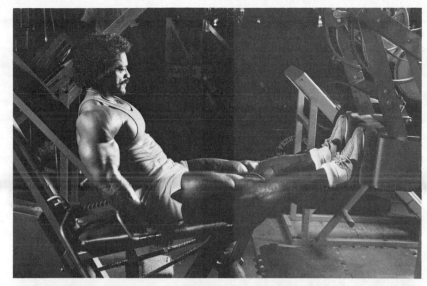

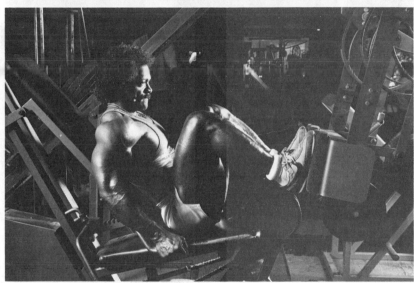

Nautilus Leg-Press Machine—start, top; finish, bottom.

justed forward and backward by lifting a lever at the right side of the seat, then lowering it when you have the seat where you want it. Sit in the seat, bend your legs, and place your feet on the pedals attached to the movement arm of the Nautilus double-leg machine. Fasten the seat belt over your lap, grasp the handles provided at the sides of the seat, and fully straighten your legs.

Starting Position (Curved-Back Leg-Press Machine): The curved-back leg-press machine is similar to the Universal and Nautilus leg-press machines. Sit down in the machine, bend your legs, and place your feet against the movement platform. Grasp the handles provided at the sides of the machine, or grasp the edges of the padded surface of the apparatus. Straighten your legs fully.

Movement Performance (All Machines): Slowly bend your legs as fully as possible. In some cases, you can achieve such an exaggerated range of motion on a leg-press machine that you must spread your legs in the bottom position so they pass on each side of your torso at the low point of the movement. Straighten your legs to return to the starting point and repeat the movement.

Training Tips: It's essential that you never hold your breath while you are exerting against the weight in a Leg-Press movement. This would build up such a high degree of blood pressure that it could be harmful to your body. With maximum weights, it is also a good practice to keep from fully straightening your legs each repetition, since this movement could eventually harm your knee joints.

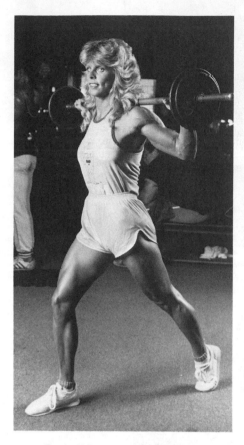

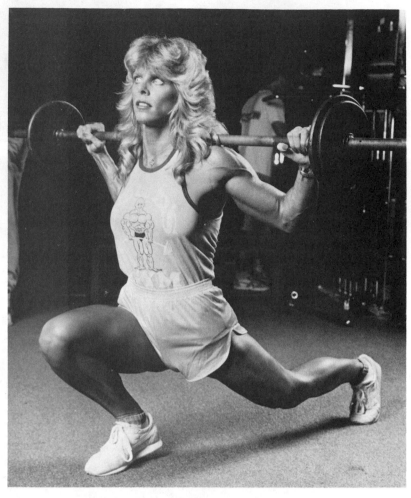

Barbell Lunge—start, above;
finish, right.

Lunges

Emphasis: This movement stresses the quadriceps (particularly the upper section of the muscle where it originates near the pelvis), buttocks, and the upper hamstrings (near where they run into the glutes). Champion competitive bodybuilders do plenty of lunges close to a major championship because the movement is excellent for carving deep cuts into the quads.

Starting Position: Place a light barbell behind your neck as for a set of Squats, holding it in place by grasping the bar on each side out near the plates. Place your feet about eight inches apart, your toes pointed directly ahead. Stand erect.

Movement Performance: Step forward 2½–3 feet with your left foot, being sure to position your foot on the floor with your toes pointed directly forward. Keeping your right leg relatively straight, slowly bend your left leg as fully as possible. This will lower your body so your right knee will be three or four inches from the floor and your left knee will be three or four inches ahead of your left ankle. In this position, you should feel a powerful stretching sensation in your left buttock and right quadriceps muscles. Push off with your left leg to return to the starting point of the movement, and do the next repetition with your right foot forward. Alternate forward feet until you have done the suggested number of repetitions with each leg.

Exercise Variations: Many bodybuilders prefer to do Lunges placing their forward foot up on a four-inch-thick block of wood. You can also do a Short Lunge in which you step only about two feet forward with your front foot and bend both legs to lower your body toward the floor.

Training Tips: Be sure to keep your torso as erect as possible as you do this movement. You may discover that it's easier to keep your torso erect if you provide resistance to the movement by holding two light dumbbells with your arms down at your sides.

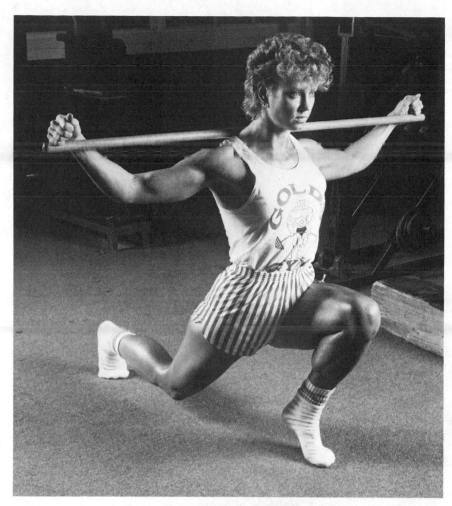

Weightless Lunge at finish.

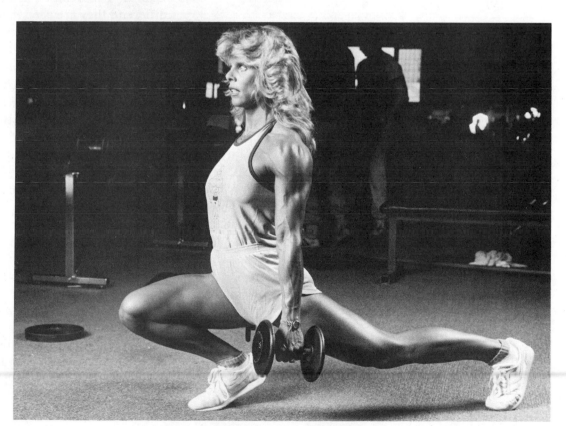

Dumbbell Lunge at finish.

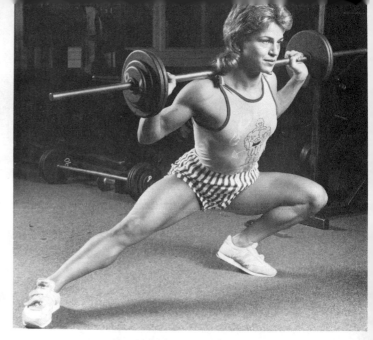

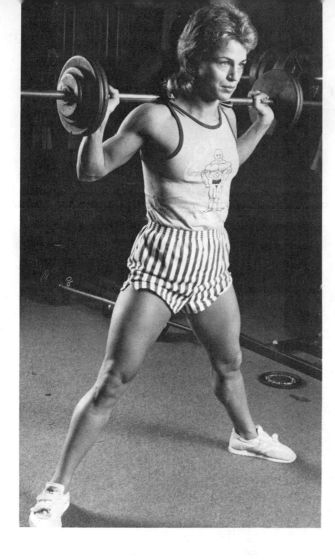

Side Lunge—start, left; finish, above.

Side Lunges

Emphasis: This version of Lunges stresses virtually all of the muscles of the thighs and hips, particularly the adductor muscles on the inner edges of the thighs.

Starting Position: Assume the same starting position as for Lunges.

Movement Performance: Without twisting your torso to one side or the other, step directly to the right with your right foot about 2½–3 feet. In the correct position, both of your legs will be straight and they will be at approximately a 60-degree angle with each other. Keeping your left leg totally straight, slowly bend your right leg as completely as you can. Push off with your right leg and return to the starting position. Do the next repetition to the left, and alternate movements to each side until you have done the required number of repetitions with each leg.

Comment: If you perform any lunging poses in your free-posing routine, this is the same type of leg movement that you use to get into and out of the lunging position.

Leg Extensions

Emphasis: Leg Extensions almost completely isolate stress on the quadriceps muscle group. There is minimal assistance in a stablizing role from the remainder of the body.

Starting Position: There are a wide variety of leg-extension machines, among them Nautilus, Brother, Corbin-Pacific, Universal Gym, and Cam II. While these machines all look somewhat different, they are used in the same way. Regardless of the type of machine, sit on it so the backs of your knees are pressed against the edge of the padded surface of the machine closest to the lever arm. Place your insteps beneath the lower set of roller pads (if there are two sets). Either sit erect or lie back against the padded back rest of the machine (if one has been provided). Grasp the handles provided at the sides of the seat or the edges of the padded surface of the machine to steady your body in position as you perform the exercise.

Movement Performance: Moving only your lower legs, slowly straighten your legs. Hold the top position of the movement with your legs straight for a moment to ensure a peak contraction in your thigh muscles. Lower your feet slowly back to the starting point and repeat the movement.

Exercise Variation: This exercise can be performed with one leg at a time, rather than with both legs simultaneously. It's particularly valuable to do one-legged exercises when, for in-

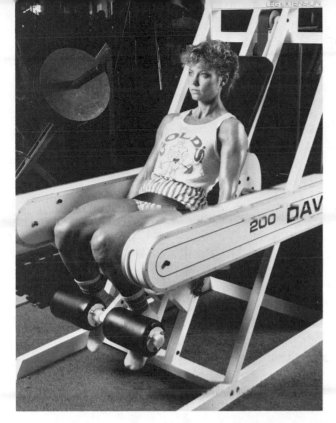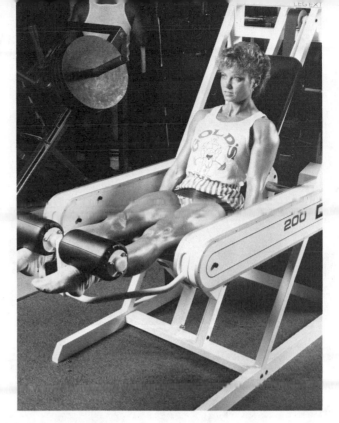

Leg Extension—start, left; finish, right.

stance, you are attempting to rehabilitate an injured knee.

Training Tip: For the ultimate thigh burn, try "21" Leg Extensions. Load a moderately heavy weight on the machine and begin with seven half reps from the bottom of the movement halfway up to the finish position. Next perform seven half reps from the midpoint to the finish of the exercise, and finally do seven complete reps. Your thighs will burn as though someone were playing a blow torch over them at the end of a set "21" Leg Extensions.

Free-Standing Machine Leg Extension—start, left; finish, right.

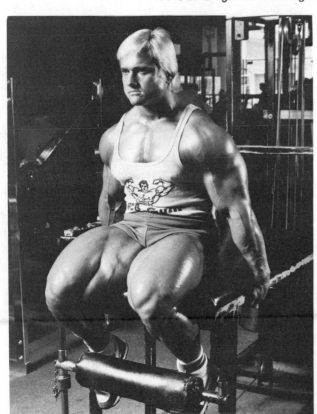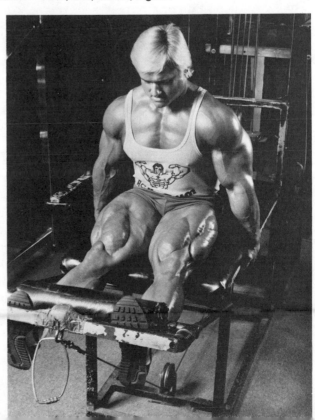

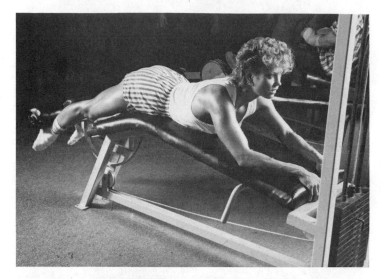

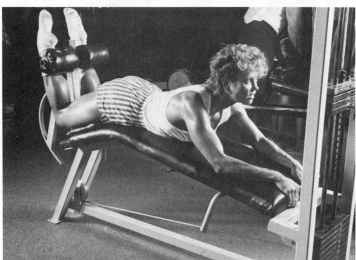

Leg Curl—start, top; finish, bottom.

or the handles provided at the head end of the padded surface to brace your body in position during your set. It is essential that you keep your pelvis in contact with the pad throughout the movement.

Movement Performance: Slowly bend your legs as fully as possible, pausing in the top position long enough to achieve a peak contraction effect in your hamstrings. Return to the starting position and repeat the movement.

Exercise Variation: As with Leg Extensions, you can perform Leg Curls one limb at a time.

Training Tip: As long as you keep your hips motionless during the movement, you can rest the weight of your torso on your elbows and elevate your hips slightly. This type of body position during Leg Curls can give you a more intense peak contraction in your hamstrings at the top point of the movement.

Standing Leg Curls

Emphasis: Like Lying Leg Curls, Standing Leg Curls stress the hamstrings in relative isolation from the remainder of your body.

Starting Position: Keeping in mind that you should do an equal number of sets and reps with each leg, let's describe how to do Standing Leg Curls with your left leg. Stand to the right side of the machine and slip your left heel against the roller pad on that side of the apparatus. Rest

Lying Leg Curls

Emphasis: Performed correctly, Leg Curls isolate stress on the hamstrings, with only minimum stress placed on the muscles that stabilize your body in position during the movement.

Starting Position: As with Leg Extensions, there are a number of brands of lying leg-curl machines, but each functions the same as the others. Regardless of the leg-curl machine, you should lie facedown on the padded surface of the apparatus with your knees set at the edge of the pad toward the lever arm of the machine. Hook the backs of your heels beneath the upper set of roller pads (if there are two sets) and completely straighten your legs. Grasp the edges of the pad

Corbin-Pacific Leg-Curl Machine at finish.

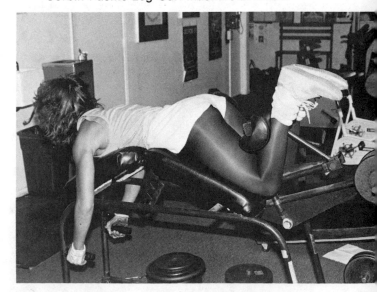

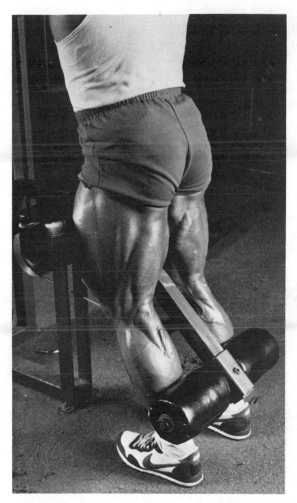

Standing Leg Curl—start, above; finish, right.

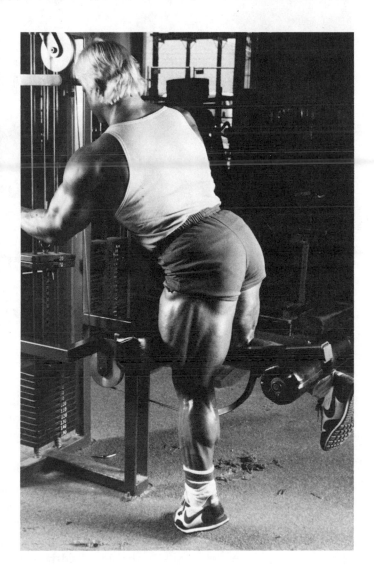

your left knee firmly against the flat pad at knee height, and keep it pressed against that pad throughout your set. Grasp either the crossbar or the uprights of the machine to steady your upper body in position as you perform the exercise.

Movement Performance: Without moving any other part of your body, slowly bend your left leg as completely as possible, attempting to touch your heel to your buttock. Lower slowly back to the starting position and repeat the movement.

Training Tip: On all Leg-Curl movements, you must be careful to do some sets with your toes pointed and some with your toes flexed.

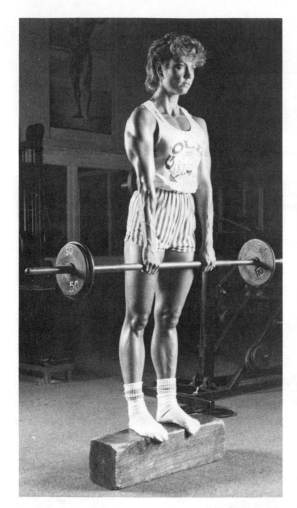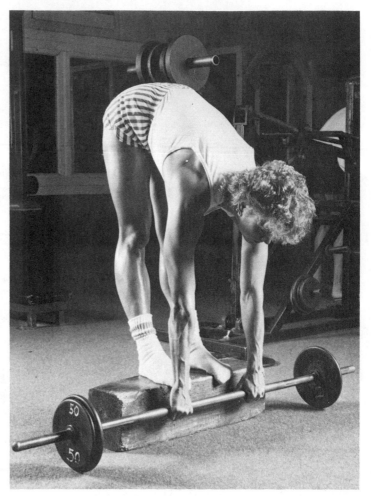

Stiff-Leg Deadlift—start, left; finish, right.

Stiff-Leg Deadlifts

Emphasis: Many bodybuilders don't realize that Stiff-Leg Deadlifts intensely stress the hamstrings. Intense stress is also placed on the lumbar muscles of the lower back and the buttocks as you do Stiff-Leg Deadlifts.

Starting Position: Place a light barbell on the floor and stand up to it with your shins touching the bar. Bend over and take a shoulder-width over-grip on the bar and stand erect, your arms straight and running down at your sides, the bar resting across your upper thighs. Stiffen your legs and hold them straight throughout the movement.

Movement Performance: Slowly bend over at the waist and lower the barbell downward until its plates touch the floor, then slowly stand erect to regain the starting position. Since your lower back is in a mechanically weak position as you perform Stiff-Leg Deadlifts, it is essential that you perform the movement very slowly.

Training Tip: To achieve a longer range of motion when performing Stiff-Leg Deadlifts, you can stand on a thick block of wood or a flat exercise bench. Standing on a bench or block allows you to move the handle of the barbell much lower without the plates contacting the floor.

Exercise Variation: For an interesting variation, you can perform your Stiff-Leg Deadlifts while holding two dumbbells in your hands rather than a barbell.

Nautilus Hip and Back Machine

Emphasis: Primary emphasis in this movement is on the buttocks and erector spinae

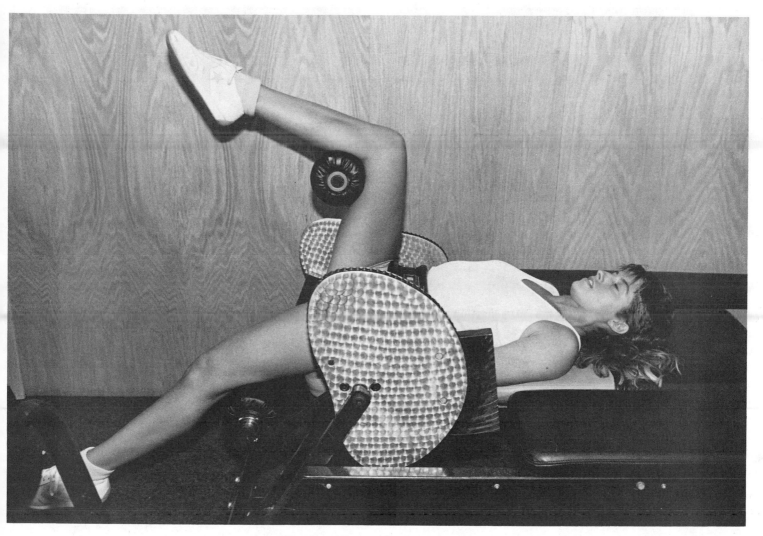

Nautilus Hip and Back Machine.

muscles of the lower back. And there is also stress on the upper part of the hamstrings.

Starting Position: Lie on your back with your hips toward the lever arms of the machine. Grasp the handles near the lever arms, curl your legs up over your chest, and pull your hips as far as possible toward the lever-arm end of the machine. As you pull yourself in that direction, place the backs of your knees against the roller pads attached to the lever arms. Once you are in this position, secure the lap belt around your hips. With most Nautilus hip and back machines, there is a small padded block provided, and you should rest that block beneath your neck and head. Arch your back and keep it arched throughout the movement. Finally, push

your knees down and simultaneously straighten your legs so your legs and torso make one long, straight line.

Movement Performance: Keeping your right leg stationary, slowly allow the weight provided by the machine to force your left knee to your chest. Return your left leg to the starting position and do the next rep with your right leg. Continue alternating legs until you have performed the required number of repetitions with each leg.

Comment: For most bodybuilders, this is an excellent buttocks exercise, but not nearly as good a lower-back movement as Hyperextensions, Good Mornings, and various types of Deadlifts.

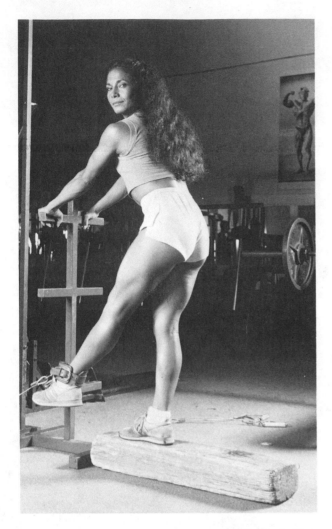 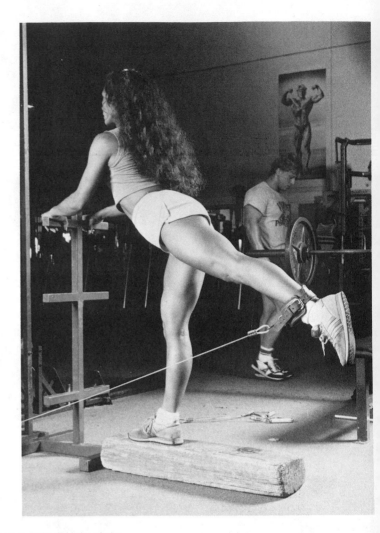

Cable Back Kick—start, left; finish, right.

Cable Back Kick

Emphasis: Cable Back Kicks directly stress the powerful gluteus maximus muscle group, giving it a rounded appearance. Secondary emphasis is placed on the lower-back and upper-hamstring muscles.

Starting Position: Attach a padded cuff to your ankle, moving the ring attached to the cuff around to the front of your ankle. Hook the end of a cable running through a floor pulley to the ring on the cuff. Stand about three feet back from the floor pulley and grasp either a sturdy upright or two tall stools to steady your body in position during the movement. (It is also possible to do all of the hip and thigh cable movements presented in this chapter without grasping

anything to steady your body, but you will get much more out of the movement when you do so in a secure position). Facing the floor pulley, straighten your leg and allow the weight at the end of the cable to pull your foot as far forward as possible.

Movement Performance: Keeping your leg straight throughout the movement, slowly move your foot in a semicircular arc as far to the rear and upward as possible. Hold this contracted position for a moment, then return your foot to the starting position. Be sure to do an equal number of reps for each leg.

Training Tip: A common error when performing this movement is allowing your torso to bend forward to help you raise your foot higher to the rear. However, you will get a lot more out of the

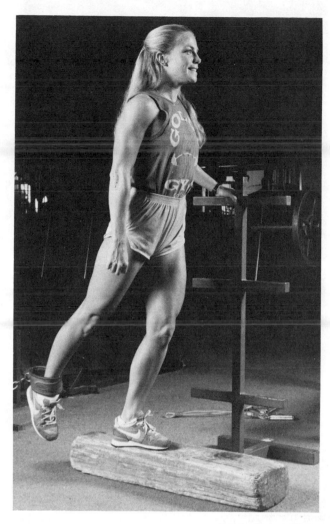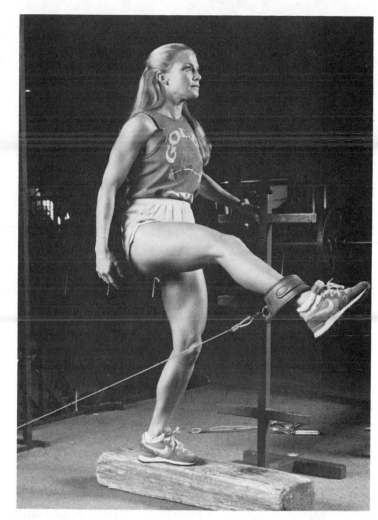

Cable Front Kick—start, left; finish, right.

movement if you keep your torso in as upright a position as possible while you do Cable Back Kicks.

Cable Front Kicks

Emphasis: With this movement, you can stress all of the quadriceps muscles, and particularly the hip flexors at the tops of the thighs where they attach to the pelvic girdle.

Starting Position: Attach the padded cuff to your ankle, but rotate the cuff so the ring is at the back of your ankle. Attach a cable through a low pulley to the ring and face away from the pulley. Move forward about three feet away from the pulley and brace your body in a secure position. Allow the weight attached to the cable

to pull your ankle as far to the rear as comfortably possible. Keep your leg straight throughout the movement.

Movement Performance: Slowly move your foot in a semicircular arc forward and upward as high as possible. Hold this top position for a moment and then return your leg to the starting position. Be sure to do an equal number of reps for each leg.

Exercise Variation: To stress the quadriceps more than the hip flexors, you should begin the movement with your leg bent at approximately a 45-degree angle, then straighten it forcefully as you finish the movement. When viewed from the side in this variation of Cable Front Kicks, your leg will look as though it is kicking a football or soccer ball.

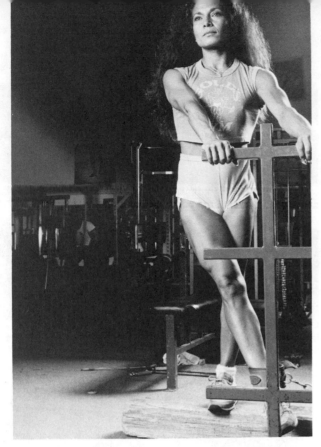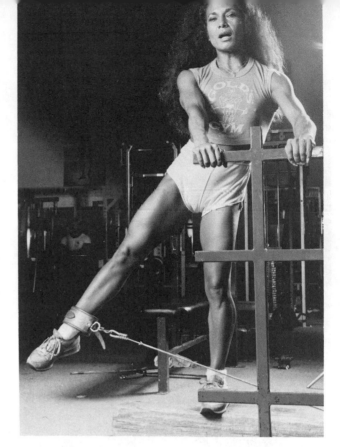

Cable Side Kick—start, left; finish, right.

Cable Side Kick

Emphasis: This unique cable movement directly stresses all of the abductor muscles of your hips and on the sides of your thighs.

Starting Position: Attach the padded cuff to your right ankle, rotating the cuff so its ring is toward the midline of your body. Attach the cable to the cuff and stand with your left side directly toward the cable so the cable runs across the front of your body. Brace your body in a secure position and allow the weight attached to the cable to pull your foot well across the midline of your body. Be sure to keep your leg held straight throughout the movement.

Movement Performance: Slowly move your right foot in a semicircular arc to the right and upward as high as you can. Hold the top position for a moment, then lower your foot back to the starting point. Be sure to do an equal number of reps for each leg.

Training Tip: With this and the other cable leg and hip movements presented in this chapter, you might find it easier to perform the exercise if you stand on a thick block of wood with your nonexercising foot.

Cable Leg Adduction

Emphasis: Cable Leg Adductions directly stress all of the adductor muscles of the thighs and hip girdle.

Starting Position: Attach the padded cuff to your right ankle, rotating the cuff so its ring is on the outside of your ankle. Attach a floor-pulley cable to the cuff and stand with your right side toward the pulley. Brace your body in a secure position and allow the weight attached to the cable to pull your foot well away from the midline of your body.

Movement Performance: Keeping your leg straight throughout the movement, slowly move your foot toward the midline of your body (and even across this midline if possible). Hold this contracted position for a moment, then allow the weight to pull your foot back to the starting position. Be sure to do an equal number of reps for each leg.

Exercise Variation: You can do Cable Leg Adductions while seated between two floor pulleys to which you have attached loop handles. Simply sit on a low bench and hold the loop handles against your knees. You can do leg adductions very effectively in this position.

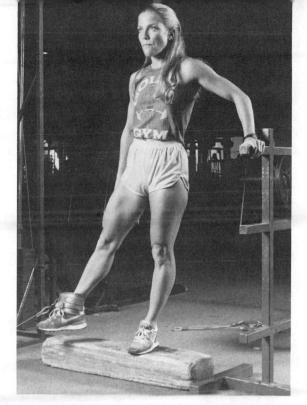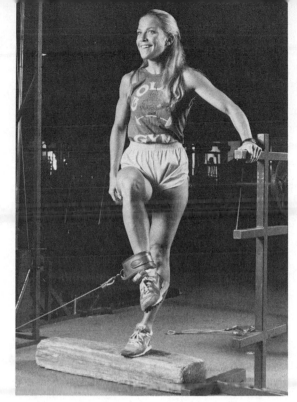

Cable Leg Adduction—start, left; finish, right.

Nautilus Adductions/Abductions

Emphasis: There is a special Nautilus machine on which you can do movements to stress both the abductors and adductors of your legs and hips.

Starting Position: Sit in the machine and rest your legs between the pads of the lever arms.

Attach the seat belt around your hips.

Movement Performance: A lever on the side of the machine allows you to select whether you will do an adduction or abduction movement. Depending on which position you select for the lever, you can either force your legs together against resistance, or push them apart against resistance provided by the machine.

Nautilus Leg Adduction.

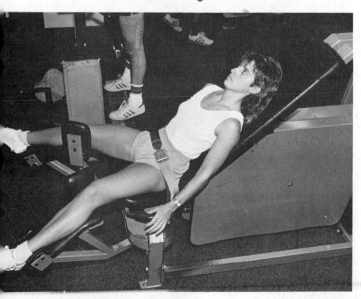

Nautilus Leg Abduction.

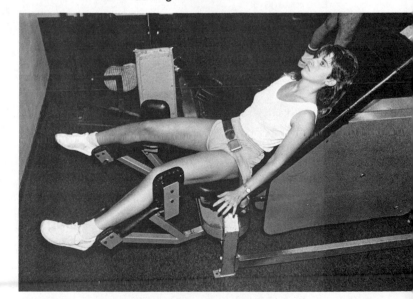

Suggested Leg Routines

If you have less than a few weeks of training behind you, the following routine can profitably be performed three nonconsecutive days per week:

Exercise	Sets	Reps
Universal Gym Leg Press	3	10–15
Nautilus Leg Extension	2	10–15
Lying Leg Curl	3	10–15

After 4–6 weeks of steady training on the foregoing program, you can use this routine three days per week:

Exercise	Sets	Reps
Squats	3	12–8*
Angled Leg Press	3	12–8*
Leg Extensions	3	10–15
Lying Leg Curls	3	10–15
Standing Leg Curls	2	10–15

* Pyramid weights and reps on exercises marked with an asterisk.

After about three months of training, you should switch to a four-day split routine in which you train each major muscle group (including the thighs and hips) twice per week. This is typically how a lower-level competitive bodybuilder will train in the off-season. Following is a sample hip and thigh training program for off-season competitive training.

Exercise	Sets	Reps
Leg Extensions	3	10–15
Front Squats	4	12–6*
Nautilus Leg Presses	4	12–6*
Lying Leg Curls	3	8–10
Standing Leg Curls	3	8–10
Squats	1	15–20

As you will see in the following section listing the leg routines of a wide variety of men and women who have trained at Gold's Gym, every bodybuilder trains differently from all others prior to a competition.

Leg Routines of the Gold's Champs

In this section, you will find a variety of thigh and hip training programs used by many of the Gold's Gym superstars who have won the sport's highest titles. Keep in mind as you examine these training programs that these men and women have been training for many years and have developed enormous recuperative powers. It is unlikely that you can make good gains using their full routines. Instead, you should use these training programs as examples of how to work your own hips and thighs. In all likelihood, you can do the same exercises as your favorite champion, but scale down the number of sets he or she does of each movement to meet your own abilities.

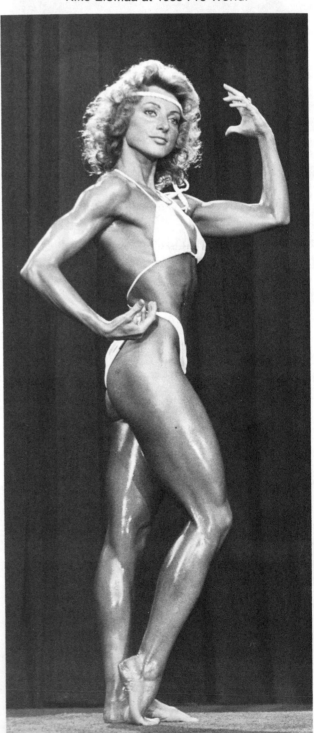

Kike Elomaa at 1983 Pro World.

TOM PLATZ
(MR. UNIVERSE)

Exercise	Sets	Reps
Squats	8–10	20–5*
Machine Hack Squats	5	10–15
Leg Extensions	5–8	10–15
Lying Leg Curls	6–10	10–15

SAMIR BANNOUT
(MR. OLYMPIA)

Exercise	Sets	Reps
Squats (warm-up)	2	15–20
Squats	5–6	6–8
Hack Squats	4	10–12
Leg Extensions	4	10–12
Lying Leg Curls	5–6	10–12

INGER ZETTERQVIST
(AMATEUR WORLD CHAMPION)

Exercise	Sets	Reps
Leg Extensions	3	10–15
Machine Hack Squat	4	10–15
Lunges	4	10–15
Standing Leg Curls	3	10–15
Stiff-Leg Deadlifts	3	10–15

CLARENCE BASS
(PAST-40 MR. USA)

Exercise	Sets	Reps
Nautilus Leg Extensions	1	8–10
Vertical Leg Presses	1	10–12
Machine Hack Squats	1	10–15
Nautilus Leg Presses	1	10–15
Nautilus Leg Curls	1	10–15

ANDREAS CAHLING
(MR. INTERNATIONAL)

Exercise	Sets	Reps
Leg Extensions	2	12–15
Front Squats	4	10–12
Angled Leg Press	2	10–12
Machine Hack Squat	2	10–12
Lying Leg Curls	2–3	10–12
Standing Leg Curls	2–3	10–12

LISA ELLIOTT-KOLAKOWSKI
(MISS EASTERN AMERICA)

Exercise	Sets	Reps
Universal Leg Presses (warm-up)	2–3	15–20
Squats	5	15–6*
Machine Hack Squats	3	10–15
Nautilus Leg Extensions	4	10–15
Nautilus Leg Curls	4–5	10–15

CHARLES GLASS
(AMATEUR WORLD CHAMPION)

Exercise	Sets	Reps
Squats	6	10
Front Squats	5	6
Leg Extensions	5–7	10
Lying Leg Curls	5–7	10
Machine Hack Squats	10	10

JON LOYD
(GOLD'S CLASSIC CHAMPION)

Exercise	Sets	Reps
Leg Extensions (warm-up)	3	12
Leg Curls (warm-up)	3	12
Front Squats	5–6	12–5*
Lunges (on block)	3	15
Machine Hack Squats	3	12
Standing Leg Curls	3	12

LISA LYON
(WORLD CHAMPION)

Exercise	Sets	Reps
Squats	4–5	10–12
Leg Presses	4–5	10–12
Leg Extensions	4–5	10–12
supersetted with		
Leg Curls	4–5	10–12

MIKE MENTZER
(MR. UNIVERSE)

Exercise	Sets	Reps
Leg Extensions	1	10
Vertical Leg Presses	1	10–15
Squats	1	10–20
Lying Leg Curls	2	10–12

Note: Forced reps are performed on both Leg Extensions and Leg Curls.

DANNY PADILLA
(MR. UNIVERSE)

Exercise	Sets	Reps
Squats	6	15–8*
Angled Leg Presses	5	10–12
Leg Extensions	5	15
Lying Leg Curls	5	15

LAURA COMBES
(MS. AMERICA)

Exercise	Sets	Reps
Leg Extensions (warm-up)	2–3	15–20
Machine Hack Squats	5	15–6*
Lunges	3	10–15
Leg Extensions	3	10–15
Lying Leg Curls	5	10–15
Lunges	3	10–15

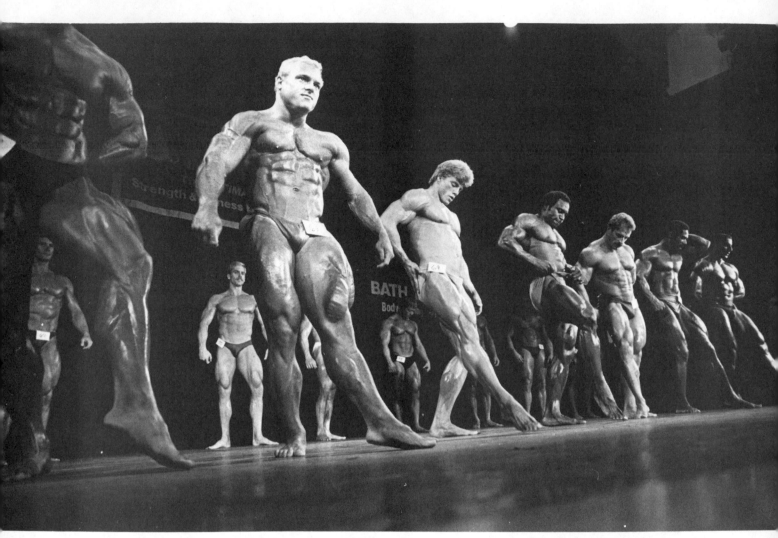

Leg exhibitions at the 1982 Nationals: (left to right) Tim Belknap, Matt Mendenhall, Lee Haney.

TONY PEARSON
(MR. UNIVERSE)

Exercise	Sets	Reps
Squats	4–6	10–20
Leg Presses	4–6	10–15
Lying Leg Curls	4–6	10–15
Lunges	4–6	10–15

PILLOW
(GOLD'S CLASSIC CHAMPION)

Exercise	Sets	Reps
Angled Leg Presses	5	12–6*
Leg Extensions	4–5	8–10
Machine Hack Squats	4–5	8–10
Lying Leg Curls	5–8	8–10
Standing Leg Curls	5–8	8–10
Cable Abductions	4–5	8–10
Cable Adductions	4–5	8–10

MIKE SABLE
(MR. WORLD)

Exercise	Sets	Reps
Leg Extensions	5	10–15
supersetted with		
Angled Leg Press	5	10–15
Machine Hack Squats	5	10–15
supersetted with		
Lying Leg Curls	5	10–15
Squats	5	10–15
Lunges	5	10–15

* All exercises marked with an asterisk should have the weights and reps pyramidded. With each succeeding set, the weight on the bar should be increased and the number of reps performed decreased.

DENNIS TINERINO
(MR. UNIVERSE)

Exercise	Sets	Reps
Leg Extensions	4-5	6-8
Squats	8-10	20-6*
Machine Hack Squats	4	6-8
Lying Leg Curls	5	6-8
Lunges	4	20

CHRIS DICKERSON
(MR. OLYMPIA)

Exercise	Sets	Reps
Angled Leg Press	6-8	8-10
Machine Hack Squats	5-6	10-15
Squats	5-6	10-15
Leg Extensions	6-8	10-15
Standing Leg Curls	4-5	10-15
Lying Leg Curls	4-5	10-15

LORI BOWEN
(MS. AMERICA)

Exercise	Sets	Reps
Front Squats (on Smith machine)	6	10-15
Lying Leg Curls	6	10-15
Leg Extensions	6	10-15
Angled Leg Presses	6	10-15
Lunges	6	10-15

ROBBY ROBINSON
(PRO GRAND PRIX CHAMPION)

Exercise	Sets	Reps
Nautilus Leg Extensions	5-8	10-15
supersetted with		
Nautilus Leg Curls	5-8	10-15
Machine Hack Squats	5-8	10-15
supersetted with		
Standing Leg Curls	5-8	10-15
Squats (very narrow stance)	5-8	10-15
Lunges	5-8	10-15

CANDY CSENCSITS
(MS. EASTERN AMERICA)

Exercise	Sets	Reps
Leg Extensions	3	8-12
Squats	3	6-8
Machine Hack Squats	3	8-10
Leg Presses	3	8-10
Lying Leg Curls	6	10
Cable Side Kicks	1-2	25
Cable Back Kicks	1-2	25

CASY VIATOR
(PRO GRAND PRIX CHAMPION)

Exercise	Sets	Reps
Standing Leg Curls	4-5	10-15
Nautilus Leg Curls	4-5	10-15
Stiff-Leg Deadlifts	4-5	15-20
Leg Extensions	6-8	10-15
Lunges	6-8	10-15
Machine Hack Squats	6-8	10-15
Sissy Squats	6-8	10-15
Squats	3-4	15-20

SCOTT WILSON
(PRO GRAND PRIX CHAMPION)

Exercise	Sets	Reps
Leg Extensions (warm-up)	2-3	15-20
Squats	6	15-6*
Machine Hack Squats	4	10-15
Leg Extensions	4	10-15
Sissy Squats	2-3	10-15
Lying Leg Curls	3-4	8-10
Standing Leg Curls	3-4	8-10

LOU FERRIGNO
(MR. UNIVERSE)

Exercise	Sets	Reps
Front Squats	5-6	10-15
Machine Hack Squats	4-5	10-15
Leg Extensions	4-5	10-15
Lying Leg Curls	5-6	10-15
Lunges	3-4	10-15

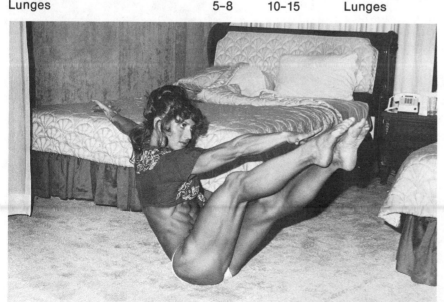

Pillow warms up in hotel room before a contest.

KIKE ELOMAA
(MISS OLYMPIA)

Exercise	Sets	Reps
Squats (warm-up)	1–2	20
Leg Presses	3–4	10–12
Leg Extensions	3–4	10–12
Lying Leg Curls	3–4	10–12
Squats	2–3	10–12

ARNOLD SCHWARZENEGGER
(MR. OLYMPIA)

Exercise	Sets	Reps
Squats	7	12–8*
Front Squats	4–5	12–8*
Lying Leg Curls	4	8–12
supersetted with		
Lunges	4	10–15

SERGIO OLIVA
(MR. OLYMPIA)

Exercise	Sets	Reps
Squats	8–10	15–2*
Leg Extensions	5–6	10–15
Lying Leg Curls	8–10	10–15
Lunges	3–5	10–15

BERTIL FOX
(MR. UNIVERSE)

Exercise	Sets	Reps
Squats	6	15–8*
Machine Hack Squats	5	15–8
supersetted with		
Leg Extensions	5	15–8*
Lying Leg Curls	5	15–8*

DR. FRANCO COLUMBU
(MR. OLYMPIA)

Exercise	Sets	Reps
Squats	8–10	15–5*
Leg Extensions	6–8	15–8*
Lying Leg Curls	5–6	10–12

RACHEL McLISH
(MISS OLYMPIA)

Exercise	Sets	Reps
Lunges	3–4	10–15
Nautilus Leg Presses	3–4	10–15
Lying Leg Curls	3–4	10–15
Leg Extensions	2–3	10–15

CHRISTER ERIKSSON
(MR. EUROPE)

Exercise	Sets	Reps
Squats	5–6	15–5*
Leg Extensions	5–6	10–15
Lying Leg Curls	5–6	10–15

Looking Ahead

In Chapter 7, we will introduce you to all of the abdominal exercises that the superstar bodybuilders at Gold's Gym use in their workouts. And we will reveal many of these champs' actual abdominal training routines.

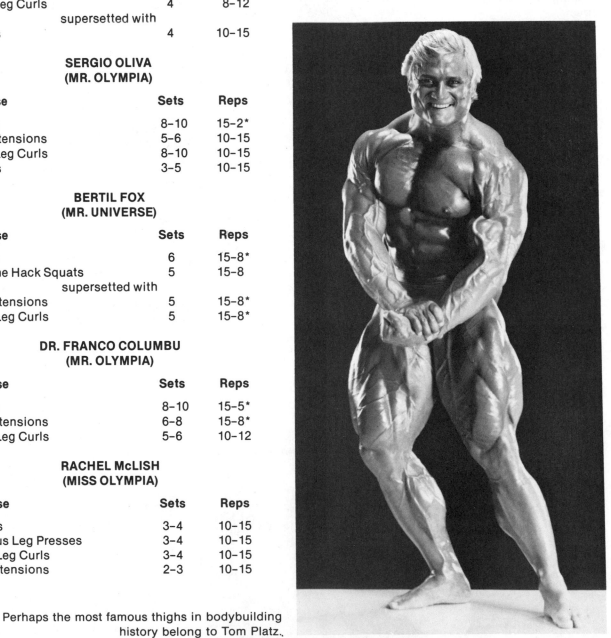

Perhaps the most famous thighs in bodybuilding history belong to Tom Platz.

7
TRICEPS TRAINING

Most bodybuilders, particularly men, are fascinated by the idea of building huge upper arms. They slave away on their biceps and often completely forget about their triceps which make up approximately two-thirds of the mass of the upper-arm musculature. Make a fastidious study of the physiques of the big-armed bodybuilders, however, and you will see that they all have tremendously thick triceps development.

A couple of good examples of men with big arms and particularly impressive triceps are Samir Bannout and Mohamed Makkawy who placed one–two at the '83 Mr. Olympia competition. They both have arm mass that compares favorably with any other bodybuilder, and that mass is complemented by the massive, deeply striated triceps muscles that each athlete has developed. And if they didn't have this type of triceps mass to go with their huge, peaked biceps muscles, their biceps would look like billiard balls lying on a flat table.

Although there is less emphasis on massive arm development in women's bodybuilding, there are still many women who have developed very thick and muscular triceps. A couple of the best are Julie McNew and Laura Combes. Julie

has yet to win a major competition because her massive arm development still overwhelms the rest of her physique, but Laura was the first American Women's Bodybuilding Champion. Laura's upper-arm development—particularly her triceps—is outstanding, but it is also in good harmony with the rest of her superb physique, which makes her a winner in any book.

You might keep in mind that many bodybuilders make the mistake of overtraining their triceps. In many chest and shoulder exercises (e.g., Bench Presses and Military Presses), your triceps work very hard, so piling a large amount of direct triceps work on top of this less-direct work can lead to overtraining the muscle group. The great French Mr. Universe title winner, Serge Nubret, has outstanding triceps development, and he rarely does any direct work for the muscle group. He feels that he gets plenty of triceps stimulation from his chest and shoulder workouts.

Anatomy and Kinesiology

The *triceps* on the back of your upper arm is a three-headed muscle that contracts to straighten your arm from a bent position. You can direct more stress to one or another triceps head (*inner head, outer head,* or *medial head*) by holding your hands in different positions and doing specific triceps exercises that seem to stress one head more than the others. So if you read the exercise descriptions in this chapter, carefully noting the **Emphasis** section, you can selectively train your three triceps heads to create any type of triceps development that you wish.

Triceps Exercises

In this section, you will find more than 20 major triceps exercises, each fully described and illustrated. Add in the numerous variations of each basic exercise, and you will have more than 40 triceps movements in your basic pool of bodybuilding exercises.

If you are relatively unfamiliar with bodybuilding exercises, you should carefully review both the written description and exercise photos of each movement before first trying it with a very light weight. Then, only when you are confident that you are correctly performing the exercise, you should use a weight that taxes the muscles you are trying to work.

Close-Grip Bench Presses

Emphasis: Close-Grip Bench Presses stress the entire triceps muscle complex in conjunction with the pectorals and anterior deltoids.

Starting Position: Load a bar lying on a bench press rack with an appropriate poundage. Lie on your back with your shoulders about three inches ahead of the uprights on the support rack and place your feet flat on the floor to balance your body on the bench. Take a narrow over-grip in the middle of the bar (there should be about six inches of space between your index fingers). Straighten your arms and lift the bar from the rack to a supported position at straight arms' length directly above your shoulder joints.

Movement Performance: Bend your arms and slowly lower the barbell down to touch the middle of your chest. Without bouncing the bar off your chest, slowly press it back to straight arms' length. Repeat the movement for the required number of repetitions.

Exercise Variations: You can also use an EZ-Curl bar for this movement. On both bars you can slightly vary the width of your grip.

Reverse-Grip Bench Presses

Emphasis: This is a very direct triceps movement that has only minimum involvement from the pectorals and anterior deltoids. You will find that Reverse-Grip Benches place significantly more stress on the long inner head of your triceps than on any other triceps head.

Starting Position: Load up a bar resting on a bench press rack. Lie back on the bench with your shoulders about three inches ahead of the rack support uprights and place your feet flat on the floor to steady your body in a secure position during the exercise. Take a shoulder-width under-grip on the barbell. Straighten your arms and bring the weight to a supported position at straight arms' length directly above your shoulder joints.

Movement Performance: Being sure that your upper arms are held in close to your torso, bend your arms and slowly lower the bar down to touch the middle of your chest. Without bouncing the bar off your chest, slowly press it back to straight arms' length. Repeat the movement for the suggested number of repetitions.

Training Tip: You'll ultimately be able to use a very heavy weight in this movement, so be sure to have a spotter standing by at the head end of the bench as you do the exercise.

Exercise Variations: You can vary the width of your grip on the bar over about a three-inch space in order to stress your triceps muscles somewhat differently.

Triceps Parallel Bar Dips

Emphasis: When performed in the manner described in this section, Parallel Bar Dips place very strong stress on your triceps. Secondary stress is on your pectorals and anterior deltoids.

Starting Position: Jump up on a set of parallel bars with your palms facing inward and your arms straight to support your body. You can bend your legs slightly, but be very careful to *keep your torso in as upright a position as*

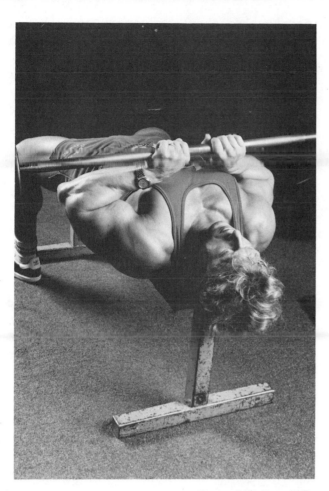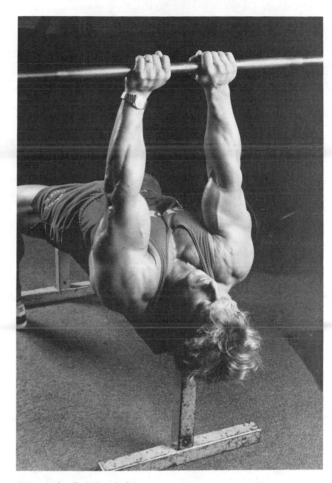

Close-Grip Bench Press—start, left; finish, right.

Reverse-Grip Bench Press—start, left; finish, right.

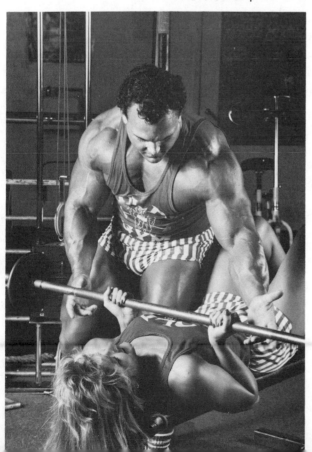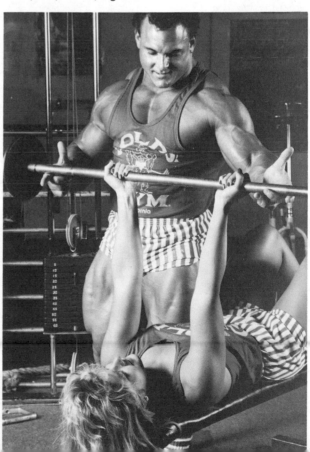

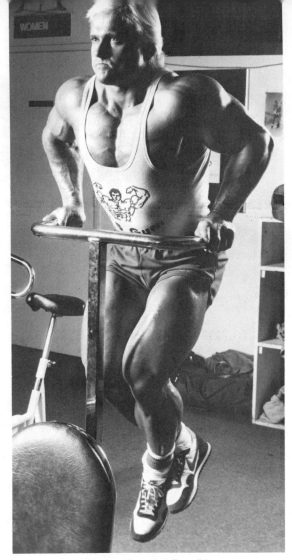

Triceps Parallel Bar Dip.

possible throughout the movement. Allowing your torso to incline forward will shift too much stress to the pectorals.

Movement Performance: Keeping your upper arms in close to your torso, slowly bend your arms and lower your body down as far below the bars as possible. Slowly push yourself back up to the starting point and repeat the movement for the desired number of repetitions.

Lying Barbell Triceps Extensions

Emphasis: This is a good triceps isolation movement that stresses primarily the inner and medial triceps heads.

Starting Position: Take a narrow over-grip in the middle of a barbell handle (there should be about six inches of space between your index fingers). Lie back on a flat exercise bench, position your feet flat on the floor to balance your body in a secure position, and extend your arms straight up from your shoulders.

Movement Performance: Keeping your upper arms motionless, slowly bend your arms and lower the barbell in a semicircular arc from the starting point down to your forehead. After lightly touching your forehead with the bar, use triceps strength to push it back along the same

Lying Barbell Triceps Extensions—start, left; finish, right.

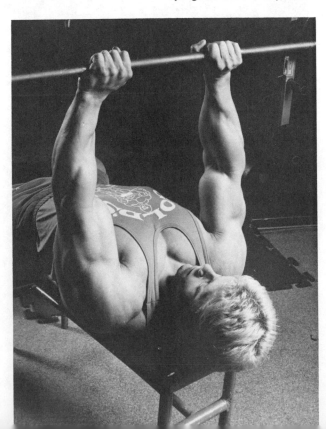

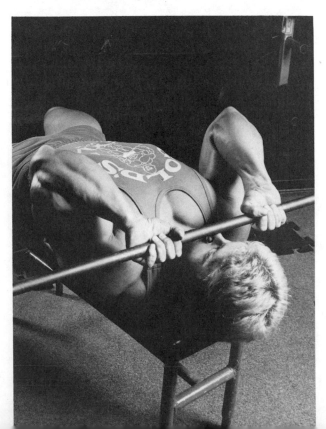

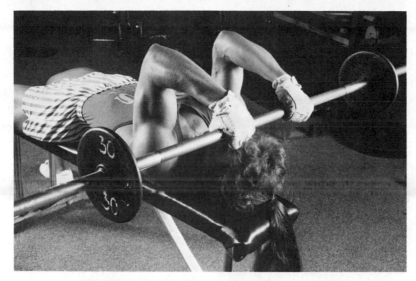

Reverse-Grip Lying Barbell Triceps Extension.

arc to the starting point. Repeat the movement for an appropriate number of repetitions.

Exercise Variations: You can vary the width of your grip on the barbell, and you can use a reversed grip on the bar. Reverse-Grip Lying Barbell Triceps Extensions place much greater stress on the long inner heads of your triceps.

Standing Barbell Triceps Extensions

Emphasis: Standing Triceps Extensions place primary stress on the inner and medial triceps heads, with secondary emphasis on the outer head of the triceps. This is a favorite upper-arm movement of Lou Ferrigno, a most successful bodybuilder and actor.

Starting Position: Take a narrow over-grip in the middle of a barbell handle (there should be about six inches of space showing between your index fingers). Place your feet a little wider than shoulder-width, flip the barbell up to straight arms' length above your head and stand erect.

Movement Performance: Keeping your upper arms motionless and in close to your ears, bend your arms and slowly lower the barbell downward in a semicircular arc until your arms are fully bent. Use triceps strength to return the barbell back along the same arc to the starting point and repeat the movement for the required number of repetitions.

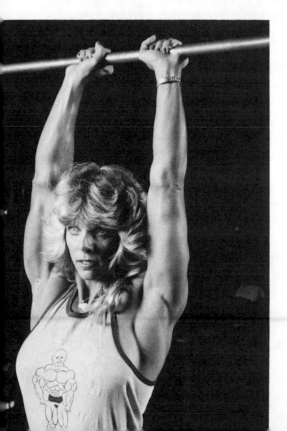

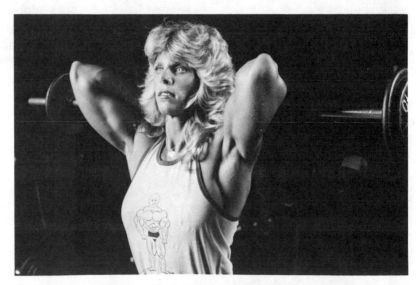

Standing Barbell Triceps Extension—start, left; finish, above.

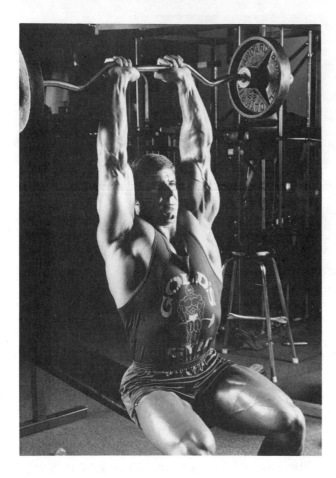

Seated Barbell Triceps Extension—start, above; finish, below.

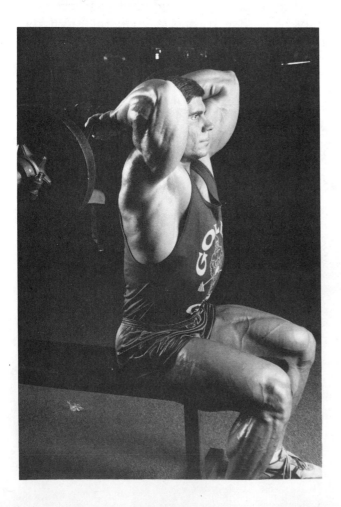

Exercise Variations: A very similar movement can be done while seated at the end of a flat exercise bench. This exercise is called Seated Triceps Extensions. With either variation of the movement, you can vary your grip inward until your hands are touching each other, or outward to about shoulder-width. You can also perform either movement with a reversed grip.

Incline/Decline Barbell Triceps Extensions

Emphasis: This movement is similar to Lying Triceps Extensions, but is performed on either an incline or decline bench. Both variations of the movement place primary stress on the inner and medial heads of your triceps and secondary emphasis on the outer head of your triceps.

Starting Position: Take a narrow over-grip in the middle of a barbell handle (there should be about six inches of space showing between your index fingers). Lie back on either an incline or decline bench and extend your arms straight up from your shoulders perpendicular to the floor.

Movement Performance: Keeping your upper arms motionless, slowly bend your arms and lower the barbell downward in a semicircular arc. With Incline Triceps Extensions, the bar can either lightly touch your forehead or the bench just behind your head; with Decline Triceps Extensions, the bar can touch either your forehead or chin. Use triceps power to push the bar back along the same arc to the starting point, and repeat the movement for the desired number of repetitions.

Exercise Variations: You can use various degrees of incline and decline benches, each giving your triceps a bit different type of stress. You can also use a variety of grip widths, as well as a reversed grip for either of these movements.

Kneeling Barbell Triceps Extension

Emphasis: This movement is very similar to Standing and Seated Barbell Triceps Extensions and it stresses primarily the inner and medial triceps heads, with secondary stress on the outer triceps heads. Kneeling makes it a very strict movement, however.

Starting Position: Take a narrow over-grip in the middle of a barbell handle (there should be about six inches of space showing between your

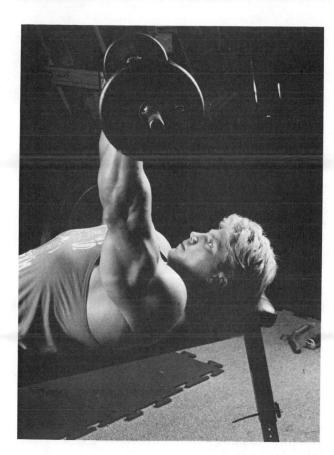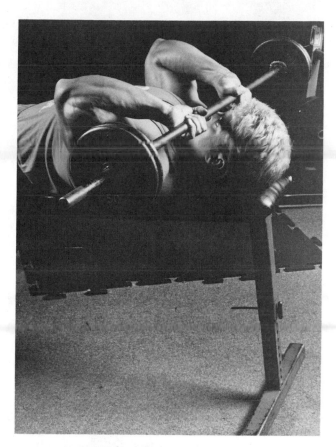

Incline Barbell Triceps Extension—start, left; finish, right.

Decline Barbell Triceps Extension.

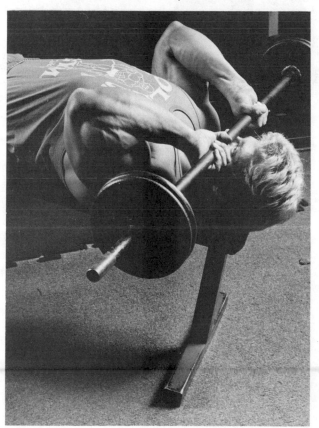

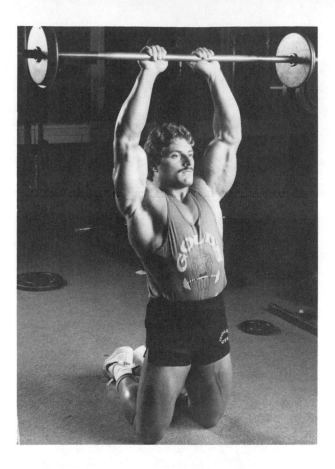

Kneeling Barbell Triceps Extension—start, above; finish, below.

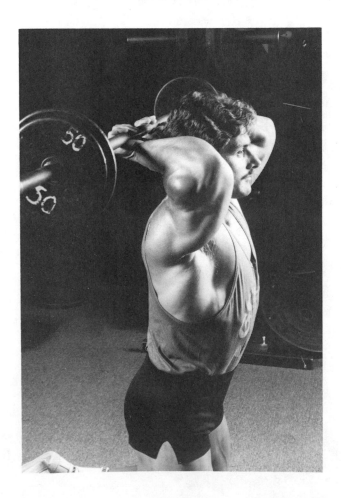

index fingers). Kneel down on the floor, either with your body erect on your knees, or sitting on your heels. Extend your arms directly above your head.

Movement Performance: Keeping your upper arms motionless and in close to your ears, bend your arms and slowly lower the barbell downward in a semicircular arc until your arms are fully bent. Use triceps strength to return the barbell back along the same arc to the starting point and repeat the movement for the suggested number of repetitions.

Exercise Variations: You can vary the width of your grip on the bar, plus use a reversed grip when you do Kneeling Barbell Triceps Extensions.

Pullover and Press

Emphasis: This is a unique compound movement that really puts the screws to the inner head of your triceps on the pullover part of the movement and to the outer head of your triceps on the pressing phase of the exercise. And throughout the movement, your medial triceps head is working. As a result, you will find the Pullover and Press movement to be one of the best all-around triceps exercises available.

Starting Position: Take a narrow over-grip on a moderately heavy barbell (there should be about six inches of space between your index fingers). Lie back on a flat exercise bench with your head at the end of the bench. Push the bar up to straight arms' length directly above your shoulder joints. Lower the bar to the middle of your chest.

Movement Performance: Keeping your elbows in toward the midline of your body, push the barbell up over your face and down in a semicircular arc to as low a position as is comfortably possible. Pull the bar back over to your chest and push it up to arms' length. Lower the bar back to your chest and repeat the movement for the suggested number of repetitions.

Training Tip: It would be most convenient if you could lift the bar off a support rack at the start of the movement, but the uprights of the rack would prevent you from doing the pullover part of the movement. Therefore, when you are using heavier weights, it's best to have a training partner hand you the bar at chest level.

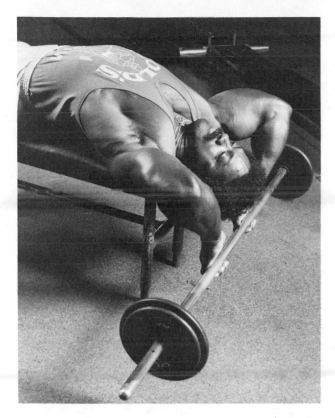 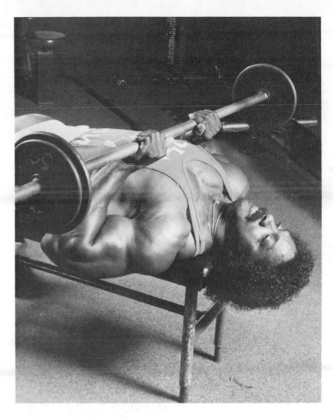

Pullover and Press—start, left; midpoint, right; finish, below.

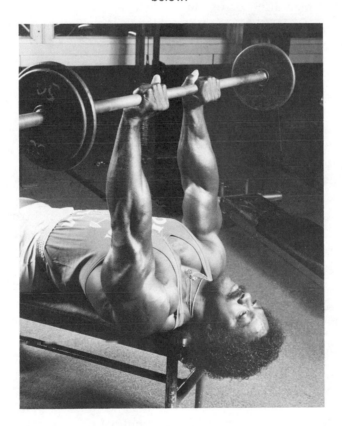

Exercise Variation: With somewhat lighter weights, you can do a similar movement with a Barbell Triceps Extension rather than the Narrow-Grip Bench Press as the second part of the movement. This Pullover and Triceps Extension is a favorite triceps movement of Andreas Cahling, the Swedish athlete who won the Mr. International title.

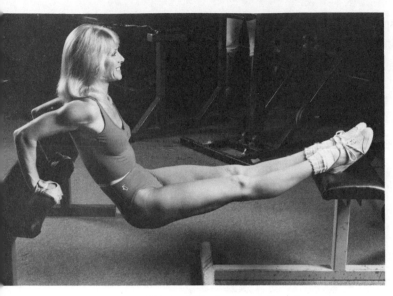

Triceps Dip between Benches.

Triceps Dips between Benches

Emphasis: This movement is good for stressing primarily the outer and medial heads of the triceps, with secondary emphasis on the inner triceps head.

Starting Position: Place two flat exercise benches about three feet apart (or, alternatively, place a flat exercise bench about three feet back from the knee restraint on a lat machine). Put your feet on one bench and your hands on the other (or the lat restraint) as illustrated. Your hands should be set about six inches apart, your fingers pointed toward your toes. Straighten your arms completely.

Movement Performance: Slowly bend your arms as fully as possible, lowering your body down between the benches. Push slowly back up to the starting point and repeat the movement for the suggested number of repetitions.

Training Tip: Obviously, this will be a relatively easy exercise to perform if you don't add resistance to it. You can add resistance to Triceps Dips by either having a training partner push down on your shoulders, or by having a light dumbbell or loose barbell plate placed in your lap for the exercise.

Dumbbell Triceps Extensions

Emphasis: All types of Dumbbell Triceps Extensions stress primarily the inner and medial heads of your triceps, with secondary emphasis on the outer head of the triceps.

Starting Position: Place your palms flat against the insides of the upper set of plates on a moderately heavy dumbbell, encircling the dumbbell handle with your thumbs to keep it from slipping out of your grasp. Set your feet about shoulder-width apart, stand erect, and extend your arms straight over your head. In the top position of the movement, the dumbbell should be hanging straight down from your hands, the handle of the dumbbell perpendicular to the floor.

Movement Performance: Without moving your upper arms and keeping them in close to your ears, slowly bend your arms and lower the dumbbell downward until your arms are completely bent. Slowly push the dumbbell back up to the starting point and repeat the movement for the required number of repetitions.

Exercise Variations: You can also do Dumbbell Triceps Extensions with a single dumbbell held in one hand. With this variation, you can lower the dumbbell both straight down to the rear and across the midline of your body. Or, you can do the movement with two light dumbbells held in your hands. All variations of Dumbbell Triceps Extensions can also be performed seated at the end of a flat exercise bench.

Lying Dumbbell Triceps Extensions

Emphasis: As with the standing or seated variations of this movement, Lying Dumbbell Triceps Extensions stress primarily the inner and medial heads of your triceps, with secondary emphasis on the outer head of the triceps.

Starting Position: Grasp two light dumbbells in your hands and lie back on a flat exercise bench, positioning your feet flat on the floor to balance your body in position on the bench during the exercise. Extend your arms straight up from your shoulders, your palms facing toward each other.

Movement Performance: Keeping your upper arms motionless, bend your arms and lower the dumbbells to the rear in semicircular arcs to as low a position as possible. Use triceps strength to return the weights back along the same arcs to the starting point. Repeat the exercise for an appropriate number of repetitions.

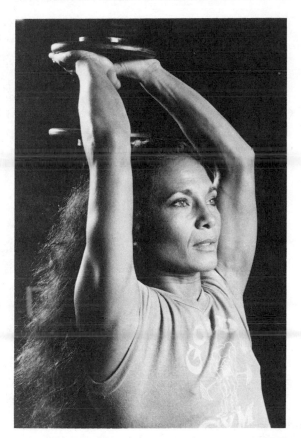
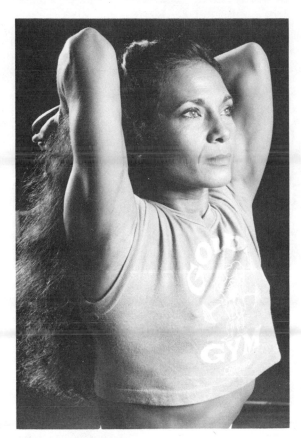

Dumbbell Triceps Extension—start, left; near finish, right.

Lying Dumbbell Triceps Extensions—start, left; finish, right.

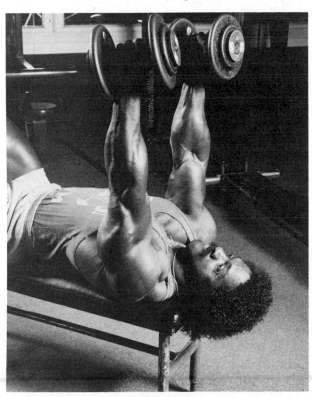
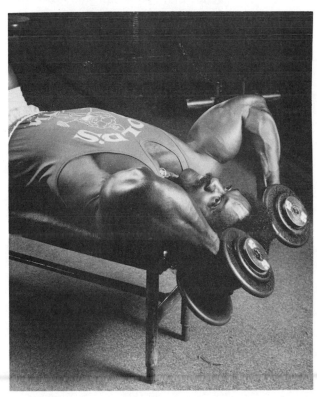

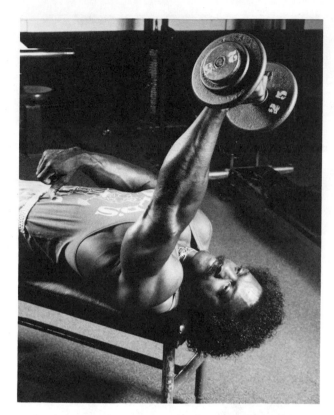 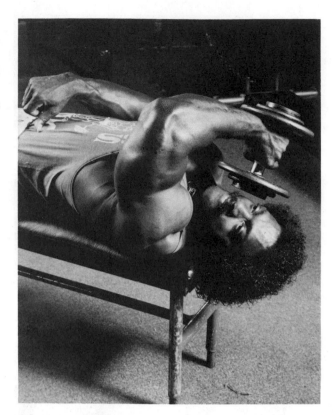

Lying Dumbbell Triceps Extension (one dumbbell)—
start, left; finish, right.

Exercise Variations: You can also do this movement with your palms facing forward at the start of the movement. Both hand variations can be accompanied by a pullover movement at the start of each repetition. Finally, you can do Lying Dumbbell Triceps Extensions one arm at a time, lowering the dumbbell across your body.

Pulley Pushdowns

Emphasis: This is one of the best movements for developing the outer head of your triceps. Secondary stress is on the medial and inner triceps heads.

Starting Position: Attach a short-angled handle to the end of a cable running through an overhead pulley. Take an overgrip on the handle with your hands as close together as possible. Step about a foot back from the pulley, bend your arms fully, press your upper arms against the sides of your torso throughout the movement, and lean slightly toward the cable.

Movement Performance: Moving only your forearms, slowly push the handle downward in a semicircular arc until it rests across your upper thighs and your arms are locked out straight. Slowly return the handle to the starting point, and repeat the movement for the suggested number of repetitions.

Exercise Variations: You can do this movement with a rope handle, which gives you a parallel grip; or you can do it with a longer, straight-bar handle. You can also use a reversed grip on the straight-bar handle. Another variation allows you to move your elbows out to the sides and completely bend your arms at the top of the movement, then push the handle downward until your arms are straight, somewhat like doing a Narrow-Grip Bench Press. This variation is particularly good when forcing out a few extra reps after you've failed a rep in the normal manner. With all variations just discussed, you can change the width of your grip. Finally, you can attach a loop handle to the end of a cable and perform One-Arm Pushdowns with either an over-grip or an under-grip.

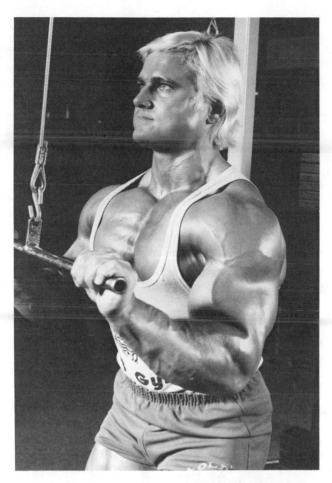 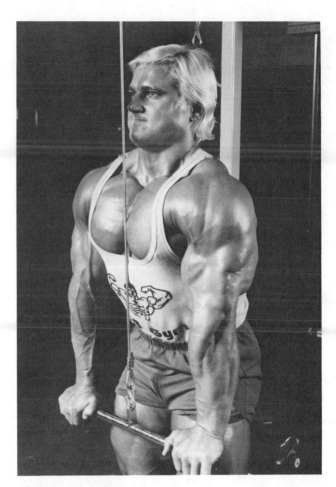

Pulley Pushdown—start, left; finish, right.

One-Arm Pulley Pushdown—start, left; finish, right.

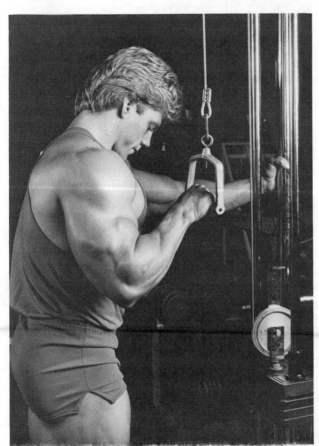 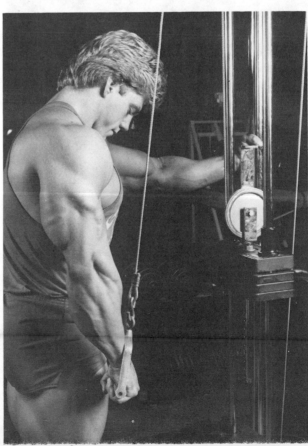

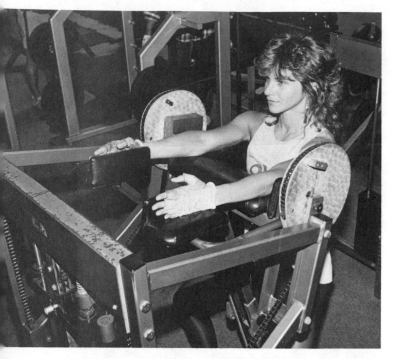

Nautilus Triceps Extension.

Nautilus Triceps Extensions

Emphasis: This exercise seems to stress all three heads of the triceps quite hard. It's one of the best triceps exercises for use with the peak-contraction training technique.

Starting Position: You will need first to adjust the seat to a height that allows your arms to assume the same angle as the large pad in front of you when you sit down. Place your wrists against the pads on the movement arm of the machine, sit down, run your upper arms up the pad in front of you, and bend your arms fully.

Movement Performance: Slowly straighten your arms fully, hold this peak-contracted position for a moment, and lower back to the starting point. Repeat the movement for the suggested number of repetitions.

Exercise Variations: You can do this movement in alternate arm fashion by first straighten-

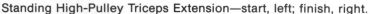

Standing High-Pulley Triceps Extension—start, left; finish, right.

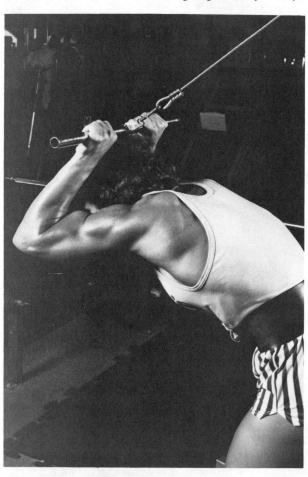

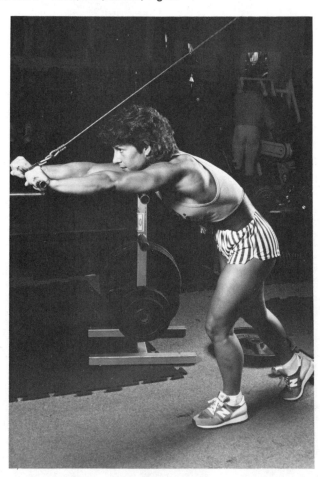

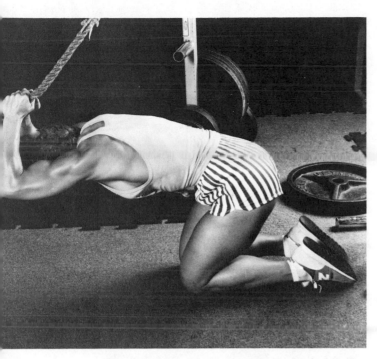

Kneeling High-Pulley Triceps Extension—start, above; finish, right.

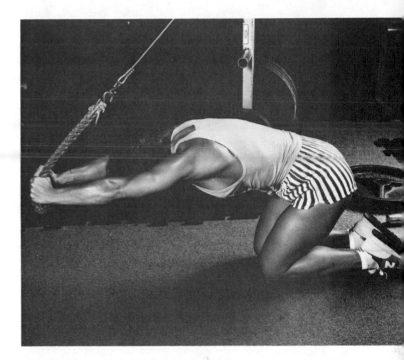

ing both arms, then by holding your right arm straight while you fully bend and then straighten your left arm. Then hold your left arm straight while you fully bend and straighten your right arm. Alternate arms in this fashion until you have fully fatigued your triceps on both arms.

Standing High-Pulley Triceps Extensions

Emphasis: This version of Pulley Triceps Extensions strongly stresses the inner and medial triceps heads. Secondary stress is on the outer heads of your triceps.

Starting Position: Attach a bar handle to a cable running through a pulley set about six feet above the floor. Take a narrow over-grip on the handle and face away from the pulley. Split your legs fore and aft to steady your body in a secure position as you perform the movement and bend

your arms completely. Lean forward to take the weight of the machine, preferably holding your torso slightly above a parallel position with the floor.

Movement Performance: Slowly straighten your arms, return to the starting position, and repeat the movement for the required number of repetitions.

Exercise Variations: You can do a very similar type of movement called Kneeling High-Pulley Triceps Extensions. With this exercise, you use the same pulley and handle, plus a flat exercise bench placed crosswise in front of you. Facing away from the pulley, grasp the pulley handle, kneel down facing the flat exercise bench, bend your arms fully, and lean forward to rest your elbows on the bench. Then you can do your Triceps Extensions quite conveniently in this position.

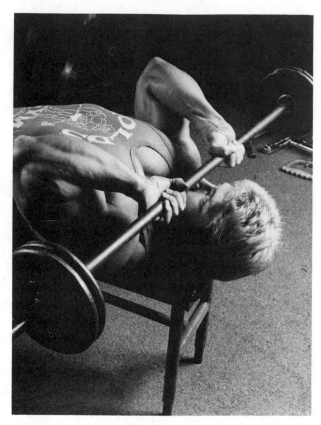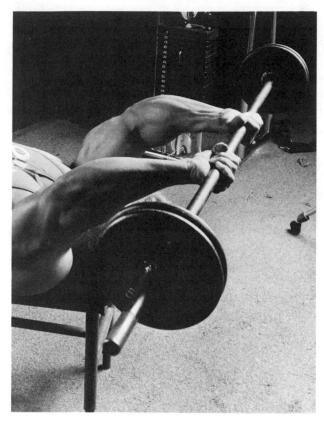

Barbell Kickback—start, left; finish, right.

Barbell Kickbacks

Emphasis: Barbell Kickbacks are an excellent outer and medial triceps exercise.

Starting Position: Take a shoulder-width over-grip on a light barbell and lie back on a flat exercise bench, balancing your body in position by placing your feet flat on the floor. Bend your arms fully and rest the barbell on your chest.

Movement Performance: Simultaneously straighten your arms and push the barbell directly back to the rear horizontal to the floor until your arms are fully straight, as in the finish position for a Stiff-Arm Pullover. Return slowly back to the starting point, and repeat the movement for an appropriate number of repetitions.

Dumbbell Kickbacks

Emphasis: Dumbbell Kickbacks are also an excellent outer and medial triceps exercise. And it's particularly good for use of peak contraction on your triceps.

Starting Position: Grasp a light dumbbell in your right hand with your palm toward your body throughout the movement. Split your left foot forward and right foot to the rear a little. Bend over until your torso is parallel to the floor and place your left hand on a flat exercise bench to maintain this torso position. Pin your right upper arm to the side of your torso with your upper arm parallel to the floor. Bend your right arm at a right angle.

Movement Performance: Slowly straighten your right arm, hold that position for a moment to intensify the peak-contraction effect, lower back to the starting point, and repeat the movement for the desired number of repetitions. Be sure to do an equal number of sets and repetitions for each arm.

Exercise Variations: You can also do this movement with two dumbbells simultaneously by simply bending over until your torso is parallel to the floor. And you can do a very similar, two-armed movement lying facedown on an incline bench.

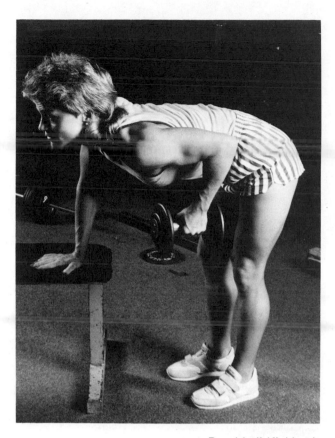 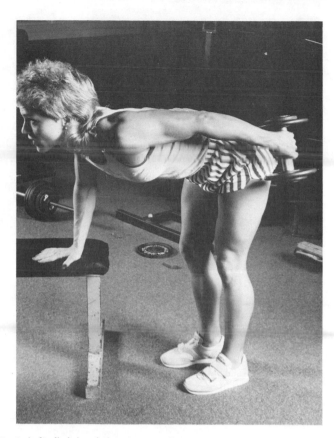

Dumbbell Kickback—start, left; finish, right.

Incline Dumbbell Kickback at finish.

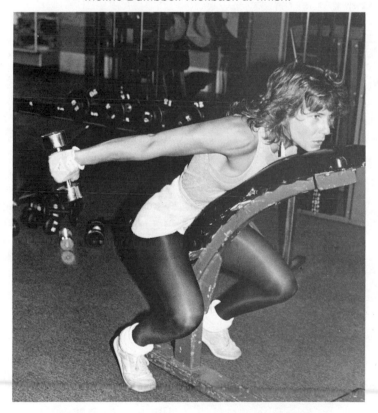

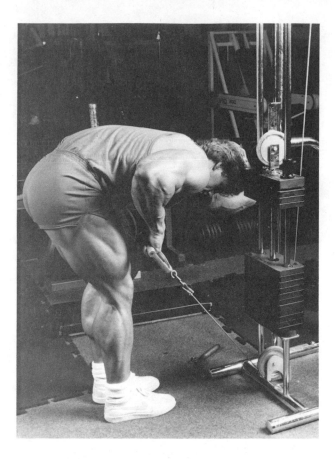

Cable Kickback—start, above; finish, below.

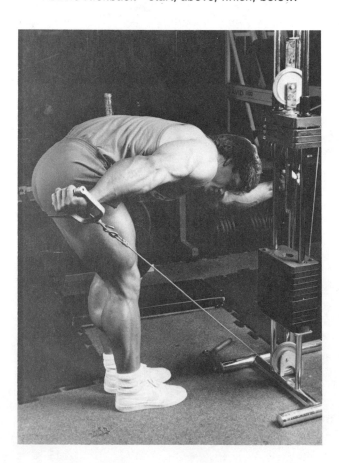

Cable Kickbacks

Emphasis: Cable Kickbacks are more of an inner-head triceps movement than one for the outer head.

Starting Position: Attach a loop handle to the cable running through a floor pulley and grasp the handle with your right hand. Back up a step and face toward the pulley. Bend over at the waist until your torso is parallel to the floor, bend your arm completely, and press your right upper arm against the side of your torso.

Movement Performance: Slowly straighten your arm, return to the starting position, and repeat the movement. Be sure to do the same number of sets and reps for each arm.

Suggested Triceps Routines

If you have less than a few weeks of training behind you, the following triceps routine can profitably be performed three nonconsecutive days per week:

Exercise	Sets	Reps
Lying Barbell Triceps Extensions	3	8–12
Pulley Pushdowns	2	8–12

After 4–6 weeks of steady training on the foregoing program, you can use this triceps routine three days per week:

Exercise	Sets	Reps
Close-Grip Bench Presses	3	6–10
Dumbbell Triceps Extensions	3	8–12
Dumbbell Kickbacks	2	8–12

After about three months of steady training, you should switch to a four-day split routine in which you train each major muscle group (including triceps) twice per week. This is typically how a lower-level competitive bodybuilder will work out in the off-season. Following is a sample triceps training program for off-season competition training:

Exercise	Sets	Reps
Triceps Parallel Bar Dips	4	6–10
Incline Barbell Triceps Extensions	3	8–12
Lying Dumbbell Triceps Extensions	3	8–12
Dumbbell Kickbacks	2	8–12

Every advanced bodybuilder trains differently from all others prior to a competition, as you will see in the following section listing the biceps routines of a wide variety of men and women who either train or have trained at Gold's Gym.

Triceps Routines of the Gold's Champs

In this section, you will find a variety of triceps training programs used by many of the Gold's Gym superstars who have won the sport's highest titles. Keep in mind as you examine these training programs that these men have been training for many years and have developed enormous recuperative powers. It is unlikely that you can make good gains using their full routines unless you have similiar experience. Instead, you should use these training programs as examples of how to work your own triceps. In all likelihood, you can do the same exercises as your favorite champion, but scale down the number of sets that he or she does of each movement to meet your own unique abilities.

ROBBY ROBINSON
(MR. UNIVERSE)

Exercise	Sets	Reps
Standing High-Pulley		
Triceps Extensions	4	8-10
One-Arm Dumbbell		
Triceps Extensions	4	8-10
One-Arm Pulley Pushdowns	4	8-10

KAY BAXTER
(GOLD'S CLASSIC CHAMP)

Exercise	Sets	Reps
Triceps Parallel Bar Dips	5	8-12
Incline Barbell Triceps		
Extensions	5	8-12
Pulley Pushdowns	4	15
Dumbbell Kickbacks	4	15
Triceps Dips between Benches	3-4	max

MIKE MENTZER
(MR. UNIVERSE)

Exercise	Sets	Reps
Pulley Pushdowns	1-2	6-8
Triceps Parallel Bar Dips	1-2	6-8
Lying Barbell Triceps		
Extensions	1-2	6-8
Nautilus Triceps Extensions	1-2	6-8

Note: On all exercises, one or two forced reps are performed at the end of each set.

TIM BELKNAP (MR. AMERICA)

Exercise	Sets	Reps
Close-Grip Bench Presses	3	10-12
Decline Barbell Triceps		
Extensions	3	10-12
Pulley Pushdowns	3	10-12

CASEY VIATOR
(MR. AMERICA)

Exercise	Sets	Reps
Lying Barbell Triceps		
Extensions	4-5	10-12
One-Arm Dumbbell Triceps		
Extensions	4	10-12
Dumbbell Kickbacks	4	10-12
Seated Barbell Triceps		
Extensions	4	10-12

COREY EVERSON
(NORTH AMERICAN CHAMPION)

Exercise	Sets	Reps
Pulley Pushdowns	3	10-15
One-Arm Pulley Extensions	3	10-15
Triceps Parallel Bar Dips	3	max
Close-Grip Bench Presses		
(sometimes)	3	8-12

ANDREAS CAHLING
(MR. INTERNATIONAL)

Exercise	Sets	Reps
Pullover and Press	3-4	8-12
Nautilus Triceps Extensions	2-4	8-12
or		
Dumbbell Kickbacks	2-4	8-12

Exercise model Julie Stangl.

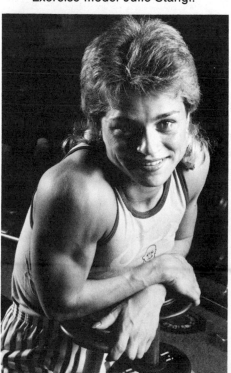

TOM PLATZ
(MR. UNIVERSE)

Exercise	Sets	Reps
Close-Grip Bench Presses	4–5	8–10
Seated Barbell Triceps Extensions	4–5	8–10
Pulley Pushdowns	4–5	8–10

LOU FERRIGNO
(MR. UNIVERSE)

Exercise	Sets	Reps
Pulley Pushdowns	5	8–10
Lying Barbell Triceps Extensions	5	8–10
Seated Barbell Triceps Extensions	5	8–10

MATT MENDENHALL
(MR. CENTRAL STATES)

Exercise	Sets	Reps
Seated Triceps Extensions (EZ-Curl bar)	4	8
Lying Triceps Extensions (EZ-Curl bar)	4	8
Pulley Pushdowns	4	8
Lying One-Arm Triceps Extensions	4	8

SAMIR BANNOUT
(MR. OLYMPIA)

Exercise	Sets	Reps
Close-Grip Bench Presses	4–5	6–10
Lying Barbell Triceps Extensions	3–4	8–10
Seated Dumbbell Triceps Extensions	3–4	8–10
Pulley Pushdowns	3	8–10
Dumbbell Kickbacks	2–3	10–12

LAURA COMBES
(MS. AMERICA)

Exercise	Sets	Reps
Pulley Pushdowns	4–5	8–12
Triceps Parallel Bar Dips	4	8–10
Standing One-Arm Dumbbell Extensions	4	8–10
Dumbbell Kickbacks	4	8–10

STEVE DAVIS
(MR. WORLD)

Exercise	Sets	Reps
Pulley Pushdowns	4	12
Lying Triceps Extensions (EZ-curl bar)	3	10
Standing High-Pulley Extensions	3	8–12
Triceps Parallel Bar Dips	3	8–12
Triceps Dips between Benches	3	15–20

JUSUP WILKOSZ
(PRO MR. UNIVERSE)

Exercise	Sets	Reps
Pulley Pushdowns	5	10–12
Triceps Parallel Bar Dips	5	10–12
One-Arm Dumbbell Triceps Extensions	5	10–12
One-Arm Cable Extensions	5	10–12

RAY MENTZER
(MR. AMERICA)

Exercise	Sets	Reps
Pulley Pushdowns	1–2	6–8
Triceps Parallel Bar Dips	1–2	6–8
Nautilus Triceps Extensions	1–2	6–8

Note: Forced reps are done at the end of each set.

RACHEL McLISH
(MISS OLYMPIA)

Exercise	Sets	Reps
Pulley Pushdowns	3	6–8
Nautilus Triceps Extensions	2–3	6–8
Seated Dumbbell Triceps Extensions	2–3	6–8

Note: Forced reps are performed at the end of each set.

RON TEUFEL
(TEENAGE MR. AMERICA)

Exercise	Sets	Reps
Close-Grip Bench Presses	5	10–12
Pulley Pushdowns	5	10–12
Standing High-Pulley Triceps Extensions	4	8–10
Lying Barbell Triceps Extensions	4	8–10

DEBORAH DIANA
(MS. USA)

Exercise	Sets	Reps
Lying Barbell Triceps Extensions	1	10–15
Triceps Parallel Bar Dips	1	10–15
Pulley Pushdowns	1	10–15

Note: These three exercises are performed as a tri set.

LISA ELLIOTT-KOLAKOWSKI
(MS. EASTERN AMERICA)

Exercise	Sets	Reps
Triceps Parallel Bar Dips	4	6–8
Lying Barbell Triceps Extensions	4	6–8
Seated Dumbbell Triceps Extensions	4	6–8
Pulley Pushdowns	4	6–8

BILL GRANT
(PRO MR. WORLD)

Exercise	Sets	Reps
Pulley Pushdowns	3	8–10
Nautilus Triceps Extensions	3	8–10
Standing Barbell Triceps Extensions	3	8–10

KENT KEUHN
(PAST-40 MR. UNIVERSE)

Exercise	Sets	Reps
Pulley Pushdowns	5	10–12
Triceps Dips between Benches	5	10–12
Lying Barbell Triceps Extensions	5	10–12
One-Arm Dumbbell Triceps Extensions	5	10–12

RORY LIEDELMEYER
(MR. CALIFORNIA)

Exercise	Sets	Reps
Pulley Pushdowns	4	10–12
One-Arm Pushdowns (reverse grip)	4	10–12
Lying Barbell Triceps Extensions	4	8–10
Standing High-Pulley Triceps Extensions	4	10–15

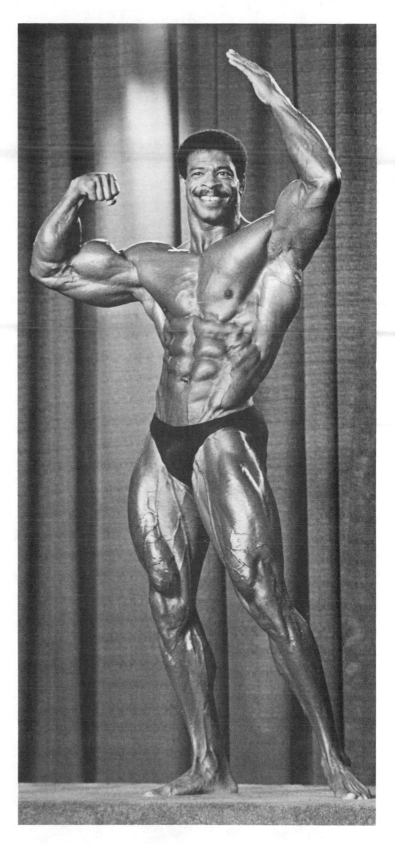

Bill Grant.

PAT NEVE
(MR. USA)

Exercise	Sets	Reps
Dumbbell Triceps Extensions	4	8–12
Lying Barbell Triceps Extensions	4	8–12
Pulley Pushdowns	4	8–12

SERGIO OLIVA
(MR. OLYMPIA)

Exercise	Sets	Reps
Standing Barbell Triceps Extensions	6	8
Pulley Pushdowns	6	8
Pulley Kickbacks	6	8

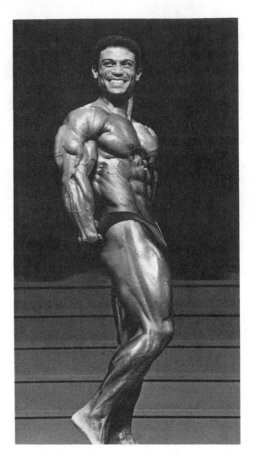

Mohamed Makkawy.

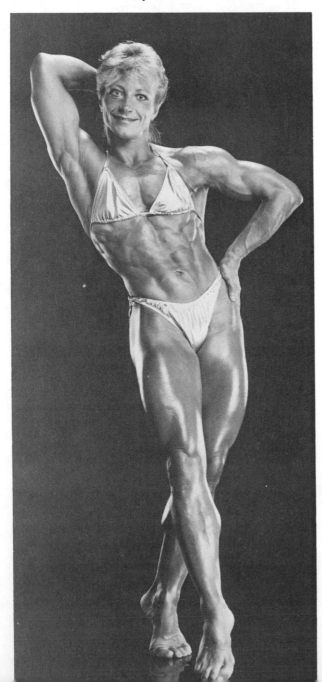

Kay Baxter.

MANUEL PERRY
(MR. USA)

Exercise	Sets	Reps
Pulley Pushdowns	5	12–15
Standing Barbell Triceps Extensions	5	12–15
One-Arm Dumbbell Triceps Extensions	5	12–15
Cable Triceps Extensions	5	12–15

DALE RUPLINGER
(MR. UNIVERSE)

Exercise	Sets	Reps
Lying Barbell Triceps Extensions	4–5	6–10
Pulley Pushdowns	4–5	8–12

Looking Ahead

In Chapter 8, we'll discuss how to train your abdominal muscles. Our discussion will include more than 20 exercises, plus more routines of the top men and women who train at the Hall of Champions, Gold's Gym!

8
ABDOMINAL TRAINING

The abdominal muscle group is very important to competitive bodybuilders because a judge's eye is naturally drawn first to the middle of a man or woman's body. And if the abs are tight and muscular, the judge gains a favorable first impression that can linger through the rest of prejudging.

The condition of your midsection is also a good indication of your health and overall physical condition. Certainly a protruding, flabby midsection does not speak well for the general health and fitness of any man or woman. But, a trim and well-muscled abdomen tells everyone who sees you that you are in outstanding shape, even if they fail to notice the massive arms, chest, back, shoulders, and legs that you carry around with you.

Most male bodybuilders, even men weighing upwards of 225 pounds in contest condition have outstanding abdominal development. While great abs weren't that important prior to about 1970, very few bodybuilders in recent years have won important titles without having superior abdominal development. Some men with truly exceptional abs are Andreas Cahling, Albert Beckles, Tim Belknap, Dr. Franco Columbu, Frank Zane, Gerard Buinoud, Steve Davis, Greg

DeFerro, Tony Emmott, Charles Glass, Bill Grant, Larry Jackson, Bob Jodkiewicz, Jon Loyd, Mohamed Makkawy, Ron Teufel, and Dennis Tinerino.

It seems to be a bit more difficult for women to achieve outstanding abdominal development, but many top women still display phenomenally sharp abs. Some of the best feminine abdominal development belongs to Shelley Gruwell, Rachel McLish, Carla Dunlap, Kike Elomaa, Laura Combes, Lynn Conkwright, Candy Csencsits, Deborah Diana, and Lisa Elliott-Kolakowski.

Anatomy and Kinesiology

There are three muscle groups in the abdominals. The first of these is the *rectus abdominis,* the wall of muscle that covers the front of the abdomen and gives your abs a washboard appearance. The rectus abdominis helps to flex your torso forward at the waist. When it contracts, it pulls your hips toward your shoulders.

The second important muscle group is the *obliques* at the sides of your waist. This group is usually called the *external obliques,* although there are really three layers of muscle there including the external, internal, and transverse oblique muscles. The obliques contract to both bend your torso to the side and to help you twist your torso in relation to your hips.

The final abdominal muscle group is the *intercostals,* which run diagonally across your sides above the obliques. Your intercostals run from the top of your obliques up to the serratus muscles of your chest, and they contract to help flex your body at the waist and twist your torso in relation to your hips and legs.

Abdominal Exercises

In this section you will find nearly 20 major abdominal movements, each fully described and illustrated. Add in the numerous variations of each basic exercise, and you will have more than 30 exercises in your basic pool of bodybuilding movements.

Sit-Ups

Emphasis: When you perform Sit-Ups, you primarily stress the rectus abdominis muscle wall. And when you do the movement with a twist, you place significant stress on your intercostals as well.

Starting Position: Lie on your back on an adjustable abdominal board, your feet at the upper end. Hook your toes under the strap or roller pads at the end of the board. Bend your legs slightly and keep them bent throughout the movement in order to protect your lower back from undue strain. Either fold your arms across your chest or interlace your fingers behind your head and neck during the exercise.

Movement Performance: Curl your torso off the board by first lifting your head, then shoulders, upper back, and lower back until your torso is perpendicular to the floor. Reverse the procedure to return to the starting point.

Training Tips: You can increase the intensity of this exercise by either holding a light barbell plate behind your head or by incrementally raising the foot end of the abdominal board.

Exercise Variations: You can do this exercise twisting to alternate sides on successive repetitions. You can also do a Sit-Up movement with continuous tension on your abdominal muscles by not letting your torso come to rest on the bench and then sitting upward only until your torso is at approximately a 60-degree angle to the floor.

Roman Chair Sit-Ups

Emphasis: Roman Chair Sit-Ups stress the entire front abdominal wall, particularly the upper section of the rectus abdominis muscle group.

Starting Position: Sit on the bench seat facing toward the toe restraint and wedge your toes and insteps beneath the restraining bar. Cross your arms over your chest and keep them in this position throughout the movement.

Movement Performance: Sit backward with your torso until it is approximately at a 30-degree angle with the floor. Sit forward only until you begin to feel tension coming off of your abdominal muscles, then move back to the low position. Rock back and forth along this short range of motion for the required number of repetitions.

Training Tips: You can increase resistance on your abdominal muscles by placing a 4 × 4-inch block of wood beneath the foot end of the apparatus, by holding a light barbell plate on your chest, or by holding over your shoulders a rope handle attached to a floor pulley behind you. This third variation of adding resistance is a favorite of Rachel McLish, winner of two Miss Olympia titles.

Exercise Variations: You can do this movement with your hands held behind your head rather than across your chest. Regardless of the hand and arm position, you can do the movement twisting alternately from side to side.

Leg Raises

Emphasis: All Leg Raise movements stress the entire front abdominal wall, particularly the lower sections of the rectus abdominis.

Starting Position: Lie on your back on an adjustable abdominal board with your head toward the upper end of the board. Reach back and grasp either the roller pads or the edges of the board to secure your upper body in position as you do the exercise. Bend your legs slightly and keep them bent throughout your set in order

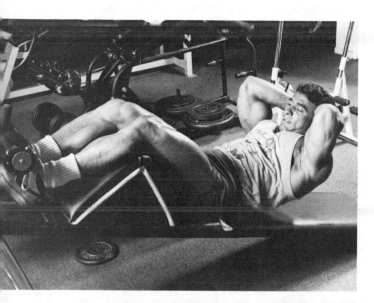
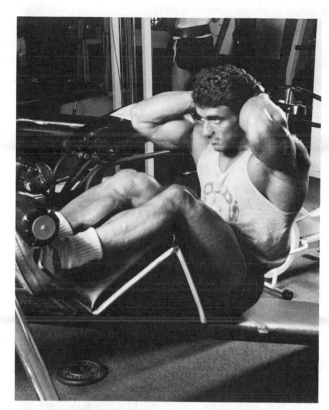

Sit-Up—start, left; finish, right.

Roman Chair Sit-Up—start, left; finish, right.

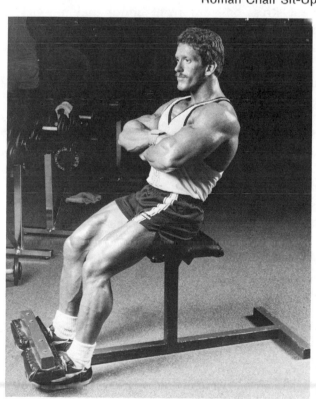
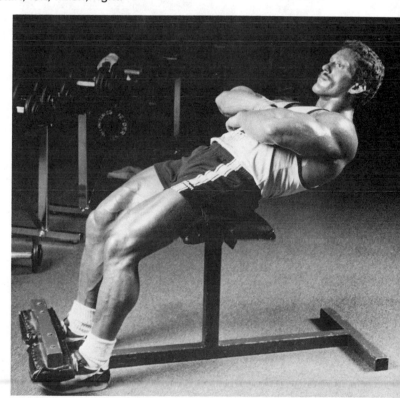

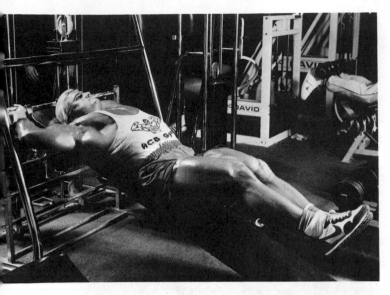

Training Tips: Not touching your heels to the abdominal board at the bottom of each rep is half of what you should do to keep continuous tension on your front abdominal muscles. The other half of the key to continuous tension is raising your legs only up to the point where your thighs are at a 45-degree angle with the floor. You can add to the intensity of Leg Raises either by incrementally raising the head end of the bench or by holding a light dumbbell between your feet.

Bench Leg Raises

Comment: This movement is similar to Leg Raises performed on an abdominal board, except that they are performed while lying back on a flat exercise bench or a pressing bench and holding the sides of the bench or the upright supports in the pressing bench to steady your torso in a secure position during the exercise. The advantage to Bench Leg Raises is that you can lower your feet below the level of your body to increase the range of motion of the exercise.

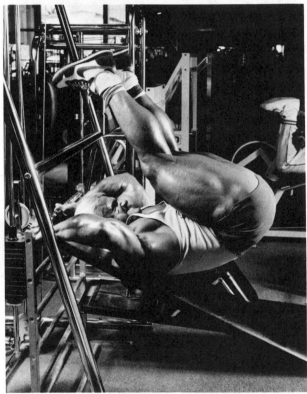

Leg Raise—start, top; finish, bottom.

Hanging Leg Raises

Emphasis: This very intense movement places great stress on your front abdominal muscles, particularly the lower third of the rectus abdominis.

Starting Position: Jump up and take a shoulder-width over-grip on a chinning bar. Hang your body straight down from the bar, but bend your legs slightly and keep them bent throughout the movement to remove undue strain from your lower back.

Movement Performance: Using abdominal strength, slowly raise your feet in a semicircular arc from the starting point to the level of your hips. At the top point of the movement, your thighs should be above a line drawn parallel to the floor through your hips. Return to the starting point and repeat the movement for the desired number of repetitions.

Training Tips: Many bodybuilders have difficulty with their body swaying back and forth beneath the bar during a set. If this is a problem for you, have a training partner steady you in position by grasping the sides of your waist or hips.

to keep undue strain off of your lower back.

Movement Performance: Use abdominal strength to move your feet in a semicircular arc from the bench to a point directly above your hips. Return your feet slowly back to a point only one inch from the abdominal board and repeat the movement for the required number of repetitions.

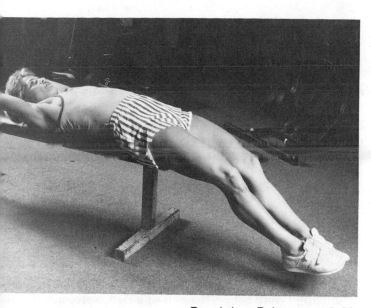
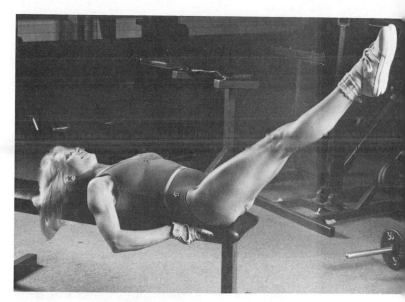

Bench Leg Raise—start (with arms at head of bench), left; finish
(with hands holding side of bench), right.

Hanging Leg Raise—start, left; finish, right.

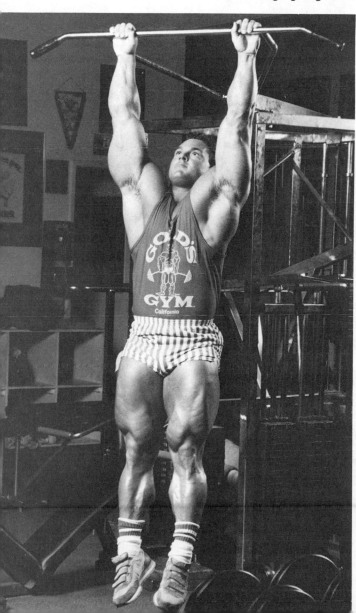
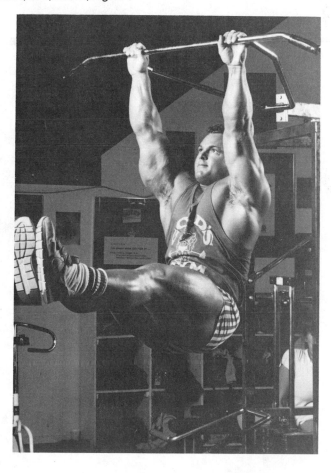

Exercise Variations: For a super-intense form of Hanging Leg Raise, try raising your feet up to the level of your shoulders or hands. On all types of Hanging Leg Raises, you can twist your legs in relation to your torso on alternate reps to add stress to your intercostals.

Parallel Bar Leg Raises

Emphasis: As with all forms of Leg Raises, this movement stresses the entire front abdominal wall, particularly the lower part of the rectus abdominis.

Starting Point: Most bigger gyms have a special apparatus for performing this movement. Step up on the foot platforms facing away from the back pad. Place your elbows and forearms on the pads provided for them, brace your back against the inclined backboard, and lift your feet from the platforms. Press your legs together and

bend them slightly during the movement to reduce potentially harmful stress on your lower back.

Movement Performance: Slowly raise your feet upward in a semicircular arc until your thighs are above an imaginary line drawn parallel to the floor through your hips. Lower your feet back to the starting point and repeat the movement for the preferred number of repetitions.

Knee-Ups

Emphasis: This low-intensity exercise places stress on your front abdominals, particularly on the lower parts of your rectus abdominis.

Starting Point: Sit on the end of a flat exercise bench and lean back until your torso is at a 45-degree angle with the floor and bench. Grasp the edges of the bench to steady your torso in the

Parallel Bar Leg Raises—start, left; finish, right.

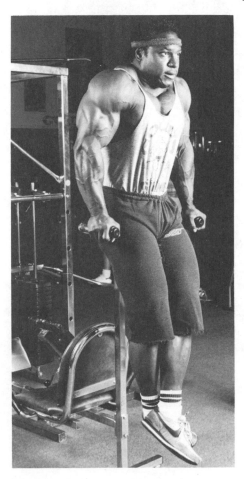
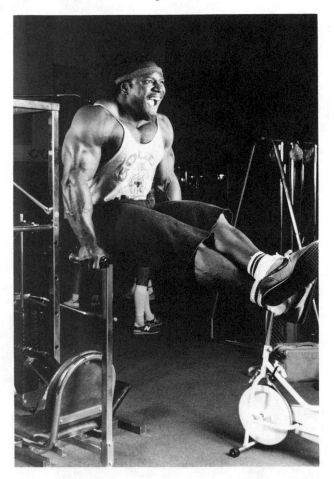

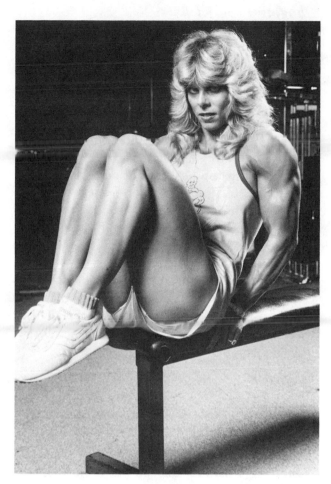

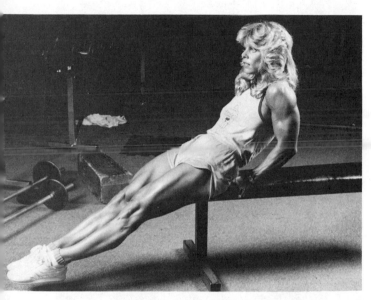

Knee-Up—start, left; finish, right.

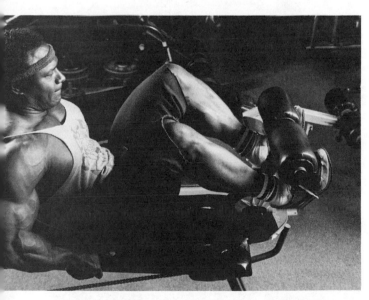

Knee-Up on Leg Extension Machine.

position throughout the movement. Extend your legs so they make one long line with your torso. Your feet should be just above the level of the floor at the start of the movement.

Movement Performance: Simultaneously pull your knees up to your chest and bend your legs completely. Just as your knees come up to your chest, incline your head toward them. Return to the starting point and repeat the movement for the required number of reps.

Training Tip: You can add resistance to this movement by holding a light dumbbell between your feet.

Exercise Variation: To add great stress to your abs, you can do this movement sitting at a leg-extension table and hooking your insteps under the roller pads. Be sure that your hips are right at the edge of the bench, then pull your knees up to your chest while dragging the weighted roller pads upward with your toes.

Hanging Frog Kicks

Emphasis: Frog Kicks are similar to Knee-Ups, but they provide significantly greater tension to your lower abdominals.

Starting Position: Jump up and take a shoulder-width over-grip on a chinning bar. Hang your body straight down from the bar.

Movement Performance: Simultaneously pull your knees up to your chest and fully bend your legs. Hold this top position for a moment, lower back to the starting point and repeat the exercise for an appropriate number of reps.

Training Tip: You can get your intercostals into the movement by twisting from side to side on successive reps.

Exercise Variation: A movement similar to Hanging Frog Kicks can be done on the same apparatus as you used for Parallel Bar Leg Raises.

Crunches

Emphasis: Crunches are one of the most direct exercises for stressing the front abdominal muscles, particularly for the upper section of your rectus abdominis.

Starting Position: Lie on your back on the gym floor and drape your lower legs over a flat exercise bench with your thighs perpendicular to the floor. Place your hands behind your head and neck and hold them there until the end of your set.

Movement Performance: You must do four things simultaneously to correctly perform the Crunch movement:

- force your shoulders toward your hips,
- use lower abdominal strength to raise your hips from the floor,
- use upper abdominal strength to raise your head and shoulders from the floor, and
- forcefully blow out all of your air.

When you perform these four tasks correctly, you will feel a very powerful contraction in your front abdominal wall. Hold this contraction for a moment, lower back to the starting point, and repeat the movement.

Exercise Variations: You can perform Wall Crunches in which you lie on the floor with your butt in the corner formed by the floor and a wall, and with your legs running straight up the wall.

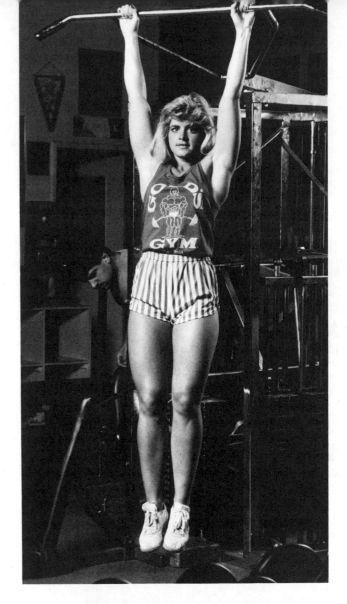

Hanging Frog Kick—start, above; finish, below.

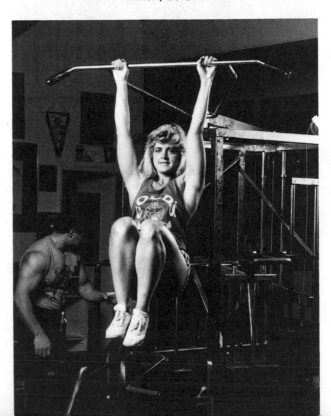

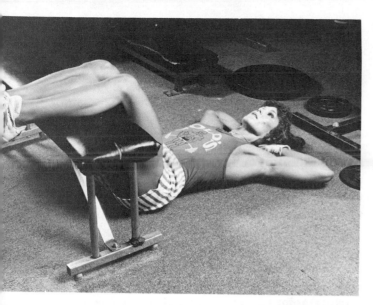
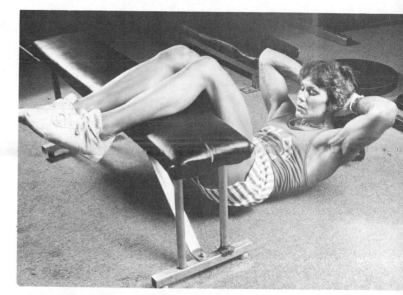

Crunch—start, left; finish, right.

Wall Crunch, left; "L" Crunch, right.

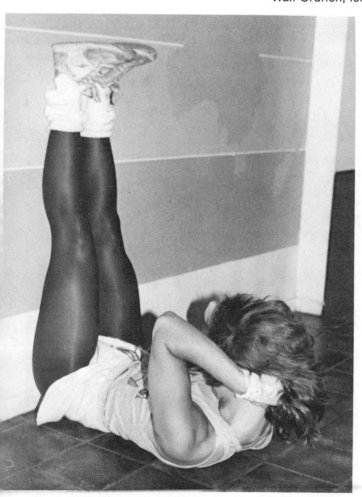
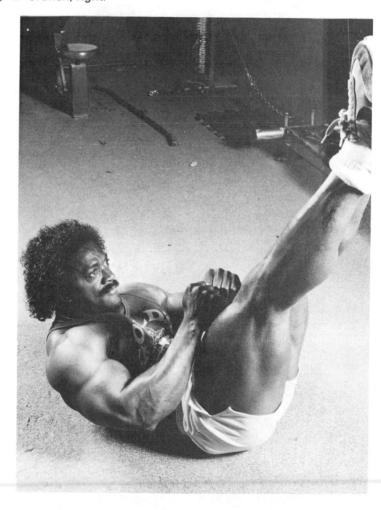

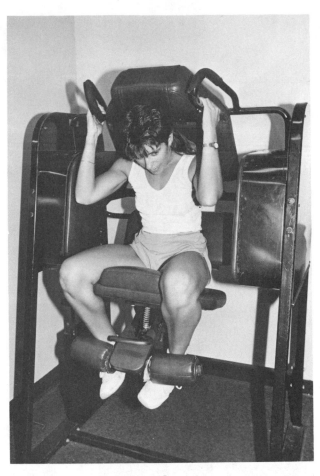

Nautilus Crunch.

You can do a similar movement while lying on your back on the floor and holding your legs straight up from your hips, making an "L" with your legs and torso.

Nautilus Crunches

Emphasis: This machine gives you a convenient method of adding heavy resistance to the Crunch movement. This allows you to place very heavy stress on your front abdominal wall, particularly the upper part of the rectus abdominis.

Starting Position: Sit on the seat and hook your insteps under the restraints beneath the seat. Reach back and grasp the handles of the machine. Put your chin on your chest at the starting point of the movement.

Movement Performance: Do the crunch movement already described, hold the top position of the movement for a moment, return to the starting point, and repeat the movement for the desired number of repetitions.

Pulley Crunches

Emphasis: Pulley Crunches stress the entire

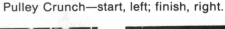

Pulley Crunch—start, left; finish, right.

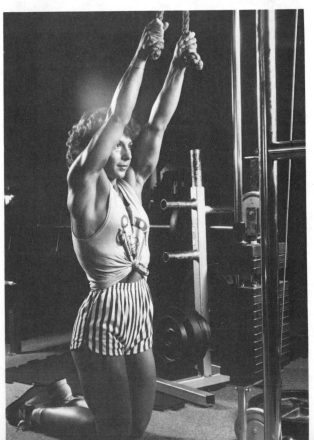

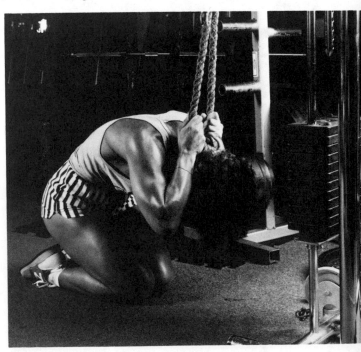

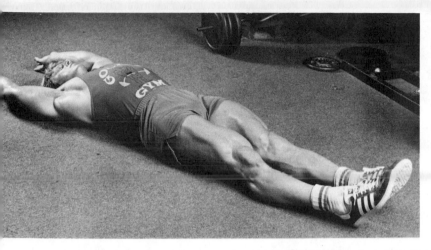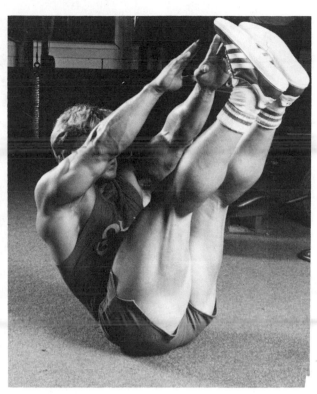

Jack Knives—start, left; finish, right.

front abdominal wall, particularly the upper section of the rectus abdominis. Strong stress is also placed on the serratus and intercostal muscles.

Starting Position: Attach a rope handle to an overhead pulley and grasp the two ropes extending from the cable in your hands. Kneel down about a foot back from the pulley and extend your body toward the pulley.

Movement Performance: You must simultaneously perform three tasks in order to do an effective Pulley Crunch movement:

- bend over at the waist until your forehead touches the floor,
- do a small, pullover movement to bring your arms from an extended position to one in which your arms are bent at 90-degree angles and your hands are on the floor just ahead of your head, and
- forcefully blow out all of your air.

When you perform these three tasks correctly, you will feel a strong contraction in your abdominal muscles. Hold this contraction for a moment, return slowly to the starting point, and repeat the movement for the suggested number of repetitions.

Exercise Variations: You can do this exercise with one arm at a time, but be sure to perform the same number of sets and reps for each side of your body. You can also do Pulley Crunches holding your hands with the rope handles in them on the sides of your neck during the exercise.

Jack Knives

Emphasis: This is an excellent movement for stressing all of the front abdominal muscles.

Starting Position: Lie on your back on the gym floor and extend your arms straight over your head along the floor. Bend your legs slightly and keep them bent throughout the movement to remove potentially harmful stress from your lower back.

Movement Performance: Simultaneously lift your torso and legs off the floor to bring yourself up so your legs and torso make a "V" with only your butt in contact with the floor. Lower slowly back to the starting point and repeat the exercise for the required number of reps.

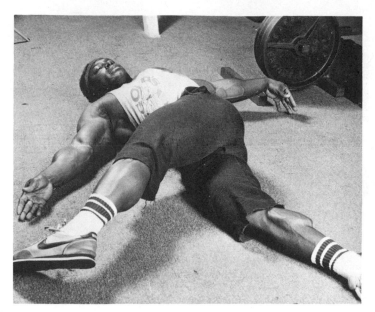
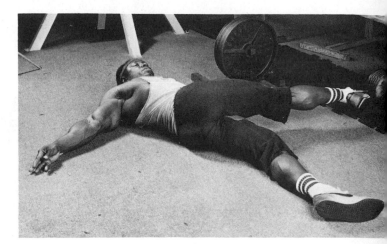

Hip Roll—start, left; finish, right.

Hip Rolls

Emphasis: This unique exercise stresses all of the muscles of the abdomen and hips.

Starting Position: Lie on your back on the gym floor and extend your arms straight out to the sides along the floor, putting yourself in a cross formation. Keeping your legs straight, spread them until they are at a 45-degree angle to each other.

Movement Performance: Lift your right leg from the floor and move your right foot up to touch your left hand. You will have to roll over on your left hip to accomplish this movement. Return to the starting position and repeat the movement to the opposite side. Keep alternating sides until you have done the suggested number of repetitions to each side.

Side Sit-Up—start, left; finish, right.

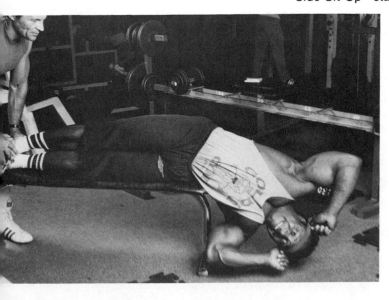
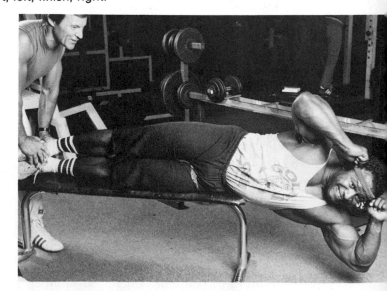

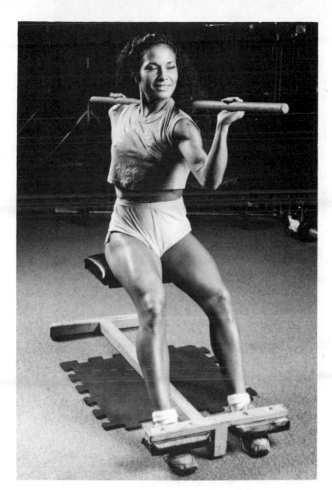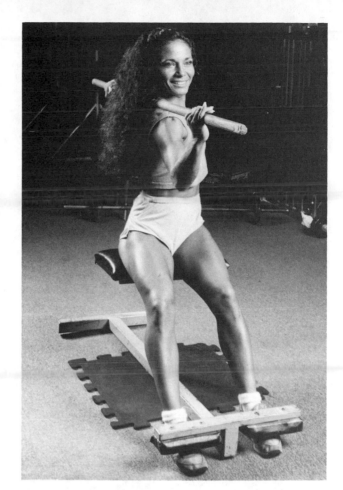

Seated Twisting—start, left; finish, right.

Side Sit-Ups

Emphasis: This is a very intense movement for stressing the oblique and serratus muscles.

Starting Position: Lie on your right side crosswise on a flat exercise bench with only your right hip in contact with the bench. Have a training partner grasp your ankles and restrain your legs during the movement. Cross your arms over your chest, or place your hands behind your head and neck during the exercise. Relax the muscles at the left side of your waist and allow your torso to bend downward toward the floor.

Movement Performance: Flex your obliques and intercostals to move your head and shoulders upward to as high a position as possible. Return slowly to the starting point and repeat the movement for the desired number of reps. Be sure to do the same number of sets and repetitions for each side of your body.

Training Tip: You can add resistance to this movement by holding a light barbell plate against your chest.

Seated Twisting

Emphasis: This movement is for the oblique muscles, although it's a fallacy to believe that doing massive numbers of twists will help to trim fat from around your waist. As a by-product, you will find that Seated Twists help to loosen up your lower back.

Starting Position: Straddle a flat exercise bench and either place your feet firmly flat on the floor or interlace your lower legs in the uprights of the bench to secure your body during the exercise. Place a broomstick or unloaded barbell bar across your shoulders and wrap your arms around the bar.

Movement Performance: Without moving your legs and hips, twist as far as you can to the left with your upper torso. Immediately twist back as far as you can to the right, and repeat the movement from one side to the other in rhythmic fashion for the suggested number of repetitions. Count one full cycle to both sides as a single rep.

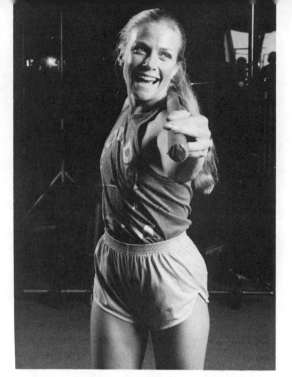
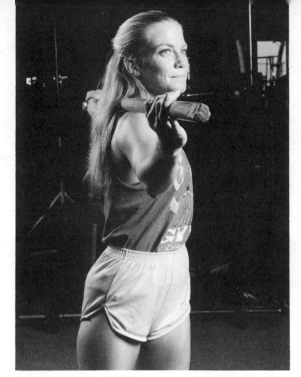

Standing Twisting—start, left; finish, right.

Bent Twisting.

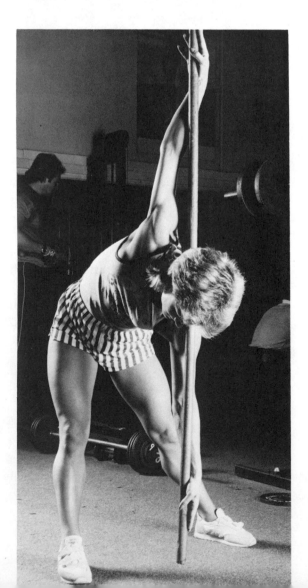

Standing Twisting

Emphasis: This movement has the same effect on your body as Seated Twisting.

Starting Position: Stand erect with your feet set slightly more than shoulder-width apart. Place a broomstick or unloaded barbell bar behind your neck and wrap your arms around it. Be sure that you don't move your legs and hips during this exercise, or you will lose much of the benefit of the movement.

Movement Performance: Twist as far as you can to the left and right in a rhythmic manner for the required number of repetitions. Count one full cycle to each side as a single rep.

Exercise Variation: You can also do Bent Twisting in a standing position. Simply start in the same position as for Standing Twisting, bend over until your torso is parallel to the floor, and perform your twisting motion from side to side with your torso in this position.

Barbell Side Bends

Emphasis: This is a direct movement for the obliques and serratus muscles.

Starting Position: Place a light barbell across your shoulders behind your neck and grasp the bar halfway between your shoulder and the end

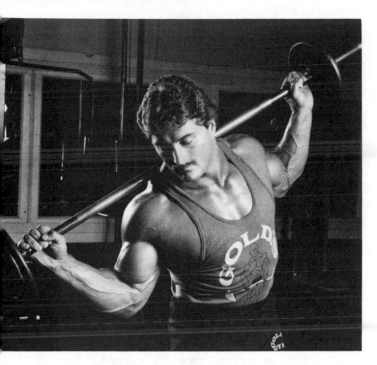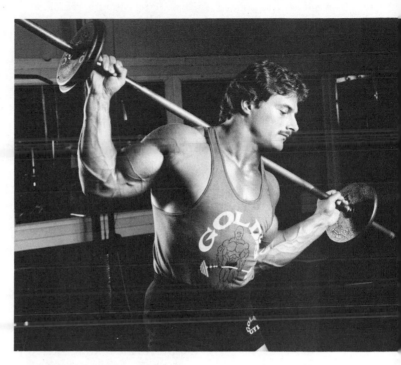

Barbell Side Bend—start, left; finish, right.

Dumbbell Side Bend.

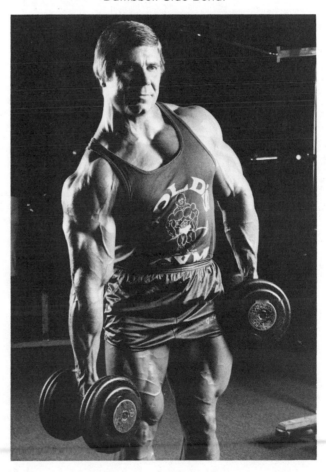

of the bar on each side. Set your feet slightly wider than the width of your shoulders and stand erect.

Movement Performance: Without shifting the bar on your shoulders, bend directly to the left as far as you comfortably can, then immediately bend back to the right as far as possible. Continue bending rhythmically from side to side until you have performed the desired number of repetitions to each side.

Training Tip: If you are using an adjustable barbell for this movement, be absolutely sure that the collars on the ends of the barbell are firmly fastened in place.

Exercise Variation: Some bodybuilders do this movement in very high reps (over 100) with a broomstick across their shoulders rather than a light barbell.

Dumbbell Side Bends

Emphasis: As with Barbell Side Bends, this dumbbell movement very directly stresses your obliques and serratus muscles.

Starting Position: Grasp a light dumbbell in your left hand and stand erect with your feet set slightly wider than the width of your shoulders. Place your right hand behind your head or neck.

Movement Performance: Bend as far to the left as you comfortably can, then immediately bend back as far as you can to the right. Return to the full, left-side bend and repeat the movement for the required number of repetitions. Be sure to do the same number of sets and repetitions with the dumbbell held in your right hand.

Exercise Variation: You can also do Dumbbell Side Bends with dumbbells held in both hands, although this variation of the movement is not as effective as the one performed with one dumbbell.

Suggested Abdominal Routines

If you have less than a few weeks of training under your belt, the following abdominal routine can profitably be performed three nonconsecutive days each week at the beginning of your regular workout:

Exercise	Sets	Reps
Sit-Ups	2	20–30
Leg Raises	2	20–30
Seated Twisting	1	50

After 4–6 weeks of steady training on the foregoing program, you can use this abdominal routine three days per week:

Exercise	Sets	Reps
Hanging Frog Kicks	3	15–20
Roman Chair Sit-Ups	3	25–30
Seated Twisting	2–3	50

After about three months of steady training, you will have switched to a four-day split routine for the rest of your body in which you train each major muscle group twice per week. However, the abdominals can profitably be worked each training day. Following is a sample two-part routine for off-season competition training:

Monday–Thursday

Exercise	Sets	Reps
Hanging Leg Raises	3	10–15
Roman Chair Sit-Ups	3	25–30
Bench Leg Raises	2	25–30
Crunches	2	25–30
Dumbbell Side Bends	2–3	20–30

Tuesday–Friday

Exercise	Sets	Reps
Incline Sit-Ups	3	20–30
Parallel Bar Leg Raises	3	20–30
Wall Crunches	2	20–30
Jack Knives	2	20–30
Bent-Over Twisting	2–3	50

Every advanced-level bodybuilder trains differently from all others prior to a competition, as you will see in the following section listing the abdominal routines of a wide variety of men and women who either train or have trained at Gold's Gym.

Abdominal Routines of the Gold's Champs

In this section, you will find a variety of abdominal training programs used by many of the Gold's Gym superstars who have won the sport's highest titles. Keep in mind as you examine these training programs that these men and women have been training for many years and have developed enormous recuperative abilities. It is unlikely that you can make good gains using their full routines. Instead, you should use these training programs as examples of how to work your own abs. In all likelihood, you can do the same exercises as your favorite champion, but scale down the number of sets that he or she does of each movement to conform to your own abilities.

LYNN CONKWRIGHT (PRO WORLD CHAMPION)

Exercise	Sets	Reps
Wall Crunch	3	20–25
Hanging Leg Raises	3	15–20
Jack Knives	3	20–25
Cable Crunches	3	20–25
Seated Twisting	3	25

MOHAMED MAKKAWY (GRAND PRIX CHAMPION)

Exercise	Sets	Reps
Hanging Leg Raises	3–5	20–30
Incline Sit-Ups (weighted)	3–5	20–30
Roman Chair Sit-Ups	3–5	100

MIKE ARMSTRONG
(MR. ALABAMA)

Exercise	Sets	Reps
Hanging Leg Raises	3	20–30
Twisting Cable Crunches	4	20–30
Weighted Sit-Ups	5	10

TIM BELKNAP
(MR. AMERICA)

Exercise	Sets	Reps
Crunches	5	20–30
supersetted with		
Cable Leg Raises	5	20–30
Side Bends	5	30–50

ANDREAS CAHLING
(MR. INTERNATIONAL)

Exercise	Sets	Reps
Hanging Leg Raises (twisting)	3–4	15–20
Roman Chair Sit-Ups	3–4	30–50
Bench Leg Raises	3–4	30–50
Seated Twisting	3–4	50
Incline Sit-Ups	3–4	20–30

Note: Foregoing exercises performed as a giant set.

LAURA COMBES
(MS. AMERICA)

Exercise	Sets	Reps
Hanging Leg Raises	4–5	15–20
Incline Sit-Ups	4–5	20–25
Crunches	4–5	20–25
Bench Leg Raises	4–5	20–25

Note: Foregoing exercises performed as a giant set.

CLIFF FORD
(PAST-40 MR. AMERICA)

Exercise	Sets	Reps
Hanging Leg Raises	4–5	15–20
Incline Sit-Ups	4–5	25–30
Seated Twisting	4–5	50
Bench Leg Raises	4–5	30
Roman Chair Sit-Ups	4–5	25–30

Note: Foregoing exercises performed as a giant set.

PAUL HILL
(MR. USA)

Exercise	Sets	Reps
Hanging Leg Raises	3–4	15–20
Incline Sit-Ups	3–4	25–30
Bench Leg Raises	3–4	25–30
Crunches	3–5	25–30

STELLA MARTINEZ
(MS. USA)

Exercise	Sets	Reps
Hanging Leg Raises	3	15–20
supersetted with		
Incline Sit-Ups	3	20–30
Incline Leg Raises	3	20–30
supersetted with		
Wall Crunches	3	20–30
Bench Leg Raises	3	20–30
supersetted with		
Cable Crunches	3	20–25

Lee Haney.

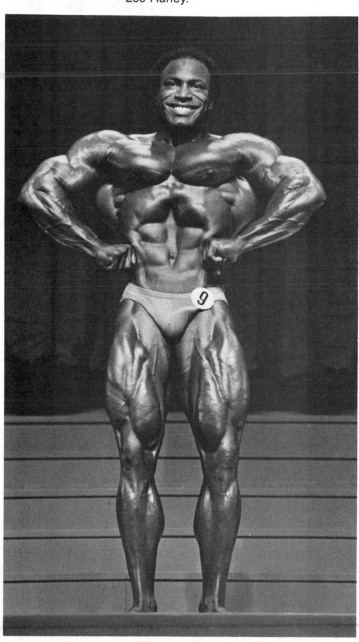

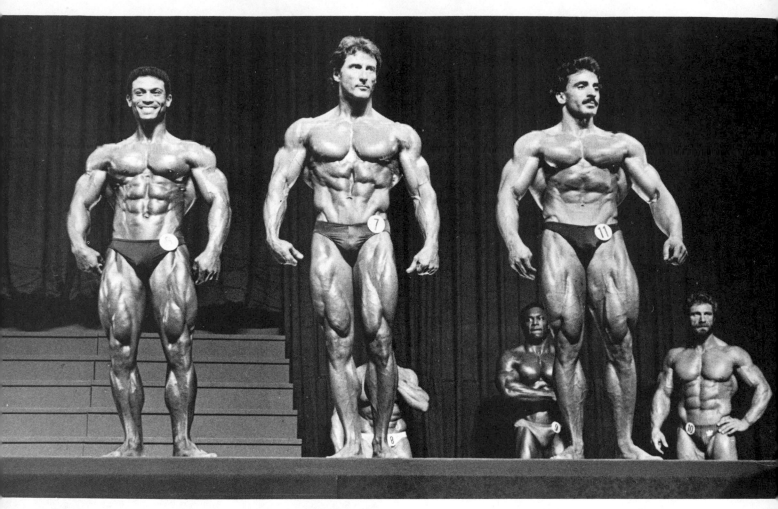

1984 Olympia: Mohamed Makkawy, Frank Zane, and Samir Bannout.

KEN PASSARIELLO
(MR. UNIVERSE)

Exercise	Sets	Reps
Hanging Leg Raises	3–4	15–20
supersetted with		
Roman Chair Sit-Ups	3–4	30
Bench Leg Raises	3–4	30
supersetted with		
Incline Sit-Ups	3–4	20–25
Incline Leg Raises	3–4	20–25
supersetted with		
Crunches	3–4	25–30

DAVID ROGERS
(MR. USA)

Exercise	Sets	Reps
Roman Chair Sit-Ups	4–6	Max
supersetted with		
Hanging Leg Raises	4–6	Max

PIERRE VAN DEN STEEN
(MR. EUROPE)

Exercise	Sets	Reps
Roman Chair Sit-Ups	1	200
Hanging Leg Raises (twisting)	2	25
Incline Sit-Ups	1	50
Twisting Leg Raises	2	80–100

COREY EVERSON
(MS. NORTH AMERICA)

Exercise	Sets	Reps
Incline Sit-Ups	3–4	20–30
Incline Leg Raises	3–4	20–30
Seated Twisting	3–4	50
Roman Chair Sit-Ups	3–4	20–30
Pulley Crunches	3–4	15–20

Note: Foregoing exercises performed as a giant set.

RON TEUFEL
(MR. USA)

Exercise	Sets	Reps
High Incline Sit-Ups	5	20–30
supersetted with		
Hanging Leg Raises	5	15–20
Crunches	4	30–40
supersetted with		
Bench Leg Raises	4	30–40
Rope Crunches	3	20–30

LOU FERRIGNO
(MR. UNIVERSE)

Exercise	Sets	Reps
Hanging Leg Raises	3–4	15–20
Roman Chair Sit-Ups	3–4	50
Crunches	3–4	30–40
Side Bends	3–4	50
Bench Leg Raises	3–4	30–40
Rope Crunches	3–4	25–30

Note: Foregoing exercises performed as a giant set.

LISA ELLIOTT-KOLAKOWSKI
(GOLD'S CLASSIC CHAMP)

Exercise	Sets	Reps
Roman Chair Sit-Ups	3	50
Hanging Leg Raises	3	15
Incline Sit-Ups	3	20
Seated Twisting	3	50
Crunches	3	25

Note: Foregoing exercises performed as a giant set.

SAMIR BANNOUT
(MR. OLYMPIA)

Exercise	Sets	Reps
Hanging Leg Raises	3–4	15–20
supersetted with		
Incline Sit-Ups	3–4	20–30
Incline Leg Raises	3–4	20–30
supersetted with		
Roman Chair Sit-Ups	3–4	50
Rope Crunches	3–4	20–30
supersetted with		
Seated Twisting	3–4	50

MIKE MENTZER
(MR. UNIVERSE)

Exercise	Sets	Reps
Roman Chair Sit-Ups (weighted)	2–3	25–10
Hanging Leg Raises	2	20–25
Side Sit-Ups	2	12–15

DENNIS TINERINO
(MR. UNIVERSE)

Exercise	Sets	Reps
Roman Chair Sit-Ups	3–4	25–30
Hanging Leg Raises	3–4	15–20
Crunches	3–4	30–40
Bench Leg Raises	3–4	30–40
Seated Twisting	3–4	100

RICHARD BALDWIN
(COLLEGIATE MR. AMERICA)

Exercise	Sets	Reps
Roman Chair Sit-Ups	3	40–50
Hanging Leg Raises	3	15–20
Crunches	3	30–40
Rope Crunches	3	25–30

Johnny Fuller.

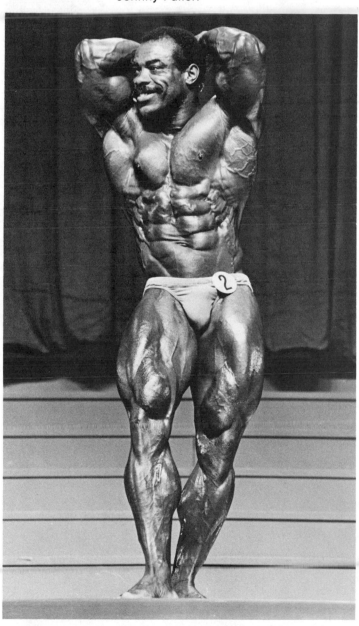

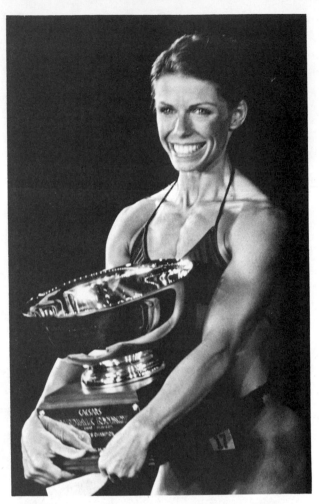

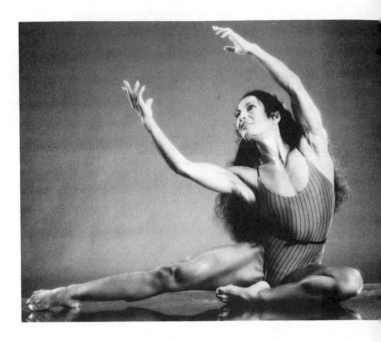

Lynn Conkwright (above) holds 1981 World Championship cup. Exercise model Maria Gonzalez (above right).

Looking Ahead

In Chapter 9, we will introduce you to all of the calf, forearm, and neck exercises that the superstar bodybuilders at Gold's Gym use in their workouts. And we will reveal many of these champs' actual training programs for these three body parts.

9
CALF, FOREARM AND NECK TRAINING

The calves, forearms and neck are body parts often neglected by bodybuilders. However, an intelligent bodybuilder will work hard to maximize his or her development in each of these areas, for a complete physique is a winning physique.

Of these three muscle groups, your calves and forearms are quite difficult to develop, while the neck is very easy to build up. In fact, your neck muscles will probably grow as big as they will ever need to be merely as a consequence of performing heavy exercises for peripheral body parts like your upper chest, traps, and deltoids. Few bodybuilders perform direct neck work, but virtually all have thick neck development, which no doubt has led to use of the derisive term "pencil necks" when referring to untrained individuals.

Your calf and forearm muscles will be difficult to develop because they are used to hard, daily work. Each time you take a step, you stress your calf muscles; and each time you grasp some object, your forearm muscles come into play. Think of how many thousands of times you have grasped something or taken a step, and you will understand that your calf and forearm muscles have been toughened to the point where they are quite resistant to the effects of bodybuilding exercise.

Due to their tough and resilient nature, you can only induce your calf and forearm muscles to respond and grow when you stress them with much higher-than-normal resistance and intensity. As a result, many bodybuilders successfully work both of these muscle groups on an almost daily basis with heavy weights and relatively high reps.

Virtually all bodybuilders have excellent neck development, and only one or two of them have performed any direct neck work to achieve it. A few male bodybuilders with superior calves are Chris Dickerson, Ken Waller, Mike Mentzer, Tim Belknap, Dan Franklin, and Bob Paris. Women with great calves are Kay Baxter, Rachel McLish, Lynn Conkwright, and Kike Elomaa. Casey Viator and Mike Mentzer have the most phenomenal forearm development among men, while Rachel McLish and Laura Combes have the most outstanding forearm development among women bodybuilders who have won top titles.

Anatomy and Kinesiology

There are two major muscle groups in your calves, plus one along the front of your shin. The largest lower-leg muscle is the gastrocnemius, which looks like an inverted heart on the upper part of your lower leg. The gastrocnemius contracts to extend your foot and toes. Beneath the gastrocnemius is a wide, flat muscle called the *soleus,* which also helps to extend the foot, but which can only be fully contracted when your leg is bent. And running over your shin bone is the *tibialis anterior* muscle, which contracts to flex your foot and toes toward your knee.

There are many muscles in your forearms, which befits their function of precisely controlling the human hand. However, you can group these smaller muscles into three larger categories—the *forearm flexors, forearm extensors,* and *forearm supinators.* The forearm flexors run up the inner sides of your forearms and contract to flex your wrists and close your fingers. The forearm extensors run along the outer sides of your forearms and contract to extend your wrists and open your fingers. And the forearm supinators lie on the upper/outer section of your forearms and contract to both help supinate your hands and to help bend your arm when you hold your hand in a pronated (palm-down) position.

There are also a large number of muscles that form the muscular column of your neck. The various muscle groups help you to move your neck to the front, back, and both sides, as well as to a myriad of directions between these four main poles. And the *sternocleidomastoid* muscles near the front of your neck allow you to rotate your neck, as when turning it to one side or the other.

Calf Exercises

In this section you will find only nine major calf exercises, each fully described and illustrated. With variations and using different machines the total of exercises nears 20. This might not sound like many movements for this body part, but you will ultimately discover that they are more than sufficient to build large, diamond-shaped calves.

Barbell Calf Raises

Emphasis: When you don't have a standing calf machine available, you can use Barbell Calf Raises to stress the gastrocnemius muscles. However, you will find it very difficult to maintain

body balance in this exercise, so it's best to do the movement on a calf machine.

Starting Position: Place a barbell across your shoulders as for a Squat movement, balancing it in position by grasping the bar out near the plates. Place your toes and the balls of your feet on a 4 × 4-inch block of wood, which will allow your heels to descend well below the level of your toes as you do the movement. Your feet should be about a foot apart on the block, and your toes should be pointed straight ahead. Keeping your legs and torso straight and erect during the exercise, relax your calves and allow your heels to travel well below the level of your toes to stretch your calves at the starting point of the movement.

Movement Performance: Use calf strength to rise up in one smooth and unbroken motion as high on your toes as you can. Lower slowly back to the starting point and repeat the movement.

Training Tips: One of the biggest keys to calf development is moving your heels over as long a range of motion as possible. Bodybuilders with poor calves tend to either not stretch very far down at the start of the movement or fail to rise completely up on their toes. Another common mistake is rising halfway up, descending a bit

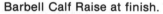

Barbell Calf Raise at finish.

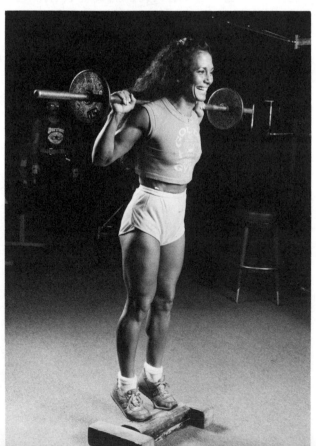

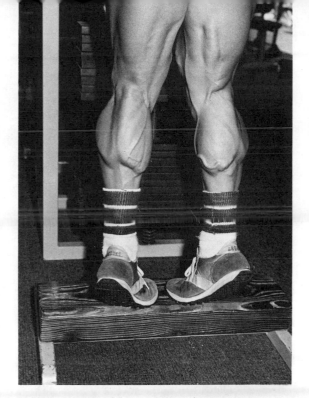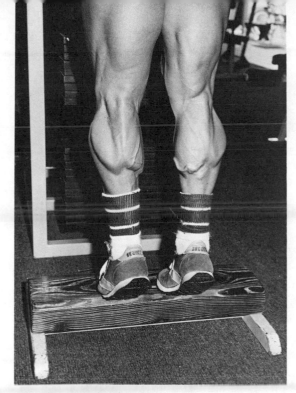

Foot positions for Toe Raises—toes in, left; toes straight ahead, right; toes out, below.

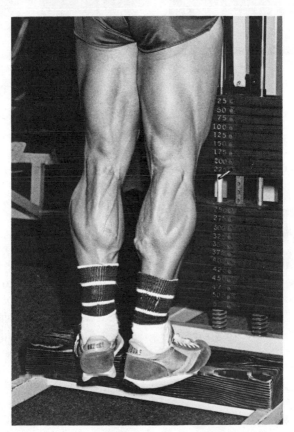

Standing Calf Machine Toe Raise—details.

and then bouncing the rest of the way to the top of the movement. You should make the exercise movement long and smooth.

Exercise Variations: On all calf exercises, you should vary the angle of your feet from set to set. Some sets should be performed with your feet angled outward at 45-degree angles, some with your toes pointed straight ahead, and some with your toes angled inward at 45-degree angles. You can also vary the width of your toe placement on the calf block as you do all types of calf exercises.

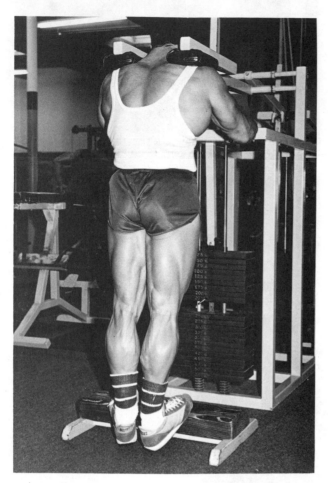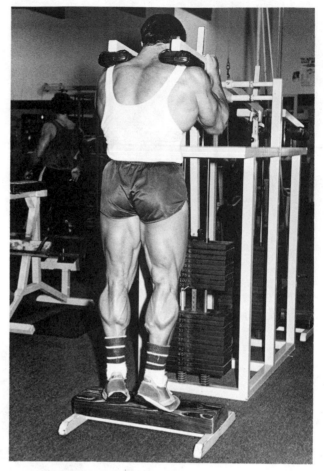

Standing Calf Machine Toe Raise—start, left; finish, right.

Standing Calf Machine Toe Raises

Emphasis: This movement allows you to very strongly stress the gastrocnemius muscles without the hassle of trying to keep your body in balance on the toe block.

Starting Position: Stand up to the machine and bend your legs enough to solidly position your shoulders under the yokes attached to the machine's lever arms. Place your toes and the balls of your feet on the calf block with your feet set about a foot apart. Straighten your body to bear the weight of the machine and allow your heels to sag as far as comfortably possible below the level of your toes.

Movement Performance: Rise up as high as possible on your toes, descend back to the starting point and repeat the exercise.

Exercise Variations: Be sure to vary both the width of your foot placement on the block and the angle of your feet from time to time. You can also do this movement with one leg at a time, a favorite variation of Rachel McLish, winner of two Miss Olympia titles.

Barbell Seated Calf Raises

Emphasis: This movement is excellent for developing the soleus muscles, which add width to the calves when viewed from the front or back. As you will remember from the kinesiology discussion earlier in this chapter, your soleus muscles can only be fully contracted when your legs are bent.

Starting Position: Roll a thick towel around the middle of a barbell bar to pad the bar. Place a calf block about two feet away from a flat exercise bench. Sit on the bench, place the balls of your feet and your toes on the calf block, have a training partner lift the barbell up to rest on your lower thighs just above your knees, and

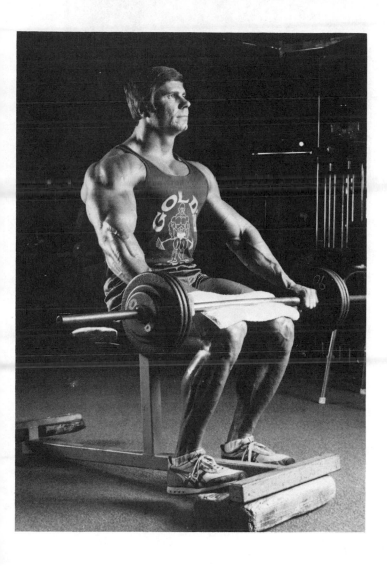

Barbell Seated Calf Raise—
start, above; finish, right.

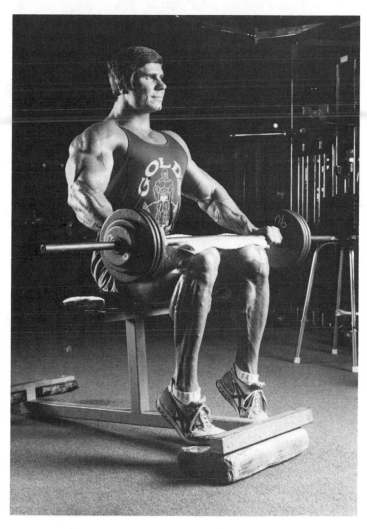

steady the barbell in this position by grasping the bar out near the plates. Allow your heels to descend as far as comfortably possible.

Movement Performance: Push down with your toes and the balls of your feet to rise up as high as you can on your toes. Lower slowly back to the starting point and repeat the movement for the required number of repetitions.

Exercise Variations: Be sure to change your foot placement as outlined in the description of Barbell Calf Raises.

Comment: This movement is intended primarily for use in a home gym situation when you don't have a seated calf machine available.

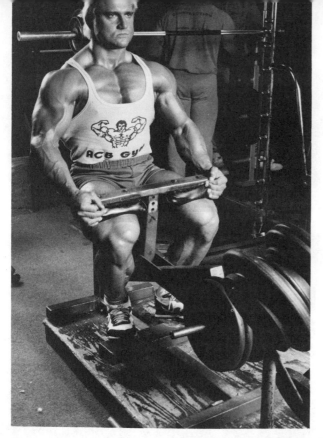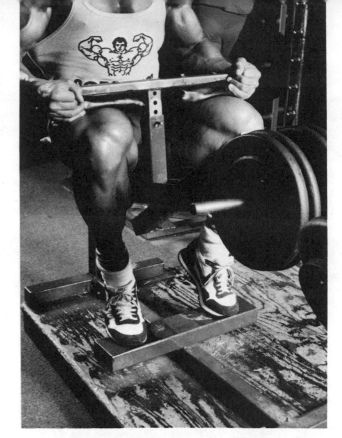

Seated Calf Machine Toe Raise—start, left; finish, right.

Seated Calf Machine Toe Raises

Emphasis: This is one of the very best soleus exercises available to you.

Starting Position: Sit on the calf machine seat and place your toes and the balls of your feet on the toe plate attached to the machine. Pull the pads attached to the machine lever arm over your knees. If the pads aren't adjusted to the correct position for this, you can adjust them by removing a pin in the column of steel that attaches the pads to the lever arm, then replacing the pin when you have the pads adjusted to the correct height. Push down on your toes to bear the weight of the machine and push the stop bar forward to release the weight (be sure to replace the stop bar before leaving the machine at the end of your set). Allow your heels to sag as far as comfortably possible below the level of your toes.

Movement Performance: Rise up on your toes as high as you can, return to the starting point, and repeat the movement for the suggested number of reps.

Exercise Variations: You should periodically vary the width of your foot placement on the toe plate, and be sure to also vary the angle of your feet from set to set.

Jump Squats

Emphasis: This is a good movement for conditioning your thighs and calves. It's particularly good if you wish to improve the height of your vertical jump.

Starting Position: Place a barbell across your shoulders behind your neck and hold it in position by grasping the bar out near the plates. Stand with your feet about shoulder-width apart, your toes slightly outward. Be sure to keep your torso upright during the exercise.

Movement Performance: Squat down to at least a position in which your thighs are parallel to the floor. Start coming back erect, but once you're halfway up, accelerate your movement and spring off the floor at the top of the exercise. As soon as you land on the floor, repeat the movement.

Exercise Variation: You can also do this movement holding a pair of moderately heavy dumbbells in your hands.

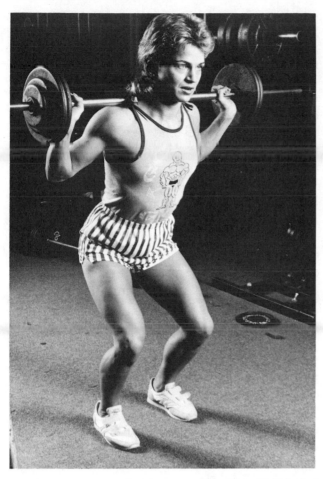
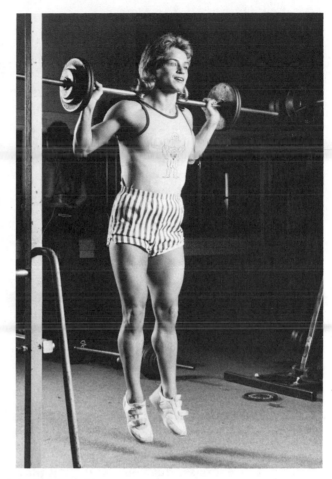

Jump Squat—start, left; finish, right.

One-Leg Dumbbell Toe Raise—start, left; finish, right.

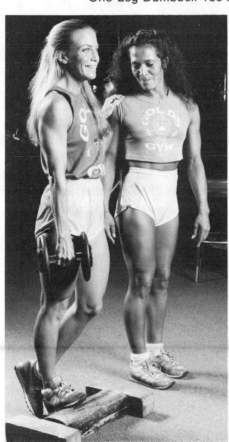
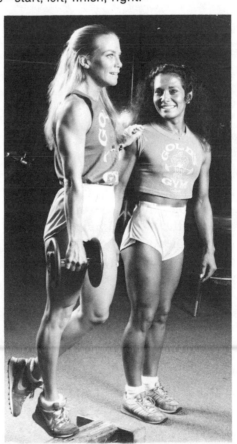

One-Leg Dumbbell Toe Raises

Emphasis: You will find this to be a very convenient exercise for placing direct stress on your gastrocnemius muscles. It can be performed both in a large public gym and a home gym equipped with nothing more than an adjustable dumbbell set.

Starting Position: Grasp a light dumbbell in your right hand, place the toes and ball of your right foot on a calf block, and grasp a sturdy upright with your left hand to steady your body in a secure position as you do the exercise. Your left leg should be bent to keep it out of the movement. Sag your heels down as far below the level of your toes as possible.

Movement Performance: Rise up as high as you can on your toes, return to the starting point, and repeat the movement for the desired number of repetitions. Do an equal amount of work with your left leg using your right arm to secure an erect position.

Training Tip: You can easily give yourself forced reps toward the end of a hard set by pulling up slightly on the upright you are holding with your left or right hand.

Exercise Variations: It's a little more difficult to do on this exercise, but you should still play with different foot angles when you do One-Leg Calf Raises.

Calf Presses

Emphasis: Calf Presses can be done on a variety of leg-press machines. Regardless of the type of leg-press machine used for the movement, the exercise very directly stresses the gastrocnemius muscles.

Starting Position: Let's describe Calf Presses as performed on a Universal Gym leg-press machine, which can be more or less adaptable to other machines. Adjust the seat as far back from the pedals as possible. Sit in the machine and place your toes and the balls of your feet on the lower set of pedals, then push your legs straight. Relax your calves and allow your heels to move as far away from the level of your toes as possible.

Movement Performance: Extend your feet and toes to push the pedals as far away from your body as possible. Return to the starting point and repeat the movement for the required number of reps.

Training Tip: This is the best exercise for using a technique called *negative emphasis* (discussed in Chapter 10) on your calves. With this technique, you will extend your feet both legs at a time, but lower the weight back to the starting point by resisting the weight with only one leg. Then after pushing the weight back out with both feet, lower it with your other leg. Alternate legs each repetition.

Exercise Variations: A very similar movement can be performed on a Nautilus leg-press machine, as well as on a vertical leg-press machine or 45-degree-angled leg-press machine.

Donkey Calf Raises

Emphasis: This is an excellent exercise for placing direct stress on the gastrocnemius muscles of your calves.

Starting Position: Place a calf block about two feet back from a flat exercise bench. Place your toes and the balls of your feet on the calf block and bend over to place your hands on the exercise bench. This will maintain your torso in a position parallel to the floor as you do this movement. To provide stress on your calves, have a training partner jump up astride your hips. If your partner isn't heavy enough, he or she can hold a dumbbell or loose barbell plate against your lower back as you perform your Donkey Calf Raises. Sag your heels as far below the level of your toes as possible.

Movement Performance: Rise up as high as possible on your toes, return to the starting position, and repeat the movement for the suggested number of repetitions.

Exercise Variations: You can also do this movement on a Nautilus multi-machine by slipping a belt attached to the lever arm around your waist. Stand on the lower set of steps of the machine and bend over a bit to support your torso at a 45-degree angle in relation to the floor as you do the movement. You should also experiment with different widths of foot placement, as well as foot angle from set to set.

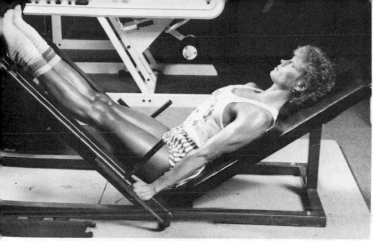

Calf Press—finish, left; detail of finish, below.

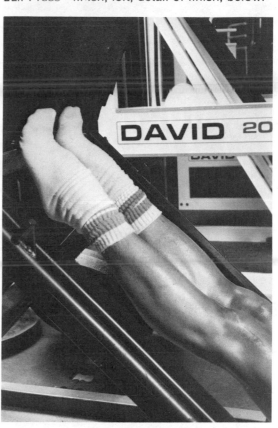

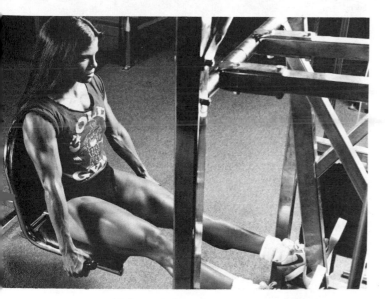

Universal Gym Machine Calf Press.

Donkey Calf Raise—start, left; finish, right.

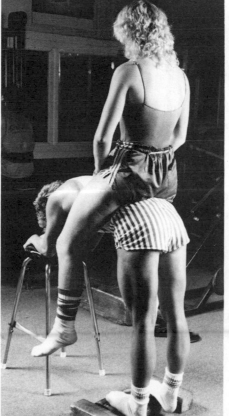

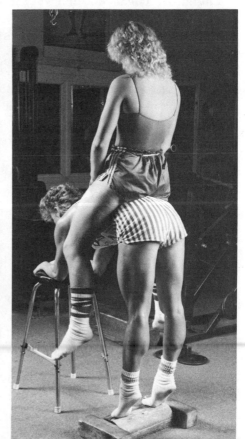

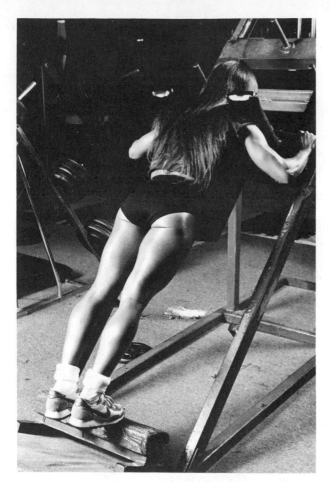 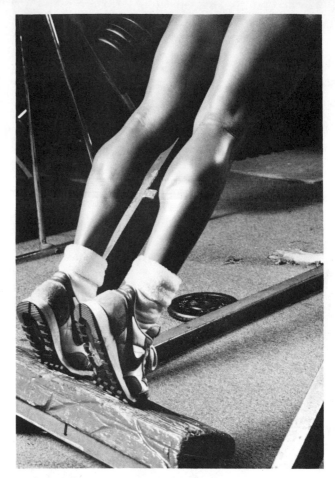

Hack Machine Toe Raise—start, left; detail of finish, right.

Hack Machine Toe Raises

Emphasis: This is another very good gastrocnemius exercise.

Starting Position: This movement is a little difficult to get into, but once you assume the correct starting position you'll find it to be a very smooth gastrocnemius exercise. Stand on the angled foot platform of a hack machine facing toward the sliding part of the machine. Either place your shoulders under the yokes, or reach down to grasp the handles at the low end of the sliding platform, resting the front of your torso on the slide. Straighten your legs and move your feet to the rear until just your toes and the balls of your feet are in contact with the angled foot platform. Relax your calves and allow your heels to travel as far as comfortably possible beneath the level of your toes.

Movement Performance: Bearing the weight of the machine, rise up as high on your toes as you can. Return slowly to the starting point and repeat the movement for an appropriate number of repetitions.

Exercise Variations: You can do this movement with one leg at a time, and you should be sure to vary the width of your foot placement on the platform, as well as your foot angle from set to set.

Forearm Exercises

In this section you will find 15 major forearm exercises, each fully described and illustrated. Add in the variations on each movement, and you will have at least 30 forearm exercises to include in your basic pool of bodybuilding movements.

Barbell Reverse Curls

Emphasis: All forms of Reverse Curls strongly stress the forearm supinator muscles in conjunction with the brachialis of the upper arm. Secondary stress is on your biceps.

Starting Position: Take a shoulder-width over-grip on a barbell, set your feet about

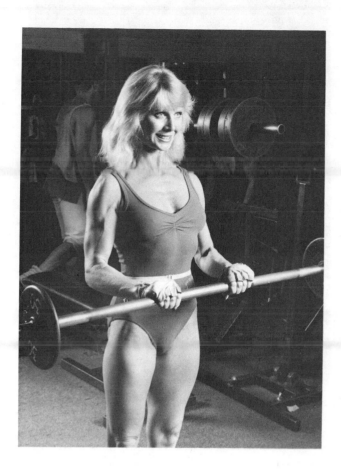

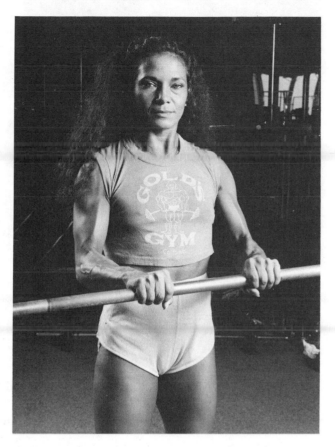

Barbell Reverse Curl—narrow grip, left;
medium grip, right; wide grip, below.

shoulder-width apart and stand erect with your
arms running straight down at your sides and the
barbell resting across your upper thighs. Pin
your upper arms against the sides of your torso
throughout the movement.

Movement Performance: Slowly curl the barbell in a semicircular arc from your thighs to a
position just under your chin. Lower the weight
slowly back along the same arc to the starting
point and repeat the movement for the required
number of repetitions.

Training Tip: If you have trouble with your
torso weaving back and forth during the exercise, you should perform the movement with
your back resting against the wall of your gym,
or against a sturdy post.

Exercise Variations: You should vary the
width of your grip on the bar from time to time.
It's anatomically difficult to use a grip wider
than shoulder-width, but you can very conveniently use a more narrow grip on the bar when
you do Reverse Curls. You can also do this
movement with an EZ-Curl bar.

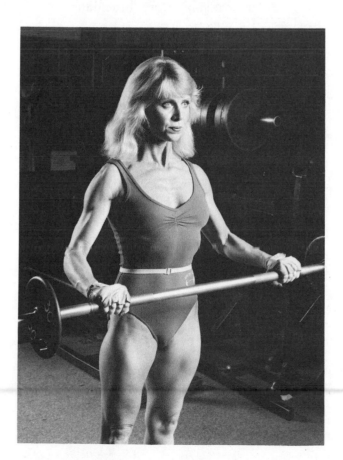

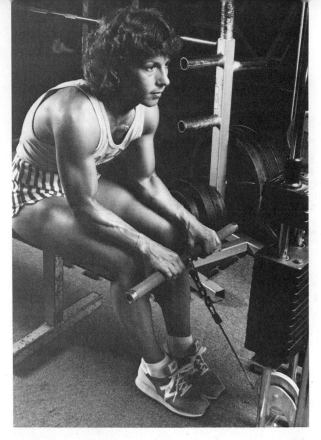
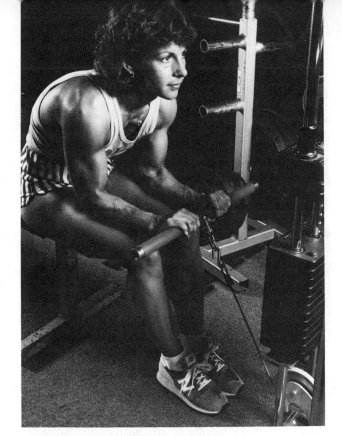

Cable Reverse Wrist Curl—start, left; finish, right.

Cable Reverse Wrist Curls

Emphasis: Cable Reverse Wrist Curls also stress the forearm supinators, brachialis muscles and biceps.

Starting Position: Attach a bar handle to the cable running through a floor pulley. Take a narrow grip on the handle, set your feet about shoulder-width apart, and stand erect with your arms running straight down at your sides and your hands with the bar in them resting across your upper thighs. Pin your upper arms against the sides of your body throughout your set.

Movement Performance: Slowly curl the pulley handle from your thighs up to a point just beneath your chin. Lower it back to the starting point and repeat the exercise.

Training Tip: Normally, you should stand about one foot back from the pulley, but you can sometimes get a better feel from the movement standing either closer to the pulley or farther away from it.

Exercise Variations: You can vary the width of your grip according to how long the bar is. You can also do this movement while lying on your back with your feet toward the pulley, a varia- tion that immobilizes your upper arms and forces you to perform a very strict movement.

Preacher-Bench Reverse Curls

Emphasis: Barbell Reverse Curls performed on a preacher bench can be an exceptionally in- tense exercise for stressing the forearm supina- tors, brachialis muscles, and biceps. This, in fact, was a favorite exercise of Larry Scott, winner of the first two Mr. Olympia titles in 1965 and 1966. Scott's biceps and forearms were unparal- leled at the time he was winning competitions, and even by today's inflated standards his over- all arm development continues to be sensational.

Starting Position: Take a shoulder-width over-grip on a moderately weighted barbell and lean over a preacher bench with the top edge of the bench wedged under your armpits. Run your upper arms down the angled surface of the bench parallel to each other and slowly straighten your arms.

Movement Performance: Use forearm and upper-arm strength to move the barbell in a semicircular arc from the starting point up to a

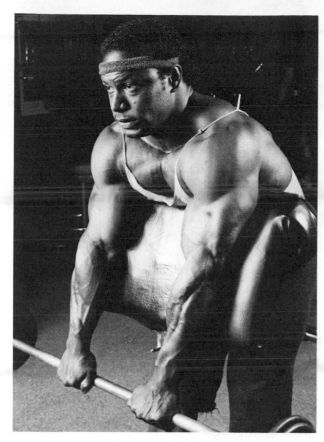
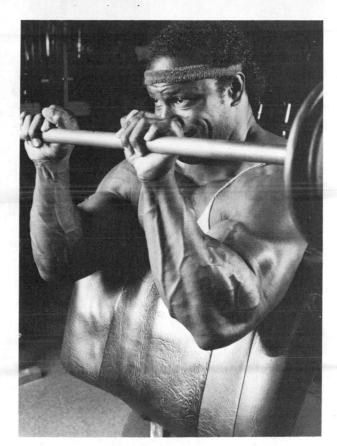

Preacher-Bench Reverse Curl—start, left; finish, right.

Hammer Curl.

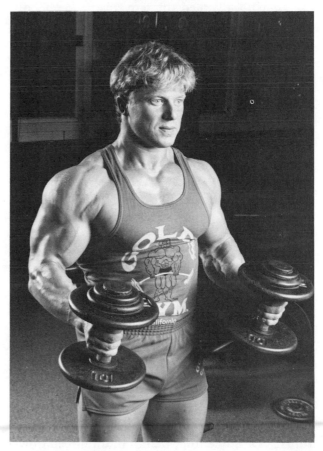

point just beneath your chin. Slowly lower the bar back to the starting point and repeat the movement for the desired number of repetitions.

Exercise Variations: You can vary the width of your grip on the barbell, plus use an EZ-Curl bar for this movement.

Hammer Curls

Emphasis: Hammer Curls are a popular arm movement that equally stresses the forearm supinators, brachialis muscles, and biceps.

Starting Position: Grasp two moderately weighted dumbbells, set your feet about shoulder-width apart, and stand erect. Your arms should be hanging straight down at your sides with your palms facing each other. Pin your upper arms to the sides of your torso throughout the movement.

Movement Performance: Keeping your palms facing each other throughout the movement (i.e., keeping your thumbs up), slowly curl the dumbbells together up to your shoulders. Lower the weights back along the same arcs to the starting point and repeat the movement for the suggested number of reps.

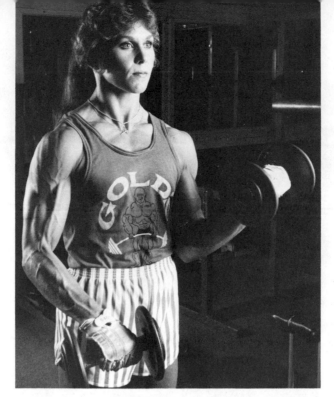

Zottman Curl.

Zottman Curls

Emphasis: This exercise was named for George Zottman, the early American strength athlete who invented the movement. With Zottman Curls, you can equally stress your biceps, brachialis muscles, and forearm supinators.

Starting Position: Grasp two moderately weighted dumbbells, set your feet about shoulder-width apart, and stand erect. Your arms should be hanging straight down at your sides with your palms facing each other. Pin your upper arms to the sides of your torso throughout the movement.

Movement Performance: Slowly curl the dumbbell in your left hand up to your shoulder, supinating your hand so your palm faces upward during the movement. Then at the top of the movement, pronate your hand so your palm faces downward as you lower the weight. Just as you start to lower the dumbbell in your left hand, start curling the weight in your right hand upward, supinating your hand. Keep alternately curling the dumbbells, supinating each hand at the bottom of the movement and pronating it at the top until you have performed the suggested number of repetitions.

Training Tip: At first this will be a somewhat confusing exercise to perform, but if you just think, "Dumbbell up, palm up; dumbbell down, palm down," you won't have any difficulty in mastering it.

Wrist Curls/Reverse Wrist Curls

Emphasis: When you perform this exercise with your palms facing upward, it stresses the flexor muscles of your forearms. And when you do it with your palms facing downward, it stresses the extensor muscles of your forearms.

Starting Position: Take a shoulder-width under-grip on a moderately weighted barbell and sit down at the end of a flat exercise bench. Place your feet shoulder-width apart and run your forearms down your thighs so your wrists and hands dangle off the ends of your knees. Allow the weight to pull your wrists downward as far as possible.

Movement Performance: Using forearm strength, flex your wrists and curl the barbell upward in a small semicircular arc to as high a position as possible. Lower the weight back to the starting point and repeat the exercise for the suggested number of repetitions. This movement is called a Barbell Wrist Curl. You can also do a Barbell Reverse Wrist Curl in precisely the same position and manner, except that your palms will be facing downward rather than upward during the movement.

Training Tip: Generally speaking, you will dis-

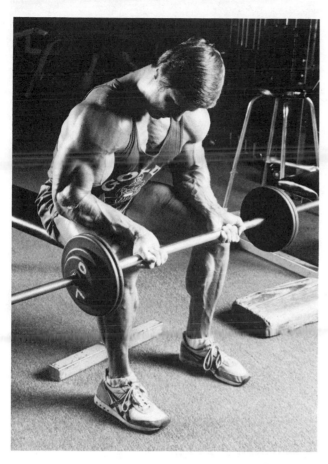
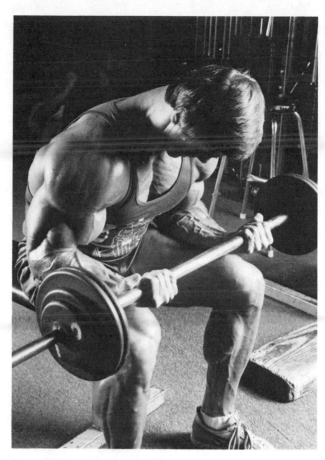

Barbell Wrist Curl—start, left; finish, right.

Dumbbell Wrist Curl—start, left; finish, right.

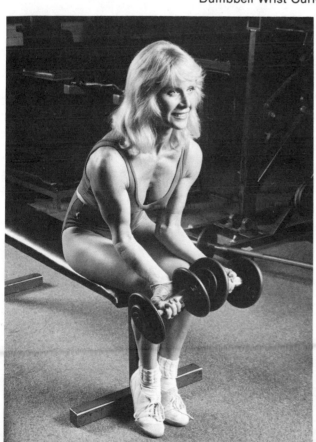
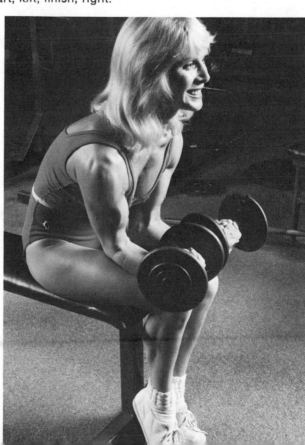

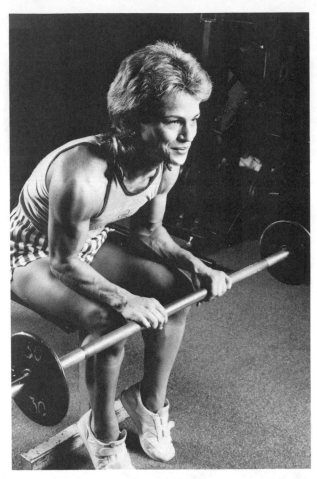 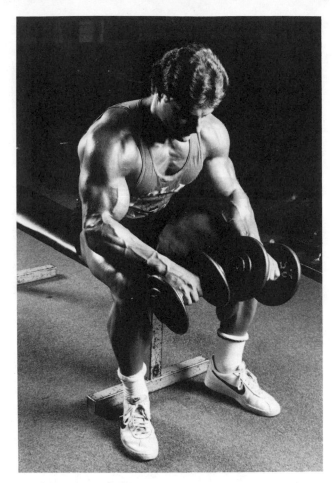

Barbell Reverse Wrist Curl, left; Dumbbell Reverse Wrist Curl, right.

cover that you can use about half as much weight in a Reverse Wrist Curl as in a Wrist Curl.

Exercise Variations: You can also perform Dumbbell Wrist Curls and Dumbbell Reverse Wrist Curls in the same manner and position, but simply while holding dumbbells in your hands.

Supported Wrist Curls

Comment: To make Barbell/Dumbbell Wrist Curls and Reverse Wrist Curls more strict, you can do them with your forearm(s) running along or across a padded, flat exercise bench. With the barbell version of this movement, it's best to kneel on one side of the bench and rest your lower forearms crosswise on the bench, being sure that your wrists and hands hang off the edge. With supported Dumbbell Wrist Curls, it's best to use a single dumbbell, straddle the bench, and run your forearm lengthwise down the bench with your wrist and hand hanging off the end of the bench. You'll most commonly see

bodybuilders doing Supported Dumbbell Wrist Curls with their palms up.

Cable Wrist Curls

Comment: You can use a bar handle attached to a cable running through a floor pulley to do Cable Wrist Curls, which are very similar to the barbell version of the movement. Simply position a flat exercise bench close enough to the floor pulley to allow you to perform the movement, holding the handle and running your forearms down your thighs. And you can also perform the pulley movement with your forearms supported by a flat exercise bench. You can do Reverse Wrist Curls using cables, too.

Nautilus Wrist Curls

Comment: As with Cable Wrist Curls, you can do both Wrist Curls and Reverse Wrist Curls on a Nautilus multi-machine by attaching the bar handle that comes with the machine to the end of the lever arm. Simply place a flat exercise

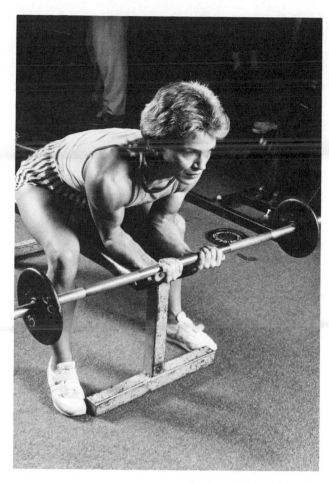
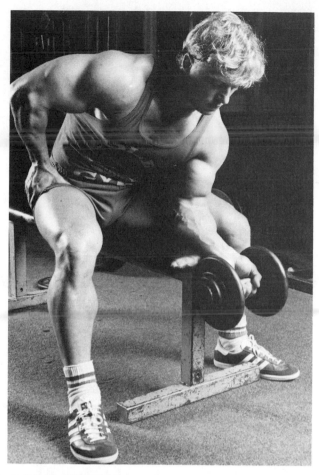

Supported Wrist Curl—barbell, left; dumbbell, right.

Nautilus Wrist Curl—start, left; finish, right.

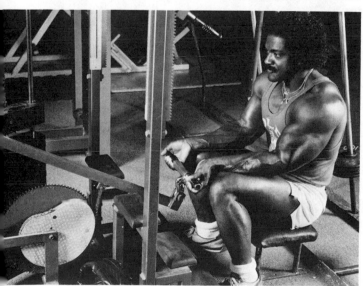
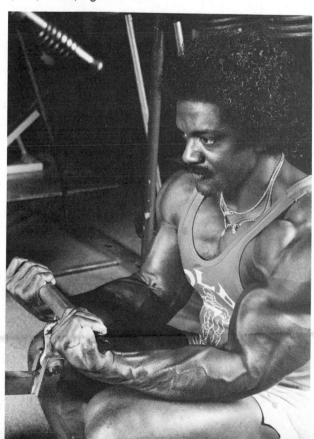

bench up close to the machine so you can run your forearms down your thighs and grasp the handle. It's easy to do both Wrist Curls and Reverse Wrist Curls in this position.

Standing Barbell Wrist Curls

Emphasis: This is a very good movement for stressing the powerful flexor muscles of your forearms.

Starting Position: Place a barbell on a rack or high exercise bench that puts it at about the level of your hips. Back up to the bar and take a shoulder-width grip on it, your palms facing toward the rear. Step away from the rack or bench, place your feet a comfortable distance apart, and stand erect with your arms hanging straight down at your sides and the barbell resting across the back of your upper thighs.

Movement Performance: Slowly flex your wrists to curl the barbell upward in a small semicircular arc to as high a position as possible. Lower back to the starting point and repeat the movement.

Exercise Variations: You can perform a similar movement, Standing Dumbbell Wrist Curls, while standing erect with your arms hanging down at your sides and two heavy dumbbells in your hands, your palms facing each other. Simply do the same type of little, wrist-curling movement in this position as you did for Standing Barbell Wrist Curls.

Wrist Roller

Emphasis: Depending on which direction you roll up the cord on this apparatus, you can stress either the forearm flexors or forearm extensors.

Starting Position: Grasp the wrist roller dowel with your palms toward your body and raise your arms upward until you are holding the dowel out at straight arms' length in front of you, your arms parallel to the floor.

Movement Performance: Move your wrists to roll the cord up completely in one direction, lower back to the starting point, and repeat the movement by rolling it up in the other direction. You can alternate directions until your forearms are completely fatigued.

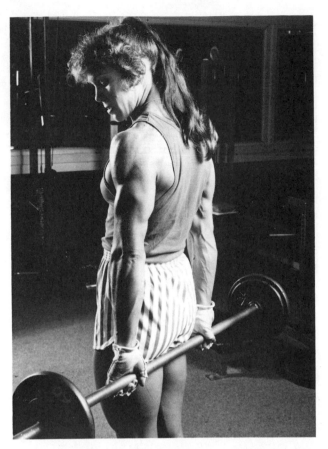

Standing Barbell Wrist Curl—start, above; finish, below.

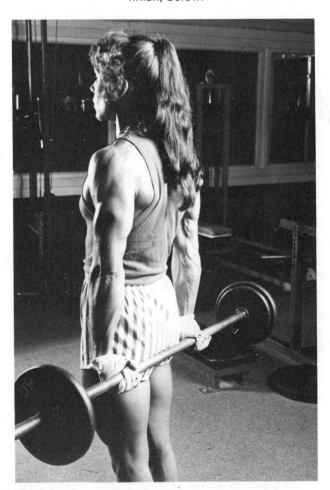

Exercise Variation: Some gyms have a wrist roller apparatus that's bolted to the wall. You can use this apparatus without placing stress on your deltoids, a practice that allows you to place greater concentration on the movement.

Spring Grips

Comment: If your forearm muscles are particularly difficult to develop, you can spend time each day squeezing on one of the commonly available spring grippers. Alternatively, you can spend time gripping a hard, rubber ball. These gripping movements will not only strengthen your gripping power, but will also build up the flexor muscles of your forearms.

Neck Exercises

In this section you will find only three neck exercises plus three variations, but they are all you will need to develop your neck muscles if they seem to be lagging behind the rest of your body. Keep in mind that your neck will probably grow very easily just from the exercises that you do for your upper chest, upper back, and shoulders. In all likelihood, you won't need to do any direct neck training.

Neck Strap Movement

Emphasis: Depending on how you wear the neck strap, you can develop all of the major muscles of your neck using this movement.

Starting Position: Load a light weight on the chair or rope attached to the neck strap and put the head dress on so the weight hangs in front of your body. Sit at the end of a flat exercise bench and rest your hands on your thighs to support your torso in a position learning slightly forward. Lower your chin to your chest.

Movement Performance: Move your head to the rear as far as possible without also moving your torso. Return to the starting point and repeat the movement.

Exercise Variation: You should also do the movement with the weight behind your torso, in which case you begin the exercise with your head tilted as far backward as possible, then move it forward until your chin is on your chest.

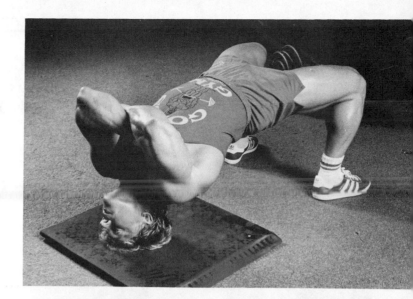

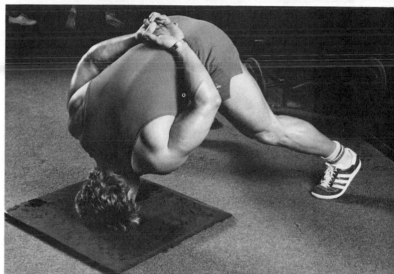

Wrestler's Bridge—back, top; front, bottom.

Wrestler's Bridges

Emphasis: This exercise also works all of the muscles of your neck.

Starting Position: Place a mat on the floor and lie on your back on the mat. Place your feet about shoulder-width apart on the mat and arc your back so only your feet and the top of your head are in contact with the mat.

Movement Performance: Rock back-and-forth, as well as from side-to-side in this position until your neck muscles are fully fatigued.

Exercise Variations: You can do a similar Wrestler's Bridge movement bent forward at the waist rather than arching backward. In Front Bridges, your forehead easily comes into contact with the mat, and you rock back-and-forth and from side-to-side in this position.

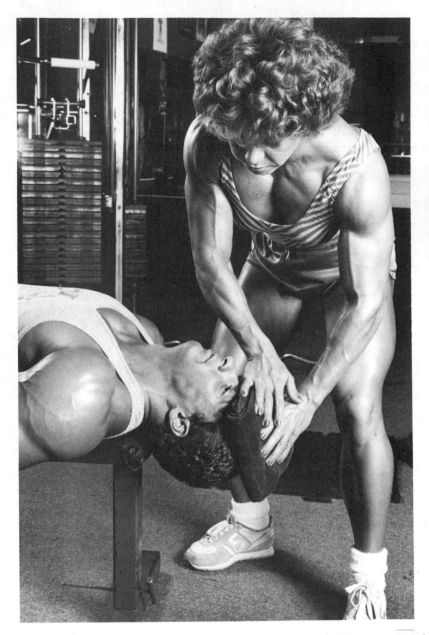
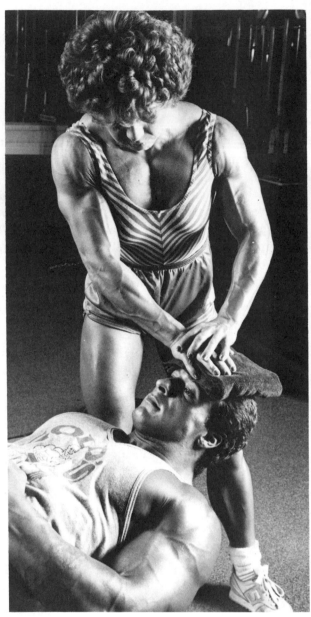

Partner Neck Movement—start, left; finish, right.

Partner Neck Movements

Emphasis: Again, this exercise stresses all the muscles of your neck.

Starting Position: Kneel on your hands and knees on the floor and have a partner stand near your head facing your body. Put your chin on your chest and have your partner apply hand pressure to the back of your head.

Movement Performance: Your partner should apply just enough hand pressure to allow you to only slowly move your head as far upward and to the rear as possible. Then he or she pushes down a bit harder and forces your head back to the starting point. Repeat the movement.

Exercise Variations: You can do a similar movement from one side to the other with your partner kneeling in front of you. Your partner can place his or her right hand against the left side of your head and grasp your right arm with his or her left hand for leverage as you do the movement. Then you can both switch to the other side and give an equal amount of stress to that side of your neck.

Suggested Calf Routines

If you have less than a few weeks of training under your belt, the following calf routine can profitably be performed three nonconsecutive days each week at the end of your regular workout:

Exercise	Sets	Reps
Standing Calf Machine		
Toe Raises	2	15–20
Seated Calf Machine		
Toe Raises	2	10–15

After 4–6 weeks of steady training on the foregoing program, you can use this calf routine three days per week:

Exercise	Sets	Reps
Donkey Call Raises	3	15–20
Calf Presses	2–3	10–15

After about three months of steady training, you will have switched to a four-day split routine for the rest of your body in which you train each major muscle group twice per week. However, the calves can profitably be worked each training day. Following is a sample two-part calf routine for off-season competition training:

Monday–Thursday

Exercise	Sets	Reps
Standing Calf Machine		
Toe Raises	3–4	10–15
One-Leg Toe Raises	3–4	15–20

Tuesday–Friday

Exercise	Sets	Reps
Seated Calf Machine		
Toe Raises	3–4	10–15
Calf Presses	3–4	15–20

Every advanced-level bodybuilder trains differently from all others prior to a competition, as you will see in the following section listing the calf routines of a wide variety of men and women who either train or have trained at Gold's Gym.

Calf Routines of the Gold's Champs

In this section, you will find a variety of calf training programs used by many of the Gold's

Gym superstars who have won the sport's highest titles. Keep in mind as you examine these training programs that these men and women have been training for many years and have developed enormous recuperative abilities. It is unlikely that you can make good gains using their full routines. Instead, you should use these training programs as examples of how to work your own calves. In all likelihood, you can do the same exercises as your favorite champion, but scale down the number of sets that he or she does of each movement to conform to your own ability level.

CHRIS DICKERSON
(MR. OLYMPIA)

Exercise	Sets	Reps
Calf Presses		
(45-degree machine)	3–5	25–30
Seated Calf Machine		
Toe Raises	3–4	25–30
Standing Calf Machine		
Toe Raises	3–4	25–30

SAMIR BANNOUT
(MR. OLYMPIA)

Day 1

Exercise	Sets	Reps
Standing Calf Machine		
Toe Raises	5–6	10–15
Donkey Calf Raises	5–6	15–20

Day 2

Exercise	Sets	Reps
Seated Calf Machine		
Toe Raises	4–5	10–15
Calf Presses		
(horizontal machine)	4–5	15–20

LAURA COMBES
(MS. AMERICA)

Day 1

Exercise	Sets	Reps
Seated Calf Machine		
Toe Raises	6–8	8–10

Day 2

Exercise	Sets	Reps
Standing Calf Machine		
Toe Raises	5–6	20–30

Day 3

Rest and repeat cycle on Day 4.

TOM PLATZ
(MR. UNIVERSE)

Exercise	Sets	Reps
Standing Calf Machine Toe Raises	3–4	10–15
Seated Calf Machine Toe Raises	3–4	10–15
Calf Presses (vertical machine)	3–4	10–15
Hack Machine Toe Raises	3–4	10–15

LOU FERRIGNO
(MR. UNIVERSE)

Day 1

Exercise	Sets	Reps
Seated Calf Machine Toe Raises	10–12	6–10

Day 2

Exercise	Sets	Reps
Standing Calf Machine Toe Raises	10–12	15–20

ROBBY ROBINSON
(PRO GRAND PRIX CHAMP)

Exercise	Sets	Reps
Standing Calf Machine Toe Raises	8	15
Calf Presses (vertical machine)	8	15
Seated Calf Machine Toe Raises	8	10
Donkey Calf Raises	8	20

RACHEL McLISH
(MISS OLYMPIA)

Day 1

Exercise	Sets	Reps
Donkey Calf Raises	3–4	10–15
Seated Calf Machine Toe Raises	3–4	10–15

Day 2

Exercise	Sets	Reps
Standing Calf Machine Toe Raises	3–4	15–20

CASEY VIATOR
(MR. AMERICA)

Exercise	Sets	Reps
Standing Calf Machine Toe Raises	6–8	10–15
Seated Calf Machine Toe Raises	6–8	10–15
Calf Presses (45-degree machine)	4–6	15–20

MIKE MENTZER
(MR. UNIVERSE)

Exercise	Sets	Reps
Calf Presses (vertical machine)	2	8–12
Seated Calf Machine Toe Raises	2	8–12
Standing Calf Machine Toe Raises	1	8–12

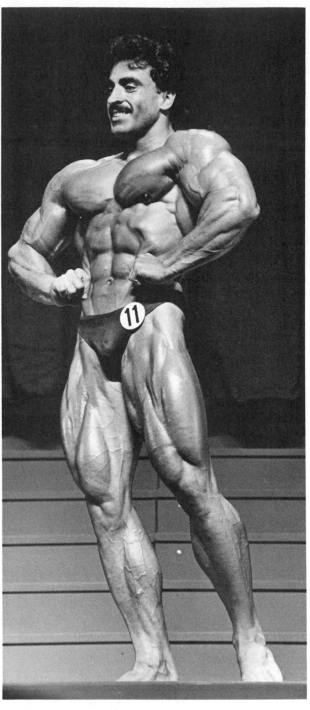

Samir Bannout.

DANNY PADILLA
(MR. UNIVERSE)

Day 1

Exercise	Sets	Reps
Seated Calf Machine Toe Raises	4	10–15
Donkey Calf Raises	4	15–20
One Leg Calf Raises	4	15–20

Day 2

Exercise	Sets	Reps
Standing Calf Machine Toe Raises	4	10–15
Donkey Calf Raises (Nautilus multi)	4	15–20
Calf Presses (vertical machine)	4	15–20

SUE ANN McKEAN
(CALIFORNIA CHAMPION)

Exercise	Sets	Reps
Standing Calf Machine Toe Raises	4–5	10–12
Calf Presses (45-degree machine)	3–4	12–15
Donkey Calf Raises	2–3	15–20

ARNOLD SCHWARZENEGGER
(MR. OLYMPIA)

Exercise	Sets	Reps
Standing Calf Machine Toe Raises	5	8–10
Donkey Calf Raises	5	15–20
Calf Presses (vertical machine)	5	10–15

DENNIS TINERINO
(PRO MR. UNIVERSE)

Exercise	Sets	Reps
Standing Calf Machine Toe Raises	4–6	15–20
Seated Calf Machine Toe Raises	4–6	15–20
Donkey Calf Raises	4–6	15–20

SHELLEY GRUWELL
(WORLD GRAND PRIX CHAMP)

Exercise	Sets	Reps
Seated Calf Machine Toe Raises	3–4	10–15
Standing Calf Machine Toe Raises	3–4	15–20
Calf Presses (horizontal machine)	3–4	20–25

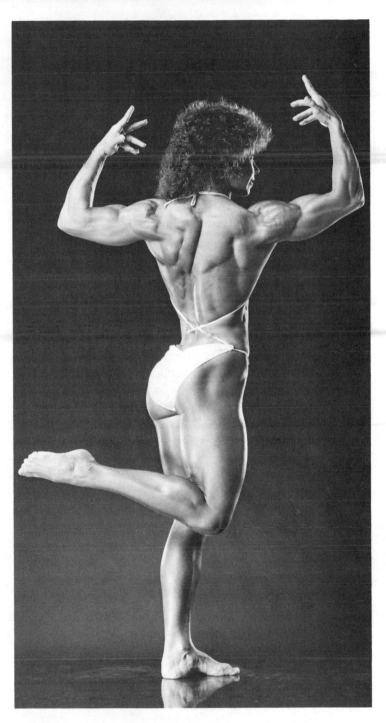

Janice Regan, Los Angeles champ and exercise model.

TIM BELKNAP
(MR. AMERICA)

Exercise	Sets	Reps
Standing Calf Machine Toe Raises	5	10–15
supersetted with		
Donkey Calf Raises	5	10–15

Suggested Forearm Routines

If you have less than a few weeks of training under your belt, the following forearm routine can profitably be performed three nonconsecutive days each week at the end of your regular workout:

Exercise	Sets	Reps
Barbell Wrist Curl	2-3	10-15

After 4-6 weeks of steady training on the foregoing program, you can use this forearm routine three days per week:

Exercise	Sets	Reps
Barbell Reverse Curls	3	8-12
Supported Dumbbell Wrist Curls	3	10-15

After about three months of steady training, you will have switched to a four-day split routine for the rest of your body in which you train each major muscle group—your forearms included—twice per week. Following is a sample forearm program for off-season competition training:

Exercise	Sets	Reps
Preacher-Bench Reverse Curls	4	8-12
Supported Dumbbell Wrist Curls	4	10-15
Barbell Reverse Wrist Curls	4	10-15

Every advanced-level bodybuilder trains differently from all others prior to a competition, as you will see in the following section listing the forearm routines of a wide variety of men and women who either train or have trained at Gold's Gym.

Forearm Routines of the Gold's Champs

In this section, you will find a variety of forearm training programs used by many of the Gold's Gym superstars who have won the sport's highest titles. Keep in mind as you examine these training programs that these men and women have been training for many years and have developed enormous recuperative abilities. It is unlikely that you can make good gains using their full routines. Instead, you should use these training programs as examples of how to work your own forearms. In all likelihood, you can do the same exercises as your favorite champion, but scale down the number of sets that he or she does of each movement to conform to your own abilities.

RACHEL McLISH
(MISS OLYMPIA)

Exercise	Sets	Reps
Barbell Wrist Curls	3-4	10-15
or		
Supported Dumbbell Wrist Curls	3-4	10-15

CASEY VIATOR
(PRO GRAND PRIX CHAMP)

Day 1

Exercise	Sets	Reps
Zottman Curls	5	6-10
Barbell Wrist Curls	5	15-20
Barbell Reverse Wrist Curls	5	15-20

Day 2

Exercise	Sets	Reps
Barbell Reverse Curls	5	6-10
Barbell Wrist Curls	5	15-20
Barbell Reverse Wrist Curls	5	15-20

BOB BIRDSONG
(PRO MR. UNIVERSE)

Monday-Wednesday-Friday

Exercise	Sets	Reps
Barbell Reverse Curls	5	8-10
Supported Dumbbell Wrist Curls	5	15
Standing Barbell Wrist Curls	5	15

Tuesday-Thursday

Exercise	Sets	Reps
Barbell Wrist Curls	5	15
Barbell Reverse Wrist Curls	5	15

MIKE MENTZER
(MR. AMERICA)

Exercise	Sets	Reps
Barbell Reverse Curls	2-3	8-10
Barbell Wrist Curls	2-3	10-15

LAURA COMBES
(MS. AMERICA)

Exercise	Sets	Reps
Hammer Curls	4	8-10
Supported Barbell Wrist Curls	4	15-20

LOU FERRIGNO
(MR. UNIVERSE)

Exercise	Sets	Reps
Barbell Wrist Curls	5	15–20
Barbell Reverse Wrist Curls	5	15–20

MATT MENDENHALL
(MR. CENTRAL STATES)

Exercise	Sets	Reps
Barbell Reverse Curls	4–5	8–10
or		
Hammer Curls	4–5	8–10
Barbell Wrist Curls	4–5	10–15
Dumbbell Wrist Curls	2–3	10–15

SAMIR BANNOUT
(MR. OLYMPIA)

Exercise	Sets	Reps
Zottman Curls	4–5	8–10
Supported Dumbbell Wrist Curls	4–5	10–15
Supported Barbell Reverse Wrist Curls	4–5	10–15

TOM PLATZ
(MR. UNIVERSE)

Exercise	Sets	Reps
Supported Barbell Wrist Curls	5–8	10–12

DANNY PADILLA
(MR. UNIVERSE)

Day 1

Exercise	Sets	Reps
Barbell Reverse Curls	4–5	8–10
Supported Barbell Wrist Curls	4–5	10–15

Day 2

Exercise	Sets	Reps
Zottman Curls	4–5	8–10
Supported Dumbbell Wrist Curls	4–5	10–15

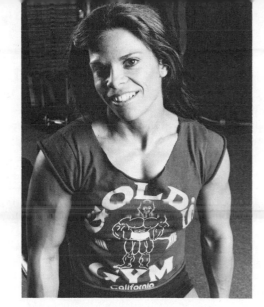

Exercise model and California Lightweight champ, Chris Glass.

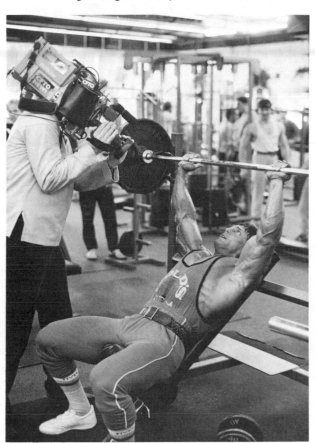

On camera at Gold's: Bob Birdsong.

Training Your Neck

As already mentioned, you probably won't have to train your neck very hard to get it to grow to very thick proportions. We suggest that you simply pick one of the listed neck exercises and use it for 5–10 minutes, or until you feel that the muscles of your neck are sufficiently pumped up. Just two or three workouts of this type each week, and you'll have a very impressively developed neck.

Looking Ahead

In the final chapter, we will discuss a number of advanced-level training techniques, including the following topics: training to failure, cheating reps, forced reps, stripping sets, compound sets, pre-exhaustion, peak-contraction, continuous tension, negative reps, rest-pause training, muscle priority training, and overtraining.

10 ADVANCED TRAINING TECHNIQUES

In this concluding chapter, we will explain more than ten advanced-level training techniques that you can use to improve your workouts. Please keep in mind that this book is intended as an encyclopedia of bodybuilding exercises rather than a manual of training techniques. Therefore, our discussions of each of these advanced workout techniques is not as detailed as similar discussions in *The Gold's Gym Book of Bodybuilding*. If you intend to get the most out of your training, it would be a good idea to read that book as well as this one.

Training to Failure

After two or three months of steady training, you will be ready to begin taking all of your post-warm-up sets to at least the point of failure, or to that point at which you can no longer complete a set under your own power. This is absolutely essential if you are to continue making good gains from your training. Virtually all superstar bodybuilders train at least to failure, and many of them do a lot of cheating reps, forced reps, and stripping sets to push their fatigued muscles to continue working *past* the failure point.

Cheating Reps

The most fundamental method of pushing a set past the failure point is doing cheating reps. We realize that you have probably been cautioned against cheating in an exercise. This is because most beginning and intermediate bodybuilders cheat to make a set *easier* on their muscles. However, as an advanced-level bodybuilder you can use cheating to make a set *harder* on your muscles.

Inexperienced bodybuilders cheat before they reach the point of failure in strict form, but you must avoid cheating before you have absolutely taken your set to failure. Only then can you inject the bare minimum of extraneous body movement (e.g., knee jerking, torso swaying, etc.) to boost the weight over the point past which you could not push it with your own muscle power. From there, you must finish the movement under your own power, then slowly lower the bar back to the starting point while powerfully resisting its downward momentum.

If you use the cheating method in this manner, you will find that you can push your muscles to the point where they burn from fatigue toxins as if someone were playing a blow torch across them. And this is a good indication that you have bombed them harder than ever before, which will force them to increase in hypertrophy unbelievably quickly.

Forced Reps

One weakness of cheating reps is that it's difficult to apply precisely the minimum amount of momentum to the weight that allows you to get it past the point where you normally fail on an exercise. With *forced reps,* however, you can have a training partner pull up on the bar with the absolute minimum amount of force necessary to help you through the sticking point.

Your training partner can stand at the head end of the bench when you perform Bench Presses, for example, and pull up on the middle of the barbell just enough to get you over the hump. And each succeeding repetition will require your partner to pull up on the bar with a little more force because your muscles will be growing progressively more fatigued.

With both cheating reps and forced reps there is a limit to how many reps you can push out past the failure point and still benefit from using either technique. With time, you will learn that anything over two or three cheating reps or forced reps is wasted effort.

Stripping Sets

Another way to remove enough weight from a barbell to allow you to grind out additional reps past the normal point of failure is *stripping sets* (sometimes called *descending sets*). With this method, you will need two training partners stationed at either end of the bar to remove a predetermined amount of weight each time you have pushed to the failure point. And you can do either one or two weight drops in the middle of each set.

Let's take Bench Presses to illustrate how to use stripping sets. Load up the bar to a weight that you can use for only five or six strict reps, but be sure you load each side with a variety of loose plates and leave the collars off the bar. Lie back on the bench with your training partners at either end of the bar. Do five or six reps to failure, and while supporting the bar have your

partners remove 15–20 pounds from each end of the bar. Continue the set to failure again, say doing three or four additional reps. And if you feel particularly motivated, make another poundage drop and force out a final few excruciating reps. That's high-intensity training!

With dumbbells, you can go "down the rack" with the weights. For example, you can begin a stripping set of Standing Dumbbell Curls with a pair of 50s in your hands, doing six reps to failure. Immediately put the 50s back on the rack and grab the 45s for as many reps as you can eke out. Put them back and grab the 40s for your final super-intense reps. No one said it was supposed to be easy, right?

Compound Sets

You can greatly increase the intensity of your training by doing two or more exercises with no rest between movements, followed by a normal rest interval of approximately 60 seconds. These compound sets are called supersets, trisets, and giant sets, and you can immediately begin to include some compound sets for your arms in your workouts.

Supersets

Supersets are groups of two movements performed one right after the other and followed by a normal rest interval. The easiest form of superset includes exercises for each of two antagonistic muscle groups (e.g., the biceps and triceps, pectorals and lats, or the quadriceps and hamstrings). In Figure 10–1 on page 239, you will find examples of this type of superset.

A more intense form of superset includes two exercises for the same muscle group. Examples of this variation of superset can be found in Figure 10–2 on page 239.

Trisets

Trisets are groups of three exercises performed one right after the other and followed by a normal rest interval. The best way to use trisets is for multifaceted muscle groups, such as the deltoids with anterior, medial, and posterior heads, or the back with traps, lats, and erectors.

Still, you *can* use trisets for any muscle group that you like. or even for two closely related muscle groups (e.g., two exercises for one body part and one for the other). You will find typical examples of trisets in Figure 10-3 below.

Biceps + Triceps = Barbell
   Curls + Pulley Pushdowns
Biceps + Triceps = Seated Dumbbell
   Curls + Lying Triceps Extensions
Pecs + Lats = Bench Presses + Chins
Pecs + Lats = Incline Presses + Seated
   Pulley Rows
Quads + Hamstrings = Leg Extensions
   + Leg Curls
Quads + Hamstrings = Squats + Stiff-
   Legged Deadlifts
Forearm Flexors + Forearm Extensors
   = Wrist Curls + Reverse Wrist Curls

**Figure 10-1: Supersets for Antagonistic Muscle
   Groups.**

Lats = Pullovers + Lat Machine
   Pulldowns
Traps = Barbell Shrugs + Upright Rows
Erectors = Deadlifts + Hyperextensions
Pecs (in general) = Bench Presses +
   Flat-Bench Flyes
Lower Pecs = Parallel Bar Dips +
   Decline Flyes
Upper Pecs = Incline Presses + Incline
   Flyes
Delts = Military Presses + Upright Rows
Delts = Presses behind the Neck + Bent
   Laterals
Quads = Squats + Leg Extensions
Calves = Seated Calf Raises + Lying
   Calf Raises
Biceps = Barbell Preacher Curls +
   Barbell Curls
Triceps = Lying Triceps Extensions +
   Pulley Pushdowns

Figure 10-2: Supersets for a Single Muscle Group.

Deltoids
Military Press (anterior head)
Bent Laterals (posterior head)
Upright Rows (medial Head + trapezius)

Arms
Lying Triceps Extensions (triceps)
Darbell Curls (biceps)
Barbell Wrist Curls (forearms)

Figure 10-3: Examples of Trisets.

Biceps + Triceps (four exercises)
Pulley Preacher Curls (lower biceps)
Lying Triceps Extensions (triceps mass)
Incline Curls (biceps shape)
Pulley Pushdowns (triceps shape)

Chest + Back (six exercises)
Bench Press (pecs, general)
Front Lat Pulldowns (lower lats)
Dips (lower–outer pecs)
Pulldowns behind the Neck (upper lats)
Incline Flyes (upper pecs)
Stiff-Arm Pulldowns (lats-
   serratus)

**Figure 10-4: Giant Sets for Antagonistic Muscle
   Groups.**

Chest (four exercises)
Incline Press (upper pecs)
Pec Deck Flyes (inner pecs)
Dips (lower–outer pecs)
Cable Crossovers (pec cuts)

Back (five exercises)
Chins (upper lats/lat width)
Hyperextensions (erectors)
Seated Pulley Rows (lat thickness)
Barbell Shrugs (traps)
Stiff-Arm Pulldowns (lats-serratus)

Figure 10-5: Giant Sets for a Single Muscle Group.

Giant Sets

Giant sets are groups of 4–6 exercises performed one right after the other and followed by a normal rest interval. Giant sets are best used for antagonistic muscle groups (see Figure 10–4 on page 239), but they can also be used for a single muscle group (see Figure 10–5 on page 239).

On a ladder of training intensity, you will find the least intense form of training to be straight sets taken to failure. Then in ascending order of intensity, you can add to your routine supersets, trisets, four-exercise giant sets, five-exercise giant sets, and finally six-exercise giant sets.

Preexhaustion

You can best stress your torso muscle groups with extreme intensity by using the *preexhaustion,* supersetting technique. To understand this technique, you must first realize that most basic exercises for your torso also involve your arm muscles. For example, when you do Bench Presses for your pectorals and anterior deltoids, you also involve your triceps; when you do Pulley Rows for your lats, you also involve your biceps; and when you do Presses behind the Neck for your delts, you also involve your triceps.

The problem with torso–arm, basic exercises is that your biceps and triceps muscles are much smaller (and hence weaker) than the larger pecs, lats, and delts. As a result, your arm muscles almost always tire and fail to move their part of the load long before your torso groups have been fully exhausted. And this is one primary reason why most uninformed bodybuilders fail to properly train their pecs, lats, traps, and delts.

The best way to stress your torso muscle groups with maximum intensity is to make your arms stronger than normal—even stronger than your torso groups—by preexhausting the torso groups with an initial set of a non-arm isolation exercise. This is immediately followed up by a basic arm-torso movement for the same body part, done with an absolute minimum of rest between exercises. Examples of this preexhaustion, supersetting technique can be found in Figure 10–6 in the next column.

If you consistently include preexhaustion su-

Upper Pecs = Incline Flyes + Incline Presses
Lower Pecs = Decline Flyes + Decline Presses
Pecs (in general) = Flat-Bench Flyes + Bench Presses
Anterior Delts = Front Raises + Dumbbell Presses
Posterior Delts = Bent Laterals + Barbell Bent Rows
Delts (in general) = Upright Rows + Presses behind the Neck
Traps = Barbell Shrugs + Upright Rows
Lats = Nautilus Pullovers + Lat Machine Pulldowns
Lats = Cross-Bench Pullovers + Chins

Figure 10–6: Examples of Preexhaustion Supersets.

persets for your torso muscle groups in your training program, you'll soon find that your pecs, traps, lats, and delts have exploded to new growth. It's the only way to attack these torso body parts with optimum training intensity.

Peak Contraction

When you fully understand how a muscle contracts, you'll know that a maximum number of muscle cells have been fired off when a muscle is in its shortest mode. And you can see this for yourself by flexing your biceps in front of a mirror and noting how much the muscle expands in thickness when you have it completely flexed.

It makes good sense, then, to place maximum resistance on a working muscle when it is completely contracted because this is when the muscle group is set up to bear the greatest load. However, many exercises don't place significant resistance on the contracted muscles. For example, when your arms are fully bent in a Barbell Curl movement, there is absolutely no stress on the biceps. Instead, your biceps are relaxed and your deltoids are holding the weight.

Placing a heavy load on a working muscle when it is totally contracted is called *peak contraction,* and you should always include peak-contraction exercises in your workouts. Some of the best peak-contraction movements are those performed on Nautilus and other machines that feature rotary resistance. Other good peak-contraction exercises include Calf Raises of all sorts, Pulldowns, Chins, all rowing movements, Barbell Concentration Curls, Leg Curls, Leg Extensions, Dumbbell Kickbacks, Hyperextensions, and Shrugs.

Continuous Tension

Continuous tension is another good workout-intensification technique, particularly when you are involved in a cycle of muscularity enhancement. With this principle, you will, first of all, move a weight relatively slowly (say, about half as fast as under normal circumstances) over a full range of motion. This places greater stress on your working muscles because it prevents momentum from robbing your muscles of some of the stress they should receive. This is particularly true over the last half of any exercise.

Second, you should flex both the working muscles and their antagonistic body parts very tightly. You'll hear top bodybuilders say, "Keep the tension up. You have to maintain maximum tension." This is what they are talking about. And keeping the antagonistic muscles tight allows you to stress a working muscle with somewhat less resistance than is normally possible.

Combined with peak contraction, quality training (a progressive reduction in the length of rest intervals between sets), and a low-calorie diet, continuous tension helps you to achieve the diamond-hard muscularity of a Mr. Olympia or Miss Olympia winner.

Negative Reps

Exercise physiologists have long since determined that the negative (downward) half of an exercise offers at least as much potential for mass and power development as the positive (upward) half. You can first take advantage of this fact by lowering a weight each rep a bit more slowly than you raise it in order to place greater stress on the negative cycle of the exercise. In any case, you should always avoid merely dropping the weight from the top point of an exercise back to the starting position.

Next, you can use either the *negative emphasis* or *forced negatives* technique. In negative emphasis reps, you will raise the weight with both arms or legs in a variety of machine exercises, then lower it slowly with only one arm or leg. Then you lift the weight up again with both limbs and lower it with the other arm or leg. It's very important that you exert yourself to the max as you attempt to slow the downward momentum of the weight during each repetition.

You can perform forced negatives on both machine and free-weight exercises. With this technique, you raise the weight under your own power and then resist additional downward force placed on the equipment by your training partner pushing against the weight. Your partner should push down with just enough force to keep you from actually stopping the downward movement of the weight.

Some bodybuilders also do pure negative reps, although it's usually next to impossible to find training partners willing to sacrifice their own workouts to keep lifting the weights up for you. With pure negatives, you can use a weight 30%–50% heavier than one with which you can perform 1–3 full, positive and negative reps. Your partners lift the weight to the top position of each movement for every rep you perform, after which you lower it by yourself. In one heavy basic exercise per muscle group 5–8 repetitions can be done.

Rest–Pause Training

Rest–pause training, which was popularized recently by long-time Gold's Gym member Mike Mentzer, is close to being the ultimate technique for building herculean mass and power. Indeed, the technique is so intense that it can only be used once each week or two for each body part, hitting only one set of 6–10 "reps."

No one familiar with bodybuilding can deny that you need to lift very heavy poundages in basic exercises in order to build a high degree of muscle mass and physical power. With the heaviest weights, though, you can only perform 1–3 reps before reaching the failure point. Therefore, you are limited to using lighter poundages that simply don't build the highest possible degree of development.

With rest–pause training, however, you *can* use maximum weights, due largely to the fact that your body recoups roughly half of its strength and endurance after only a very short, 15-second rest interval. So with rest–pause training, you choose a basic exercise and load a weight on the bar that limits you to only 1–3 reps. Grind out these reps, place the bar on a rack, rest only 10–15 seconds, then pick up the bar and get another one or two reps.

You'll usually have to reduce the weight on the bar by 10%–15% after this second mini-set, but don't take more than 15 seconds to do so, even if you must have two training partners make the weight change for you. Take the reduced weight and grind out two or three more reps, followed by a 15-second rest–pause, and a final supermacho one or two reps. This will give you 6–10 "reps" of the basic exercise with maximum poundages.

Use caution with rest–pause training. Do no more than one set of each movement, 6–10 reps, each 3–5 workouts. Doing any more than this amount of rest–pause work will quickly lead to overtraining, a topic that is covered later in this chapter.

Muscle Priority Training

Poll several experienced, bodybuilding competition judges, and you'll discover that they place very high importance on equal proportions from one body part to another. But talk to any experienced bodybuilder, and he or she will tell you that every person's body responds unevenly to training. Some muscle groups come up very quickly, while others seem to resist all of your efforts to improve them. So, from the very beginning of your involvement in bodybuilding, you should seek to maintain good proportional balance.

It takes plenty of specialized high-intensity training to improve a weak muscle group, as well as use of a technique called *muscle priority training*. This latter technique primarily involves performing your routine for a lagging muscle group first in your workout when you have available maximum physical and mental energy.

Only then can you bomb your lagging body part with sufficient intensity to force it to grow in mass and power.

Muscle priority training also involves cutting back on the amount and intensity of stress that you put on a relatively strong body part. It certainly doesn't make much sense to continue improving a muscle group that is already far ahead in development, does it? So, you should use muscle priority training to save energy for expenditure on a lagging body part.

Overtraining

One of the most common mistakes made by inexperienced bodybuilders is overtraining, or doing too much work in each training session, driving the body so deeply into an energy debt that it is unable to recuperate between training sessions. Overtraining is death to a bodybuilder because it prevents you from making gains from your workouts. In more serious cases, it can actually cause a regression in the amount and quality of your muscle tissue.

Your body is a dynamic energy system in which energy is stored and then expended in each workout. It's very much like a bank account in that you can't expend more energy than you have deposited without going "energy broke," or overtraining. And it's important to note that short, high-intensity workouts don't lead to overtraining. Instead, it is an accumulation of long, low-intensity training sessions that ultimately leads to an overtrained state.

If you display more than one of the following nine symptoms, it is probable that you are entering an overtrained state:

- Lethargy; a feeling of always being fatigued.
- Persistently sore joints and/or muscles.
- Loss of appetite.
- Insomnia.
- Illness and/or chronic infections.
- Lack of enthusiasm for your workouts.
- Regression in neuromuscular control.
- Elevated morning pulse rate.
- Elevated blood pressure not accounted for in another fashion (i.e., not due to an increase in body weight, salt consumption, etc.).

The best solution to overtraining is to prevent it from occurring in the first place. You can prevent overtraining by avoiding high-set workouts. Without a doubt, the most common reason why young bodybuilders fail to make good gains from their training is that they perform far too many total sets for each muscle group, thereby making it difficult or even impossible for their bodies to recuperate sufficiently between training sessions.

If you have less than three months of steady training under your belt, you should do no more than six total sets for large muscle groups (e.g., thighs, back, chest, deltoids) and no more than four total sets for smaller body parts (e.g., biceps, triceps, forearms, abdominals, calves). With up to six months of training, you can do 8–10 total sets for large muscle groups and up to six total sets for smaller ones. With up to a year of training, do no more than 12 sets for large muscle groups and up to seven or eight for smaller body parts. And with more than a year of gym experience, you will have developed a sufficient knowledge of how your body responds to exercise to accurately determine for yourself how much total work you should perform in each training session.

Two other factors are important in preventing overtraining. First of all, you must get adequate high-quality sleep each night to completely rest your body. And secondly, you must maintain a healthy bodybuilding diet devoid of energy-robbing junk foods.

If you do enter an overtrained state, the best solution for the condition begins with a 1–2-week total layoff from bodybuilding training (you can still engage in recreational physical pursuits, however). Then once you are back in the gym, be sure to take only short, high-intensity workouts.

Our Last Set Together

It's up to you now. One of the best things about bodybuilding is that you can sculpt your body in any way you like. And when you are successful, only you are responsible for your achievement. But on the other side of the coin, you can blame no one but yourself if you fail to reach your goals. Which do you want, success or failure? We're sure you will shoot for success, so go for the gold the Gold's Gym way!

GLOSSARY

AEROBIC EXERCISE—Long-lasting, low-intensity exercise that can be carried on within the body's ability to consume and process enough oxygen to support the activity. The word *aerobic* means literally *with air*. Typical aerobic exercise activities include running, swimming, and cycling. Aerobic exercise leads to cardiorespiratory fitness.

AFWB—The American Federation of Women Bodybuilders, the sports federation responsible for administering women's amateur bodybuilding in America. The AFWB is affiliated internationally with the IFBB.

AMDR—The Adult Minimum Daily Requirement for various nutrients, as established by the U.S. Food and Drug Administration.

ANAEROBIC EXERCISE—High-intensity exercise that exceeds the body's aerobic capacity and builds up an oxygen debt. Because of its high intensity, anaerobic exercise can be continued for only a short time. A typical anaerobic exercise would be full-speed sprinting on a track.

BALANCE—Referring to even body proportions, as in, "He has nice balance to his physique."

BAR—The iron or steel shaft that forms the handle of a barbell or dumbbell. Barbell bars vary in length from about four to seven feet, while dumbbell bars are 12–16 inches long. Bars are usually one inch in diameter, and they are often encased in a revolving sleeve.

BARBELL—This is the basic piece of equipment for weight training and bodybuilding. It consists of a bar, sleeve, collars, and plates. The weight of an adjustable barbell without plates averages five pounds per foot of bar length. The weight of this basic barbell unit must be considered when adding plates to the barbell to form a required training poundage. Barbells in large gyms are usually "fixed," with the plates welded or otherwise semipermanently fastened to the bars in a variety of poundages. These poundages are designated by numerals painted or engraved on the sides of the plates of each barbell.

BMR—The Basal Metabolic Rate, or the natural speed at which the body burns calories when at rest to provide its basic survival energy needs.

BODYBUILDING—A subdivision of the general category of weight training in which the main objective is to change the appearance of the human body via heavy weight training and applied nutrition. For most men and women bodybuilding consists merely of reducing a fleshy area or two and/or building up one or two thin body parts. In its purest form, bodybuilding for men and women is a competitive sport, both nationally and internationally, in amateur and professional categories.

BODYSCULPTING—This term is occasionally used in a feminine context to mean *bodybuilding*.

BURN—The feeling a muscle gets when it has really been pushed to its limits.

CHEATING—A method of swinging the weights or body to complete a rep that would have otherwise been impossible.

CIRCUIT TRAINING—A specialized form of weight training that develops body strength and aerobic endurance simultaneously. In circuit training a bodybuilder plans a circuit of 10–20 exercises covering all of the body's major muscle groups, then proceeds around the circuit in order while resting minimally between sets. Many bodybuilders use circuit training to improve their muscularity prior to a competition. As such, it is a good form of quality training.

CLEAN—The act of raising a barbell or dumbbell to shoulder height.

COLLAR—The cylindrical metal clamp used to hold plates in position on a barbell. Usually these collars are secured in place with a "set screw" threaded through the collar and tightened against the bar with a wrench. *Inside collars* keep plates from sliding inward and injuring a bodybuilder's hands, while *outside collars* keep the plates from sliding off the end of the bar. For safety's sake, you should never lift a barbell unless the collars are tightly fastened in place.

COUPLES' COMPETITION—Sometimes called "Mixed Pairs Competition," this is a new form of bodybuilding competition in which man–woman teams compete against each other. Couples' competition is becoming very popular with bodybuilding fans all over the world. It is now part of competitions even on the international level.

CUT UP—A term used to denote a well-defined bodybuilder. Usually this is a complimentary term, as in saying, "He's really cut up for this show!"

DEFINITION—This term is used to denote an absence of body fat in a bodybuilding competitor, so that every muscle is fully delineated. When a competitor has achieved ideal definition, his or her muscles will show striations, or individual fibers visible along a muscle mass. Definition is often called *muscularity*.

DENSITY—The hardness of muscle tissue, denoting complete muscularity, even to the point where fat within a muscle mass has been eliminated.

DUMBBELL—This is simply a shorter version of a barbell, which is intended for use in one hand, or more commonly with equally weighted dumbbells in each hand. All of the characteristics and terminology of a barbell are the same in a dumbbell.

EXERCISE—Used as a noun, this is the actual bodybuilding movement being done (e.g., a Bench Press or a Concentration Curl). An exercise is often called a *movement*. Used as a verb, *to exercise* is to work out physically and recreationally with weight training or any number of other forms of exercise (e.g., running, playing softball, etc.).

FLEXIBILITY—A suppleness of muscles and connective tissue that allows any man or woman to move his or her limbs and torso over a complete—or even exaggerated—range of motion.

FORCED REPS—A method of training whereby a training partner helps lift a weight just enough so the movement can be completed for two or three repetitions once the trainee has reached a point where he cannot complete it on his own.

HYPERTROPHY—The increase due to an overload on a muscle in that muscle's mass and strength. This is usually referred to by bodybuilders as *muscle growth*, though muscles do not grow in the sense of adding new cells to their mass.

IFBB—The International Federation of Bodybuilders, which was founded in 1946 by Ben and Joe Weider. It is the parent international federation overseeing worldwide, men's and women's amateur and professional bodybuilding. More than 115 national bodybuilding federations are affiliated with the IFBB, making bodybuilding the world's fifth most popular sport.

INTENSITY—The degree of difficulty built into weight training exercise. Intensity can be increased by adding resistance, increasing the number of repetitions done of an exercise, or decreasing the rest interval between sets. The greater the intensity of bodybuilding exercise placed on a muscle, the greater will be that muscle's rate of hypertrophy.

JUDGING ROUNDS—In the internationally accepted IFBB system of bodybuilding judging, three judging rounds are contested, plus a final posedown in which the top five contestants compete in a free-posing manner for added points. In Round I each bodybuilder is viewed standing relaxed with his or her front, left side, back, and right side toward the judging panel. Round II consists of a set of standardized "compulsory poses," while Round III is devoted to creative individual "free posing" to each contestant's own choice of music.

LIFTING BELT—A leather belt four to six inches wide at the back that is worn around the waist to protect a trainee's lower back and abdomen from injuries. The six-inch belt can be used in training, but only the four-inch belt can be used in actual weightlifting competition.

MASS—The size or fullness of muscles. Massiveness is highly prized in bodybuilding competition, especially by the male competitors.

MUSCULARITY—Another term for *definition*, it denotes an absence of body fat, so that every muscle is fully delineated.

NPC—The National Physique Committee, Inc., the sports federation responsible for administering men's amateur bodybuilding in America. Like the AFWB, the NPC is affiliated internationally with the IFBB.

NUTRITION—The various practices of taking food into the human body. Bodybuilders have made a science of nutrition by applying it either to add muscle mass or to totally strip fat from their bodies to achieve optimum muscle definition.

OLYMPIAN—An appellation given to those men and women who have competed in the Mr. Olympia or Miss Olympia contests. Olympians are elite bodybuilders.

OLYMPIC BARBELL—A highly specialized and finely machined barbell used in weightlifting competition and heavy bodybuilding training. An Olympic barbell weighs 20 kilograms (slightly less than 45 pounds), and each of its collars weighs 2½ kilograms (5.5 pounds).

OLYMPIC LIFTING—A form of competitive weightlifting included in the Olympic Games program since the revival of the modern Olympics at Athens in 1896. Until 1972 this form of weightlifting consisted of three lifts: the Press, Snatch, and Clean and Jerk. Because of officiating difficulties, however, the Press was dropped from use following the 1972 Olympic Games, leaving the Snatch and Clean and Jerk as the two competitive Olympic lifts.

OVERLOAD—A degree of stress placed on the muscle that is over and above the amount the muscle is ordinarily used to handling. In bodybuilding this overload is applied by lifting heavier and heavier weights.

PEAK—Used two ways in bodybuilding jargon—to indicate the top of a muscle (usually the biceps) and to describe the process of reaching top physical condition before a contest.

PHA—An abbreviation for *peripheral heart action,* in which each skeletal muscle acts as an auxiliary heart by milking blood past one-way valves in the arterial system. Without PHA the heart itself would have difficulty circulating blood throughout the body. PHA is also a term assigned to a system of circuit training in which shorter series of four to six exercises are used in circuits. This system was pioneered by Bob Gajda, the 1966 Mr. America winner.

PLATES—The flat discs pierced with holes in the middle that are fitted on barbells and dumbbells to increase the weight of these apparatus. Plates are made of either cast metal or vinyl-covered concrete. They come in a wide range of graduated weights from as little as 1¼ pounds to more than 100 pounds each.

POUNDAGE—The actual weight of a barbell, dumbbell, or weight machine resistance used in an exercise.

POWERLIFTING—A form of competitive weightlifting using three lifts: the Squat, Bench Press, and Deadlift. The sport has both national and international competitions. Unlike in Olympic lifting, special women's competitions are held in powerlifting.

PROGRESSION—The act of gradually and steadily adding to the resistance used to overload a muscle group stressed by an exercise.

PROPORTION—A competitive bodybuilding term referring to the size relationships between various body parts. A contestant with good proportions will have no over- or under-developed muscle groups.

PUMP—To achieve a *pump* or to get *pumped* is to exercise a muscle until it is heavily engorged with blood.

QUALITY TRAINING—A type of workout in which the rest intervals between sets are drastically shortened prior to a competition. Quality training in combination with a low-calorie diet results in the best possible combination of muscle mass and muscle density.

REPETITION—Often abbreviated as *rep,* this is each individual full cycle of an exercise from the starting point of the movement to the midpoint and back again to the starting point. Usually, a series of several repetitions are done for each exercise.

RESISTANCE—As with poundage, this is the actual weight being used in an exercise.

REST INTERVAL—The pause between sets of an exercise during which the worked muscles are allowed to recuperate partially before the succeeding set is begun. Rest intervals vary from as little as 10–15 seconds to as much as five minutes. An average rest interval is about 60 seconds.

RIPPED—A term synonymous with *cut up,* as in "He's really ripped."

ROUTINE—Sometimes called a *program* or *schedule,* this is the complete accumulation of exercises, sets, and reps done in one training session. A routine is usually repeated two or three times each week.

SET—A distinct grouping of repetitions, followed by a brief rest interval and another set. Usually, several sets are done for each exercise in a training program.

.SLEEVE—A hollow metal tube fitted over the bar of a barbell. The sleeve allows a bar to rotate more freely in your hands. Ordinarily, grooved knurlings are scored into the sleeve to aid in gripping the barbell when the hands have become sweaty during a training session.

SPOTTERS—Training partners who stand by as a safety factor to prevent you from being pinned under a heavy barbell during an exercise. Spotters are particularly necessary when you are doing limit Bench Presses and Squats.

STEROIDS—Prescription artificial male hormones that some bodybuilders use to increase muscle mass. Anabolic steroids are very dangerous drugs, however, and we strongly discourage their use.

STICKING POINT—Any part of a movement that is very difficult to get past in order to complete the movement.

STRETCHING—A type of exercise program used to promote body flexibility. It involves assuming and then holding postures in which certain muscle groups and body joints are stretched.

STRIATIONS—This is the ultimate degree of muscle definition. When a muscle mass like the pectoral is fully defined, it will have myriad small individual grooves across it, almost as if a cat had repeatedly scratched the surface of a wax statue's pectoral muscles. These tiny muscular details are called striations.

SUPPLEMENTS—Concentrated vitamins, minerals, and proteins, usually in tablet/capsule or powder form. Food supplements are widely used by competitive bodybuilders, weightlifters, and other athletes to optimize their overall nutritional intake.

SYMMETRY—In competitive bodybuilding parlance, this is the shape or general outline of the body, as if it were seen in silhouette. Symmetry is enhanced in both male and female bodybuilders by a wide shoulder structure; a small waist–hip structure; small knees, ankles, and wrists; and large muscle volumes surrounding these small joints.

TRAINING TO FAILURE—Method of training whereby the trainee has continued a set to a point where it is impossible for him to complete another rep without assistance.

VASCULARITY—The appearance of surface veins and arteries in any bodybuilder who has achieved a low level of body fat. Women tend to have vascularity primarily in their arms, while male bodybuilders can have surface vascularity all over their bodies.

WEIGHT—Another term for *poundage* or *resistance*. Sometimes this term is used generally to refer to the apparatus (barbell, dumbbell, etc.) being used in an exercise, versus the exact poundage being used in an exercise.

WEIGHT CLASS—So that smaller athletes are not overwhelmed by larger ones, both competitive bodybuilding and weightlifting use weight classes. In women's bodybuilding the classes (at the time of this writing) were under 52½ kilograms (114 lbs.) and over 52½ kilos, while men's bodybuilding weight classes are set at 70 kilograms (154 pounds), 80 kilograms (176 pounds), 90 kilograms (198 pounds), and over 90 kilograms, or "unlimited," Powerlifting and Olympic lifting are contested in a much wider variety of weight classes. Converted to pounds from international metric equivalents, these are 114, 123, 132, 148, 165, 181, 198, 220, 242, 275, and over 275 pounds.

WEIGHTLIFTING—The subdivision of weight training in which men and women compete in weight classes both nationally and internationally to see who can lift the heaviest weights for single repetitions in prescribed exercises. Two types of weightlifting—Olympic lifting and powerlifting—are contested.

WEIGHT TRAINING—The various acts of using resistance training equipment either to exercise the body or for competitive purposes.

WORKOUT—A bodybuilding training session. "To work out" is to take a bodybuilding training session.

YOGA—An Eastern physical discipline that promotes body flexibility. Yoga also is a particularly tranquil philosophy of life.

INDEX

251